SPECIAL PROBLEMS IN REHABILITATION

Number 885

AMERICAN LECTURE SERIES

A Publication in

The BANNERSTONE DIVISION *of*
AMERICAN LECTURES IN SOCIAL
AND REHABILITATION PSYCHOLOGY

Consulting Editors

JOHN G. CULL, Ph.D.
Director, Regional Training Program
Department of Rehabilitation Counseling
Virginia Commonwealth University
Fisherville, Virginia

and

RICHARD E. HARDY, Ed.D.
Chairman, Department of Rehabilitation Counseling
Virginia Commonwealth University
Richmond, Virginia

The American Lecture Series in Social and Rehabilitation Psychology offers books which are concerned with man's role in his milieu. Emphasis is placed on how this role can be made more effective in a time of social conflict and a deteriorating physical environment. The books are oriented toward descriptions of what future roles should be and are not concerned exclusively with the delineation and definition of contemporary behavior. Contributors are concerned to a considerable extent with prediction through the use of a functional view of man as opposed to a descriptive, anatomical point of view.

Books in this series are written mainly for the professional practitioner; however, academicians will find them of considerable value in both undergraduate and graduate courses in the helping services.

SPECIAL PROBLEMS
IN REHABILITATION

Edited by

A. BEATRIX COBB, Ph.D.

Horn Professor of Psychology
Former Director, Research and Training Center in Mental Retardation
Texas Tech University
Lubbock, Texas

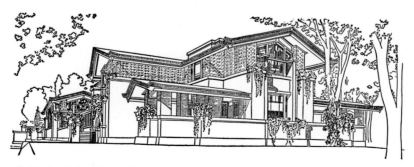

C H A R L E S   C   T H O M A S   •   P U B L I S H E R
Springfield • *Illinois* • *U.S.A.*

Published and Distributed Throughout the World by

CHARLES C THOMAS • PUBLISHER

Bannerstone House

301-327 East Lawrence Avenue, Springfield, Illinois, U.S.A.

©*1974, by* CHARLES C THOMAS • PUBLISHER

ISBN 0-398-02787-0

Library of Congress Catalog Card Number: 72-11609

With *THOMAS BOOKS careful attention is given to all details of
manufacturing and design. It is the Publisher's desire to present books that are
satisfactory as to their physical qualities and artistic possibilities and
appropriate for their particular use. THOMAS BOOKS will be true to those
laws of quality that assure a good name and good will.*

Printed in the United States of America

A-2

This Book Is Dedicated

to

*My Rehabilitation Counseling Students,
whose friendship and accomplishments
through the years have enriched
my life*

and

*My Co-Worker and Friend, Martha,
whose real assistance and encouragement
made the compilation of the book possible.*

CONTRIBUTORS

Anne L. Bloxom, M.A.: Research Associate, Department of Psychology, Vanderbilt University, Nashville, Tennessee.

Charles L. Bowden, M.D.: Assistant Professor, Department of Psychiatry, The University of Texas Medical School at San Antonio, Texas, Clinical and Research Psychiatrist, Drug Dependence Program of The Bexar County Mental Health, Mental Retardation Center, San Antonio, Texas.

James B. Caylor, II, M.A.: Psychologist, Criss Cole Rehabilitation Center, State Commission for the Blind, Austin, Texas.

George V. Clark, B.A., B.D.: Program Specialist, Alcoholism, Mental Health, Drug Abuse, Tuberculosis and Respiratory Diseases, Texas Rehabilitation Commission, Austin, Texas.

A. Beatrix Cobb, Ph.D.: Horn Professor of Psychology, Texas Tech University, Lubbock, Texas.

Thomas R. Collingwood, Ph.D.: Senior Research Scientist, Arkansas Rehabilitation Research and Training Center, Hot Springs, Arkansas.

Harry G. Davis, Ph.D.: Chief of Psychology, Big Spring State Hospital, Big Spring, Texas.

John A. Fenoglio, M.A.: Director, General Programs, Texas Rehabilitation Commission, Austin, Texas.

Victor J. Ganzer, Ph.D.: Staff Psychologist, Child Study and Treatment Center, Fort Steilacoom, Washington.

John W. Gladden, Ph.D.: Superintendent, State School for the Mentally Retarded, Lubbock, Texas.

Randolph H. Greene, M.A.: Director, Criss Cole Rehabilitation Center, State Commission for the Blind, Austin, Texas.

Roy C. Grzesiak, M.A.: Ph.D. Intern in Psychology, Institute of Rehabilitation Medicine, New York University Medical Center, New York, N.Y.

Preston E. Harrison, M.D., Ph.D.: Director, Big Spring State Hospital, Big Spring, Texas.

Randy Jennings, M.S.: Program Specialist, Juvenile Corrections, Texas Rehabilitation Commission, Austin, Texas.

Clifford S. Knape, Ph.D.: Chief of Psychology Service, Veterans Administration Hospital, Waco, Texas; Board Member, Texas Rehabilitation Commission, Austin, Texas.

Kenneth Krause, Ph.D., ACSW: Associate Professor, The Jane Addams Graduate School of Social Work, University of Illinois at Chicago Circle.

G. Frank Lawlis, Ph.D.: Director of Rehabilitation Counseling, Texas Tech University, Lubbock, Texas.

James F. Maddux, M.D.: Professor, Department of Psychiatry, The University of Texas Medical School at San Antonio, San Antonio, Texas: Director, Drug Dependence Program of Bexar County Mental Health Retardation Center, San Antonio, Texas.

Frank B. Perdue, M.Ed.: Program Specialist, Division of Vocational Rehabilitation,

Texas Rehabilitation Commission, Austin, Texas.

Dale H. Place, M.S.: Welfare Program Specialist, Texas Rehabilitation Commission, Austin, Texas.

Larry C. Rhoades, M.A.: Program Specialist, Mental Health, Drug Abuse, Alcoholism, Tuberculosis and Respiratory Diseases, Texas Rehabilitation Commission, Austin, Texas.

Paul L. Rosenberg, M.D.: Resident in Psychiatry, Camarillo State Hospital, Camarillo, California; School Consultant, Santa Monica, California; Consultant to the Santa Monica Child Care Centers; Co-Founder of the Los Angeles Free Clinic, Los Angeles, California.

Richard Russell, M.Ed.: Program Specialist, Adult Corrections, Texas Rehabilitation Commission, Austin, Texas.

John Goss Skelton, Jr., Ph.D.: Private Practice, Chairman, Department of Psychology, Park North General Hospital, San Antonio, Texas; Consultant to the Northside and San Antonio Independent School Districts, San Antonio, Texas.

Hans H. Strupp, Ph.D.: Project Director, Department of Psychology, Vanderbilt University, Nashville, Tennessee.

EDITORS' FOREWORD

R ARELY in the area of rehabilitation have two volumes covered the clients whom we serve as thoroughly and as succinctly as do the two volumes which Doctor Cobb has completed. The major thrust of these two books, which are companion volumes, is a treatment of the psychological, social, medical, and vocational aspects of disability. Doctor Cobb and her co-authors have zeroed in on the major problem areas confronting contemporary rehabilitation counseling.

Volumes such as this are written only after many years of experience in the profession of rehabilitation counseling and after extended consideration of the concerns confronting the profession and thorough consideration of an organization for the lucid treatment of these problem areas in textbook form.

We, the editors of *The Social and Rehabilitation Psychology Series,* are quite pleased to have these two books included in our series. We feel that they will make a very basic contribution to the professional literature and will become landmark publications in years to come. Not only will these texts be of great value to university professors who are confronted with the task of teaching in the area of disability, but they will serve as a basic reference text to practitioners in all phases of rehabilitation.

John G. Cull, Ph. D.
Richard E. Hardy, Ed. D.

Stuarts Draft, Virginia

The following books have appeared thus far in this Series:

SOCIAL AND REHABILITATION SERVICES FOR THE BLIND—Richard E. Hardy and John G. Cull

MENTAL RETARDATION AND PHYSICAL DISABILITY—Richard E. Hardy and John G. Cull

UNDERSTANDING DISABILITY FOR SOCIAL AND REHABILITATION SERVICES—John G. Cull and Richard E. Hardy

VOLUNTEERISM AN EMERGING PROFESSION—John G. Cull and Richard E. Hardy

THE NEGLECTED OLDER AMERICAN—SOCIAL AND REHABILITATION SERVICES—John G. Cull and Richard E. Hardy

FUNDAMENTALS OF CRIMINAL BEHAVIOR AND CORRECTIONAL SYSTEMS—John G. Cull and Richard E. Hardy

THE BIG WELFARE MESS—PUBLIC ASSISTANCE AND REHABILITATION APPROACHES—John G. Cull and Richard E. Hardy

ADJUSTMENT TO WORK—John G. Cull and Richard E. Hardy

VOCATIONAL EVALUATION FOR REHABILITATION SERVICES—Richard E. Hardy and John G. Cull

REHABILITATION OF THE DRUG ABUSER WITH DELINQUENT BEHAVIOR—Richard E. Hardy and John G. Cull

APPLIED PSYCHOLOGY IN LAW ENFORCEMENT AND CORRECTIONS—Richard E. Hardy and John G. Cull

INTRODUCTION TO CORRECTIONAL REHABILITATION—Richard E. Hardy and John G. Cull

DRUG DEPENDENCE AND REHABILITATION APPROACHES—Richard E. Hardy and John G. Cull

CLIMBING GHETTO WALLS—Richard E. Hardy and John G. Cull

APPLIED VOLUNTEERISM IN COMMUNITY DEVELOPMENT—Richard E. Hardy and John G. Cull

CONTEMPORARY FIELD WORK PRACTICES IN REHABILITATION—John G. Cull and Craig R. Colvin

VOCATIONAL REHABILITATION: PROFESSION AND PROCESS—John G. Cull and Richard E. Hardy

MEDICAL AND PSYCHOLOGICAL ASPECTS OF DISABILITY—A. Beatrix Cobb

LAW ENFORCEMENT AND CORRECTIONAL REHABILITATION—John G. Cull and Richard E. Hardy

EVALUATION FOR REHABILITATION SERVICES—Richard E. Hardy and John G. Cull

COUNSELING HIGH SCHOOL STUDENTS—John G. Cull and Richard E. Hardy

PREFACE

OVER THE PAST fifteen years, the clientele served by the state rehabilitation agencies of the nation has fulminated from a compact basic service to the physically handicapped to include an ever increasing number of diverse and complex disabilities. In the past decade alone, such entities as the public offender, the disabled disadvantaged, the addicted (alcoholic and chemical), and those suffering from stroke and cancer have been added to the service roster.

This breathtaking expansion of the nature and the number to be served created a two-fold emergency. First, there was the problem of staff expansion to meet the new demand for service. Professionally trained individuals were not available; indeed, so new were some of the problems of the categories that very little information was available for in-service training to meet the emergency. This dearth of essential information brought into focus the second portion of the challenge: the preparation of data on medical, psychological and rehabilitation problems related to the specific needs of the new clientele.

To date, for the most part, it would seem that this information has been collected on an individual basis by each state, or each staff member assigned to the new case loads. Dedicated search and experience have resulted in extension of knowledge and skills pertinent to the new categories of service.

This book seeks to bring together basic operational data and pertinent psychosocial, medical, and employment information related to the special problems in rehabilitation. Program specialists from the Texas State Rehabilitation Commission were persuaded to present the basic chapter in each category. These chapters hold a wealth of realistic knowledge gleaned by these dedicated professionals as they accepted the challenge of service and moved in to set up service programs. This over-all approach in each bracket is followed by specific psychosocial, medical and placement information compiled by other workers in the field who attempt to integrate knowledge now available in these new areas of endeavor. This book does not pose as a panacea of answers to the many problems encountered in the process of rehabilitation of these new and diversified types of clients. It does attempt a synthesis of material developed as dedicated individuals met the tremendous demand for new services. Other states and individuals may have developed other procedures, but the basic problems are common. It is hoped that this initial sharing of approaches may lead to further integration of materials at the national level.

The two-fold purpose of this book, then, is to provide basic information and an operational framework for delivery of services to the new categories of clients posing special problems in rehabilitation. First, the book has been developed in such a way as to lend itself to utilization as a textbook for counselors-in-training in university settings. Second, the material has been organized and presented in a fashion that would make it useful to the rehabilitation agency personnel as an in-service training manual for new counselors in the new areas, or to newly assigned special programs counselors. Still another valuable use of the information could be in the area of family and client education relative to the problems and opportunities for help available to those who must live with these traumatic difficulties.

This book, then, is the result of generous and expert efforts on the part of many dedicated individuals in the field of Rehabilitation. Each contributor is acknowledged with pride and appreciation. Particular gratitude is due the members of the staff of the Texas Commission for the Blind, and Burt L. Risley, Executive Director, for the comprehensive coverage of rehabilitation approaches in working with the visually disabled. Specific appreciation and acknowledgment is made of the invaluable contribution made by the program specialists responsible for the rehabilitation of the public offender, the disabled disadvantaged, the addicted, the mentally retarded, and the severely disabled in the Texas Rehabilitation Commission, and the Director of that Commission, Jess M. Irwin, Jr. Without the realistic and innovative accounts of actual approaches to the rehabilitation of clients in these special categories, this book could not have met the criterion of realism essential to the training of counselors in the field.

A.B.C.

CONTENTS

	Page
Contributors	vii
Editors' Foreword	ix
Preface	xi

PART ONE
THE PUBLIC OFFENDER

Chapter
1. VOCATIONAL REHABILITATION OF THE PUBLIC OFFENDER— *Randy Jennings and Richard Russell* ... 5
2. THE USE OF MODELING TECHNIQUES IN REHABILITATION OF THE PUBLIC OFFENDER—*Victor J. Ganzer* ... 20
3. SURVIVAL CAMPING: A THERAPEUTIC TECHNIQUE TO AID THE REHABILITATION OF THE YOUTHFUL OFFENDER— *Thomas R. Collingwood* ... 41

PART TWO
THE DISABLED DISADVANTAGED

4. VOCATIONAL REHABILITATION OF THE DISABLED DISADVANTAGED— *Dale H. Place* ... 59
5. THE DISABLED DISADVANTAGED—*Kenneth Krause* ... 83
6. ROLE INDUCTION FOR PSYCHOTHERAPY: A PROMISING TECHNIQUE FOR THE REHABILITATION CLIENT—*Hans H. Strupp and Anne L. Bloxom* ... 98
7. MOTIVATING THE CULTURALLY DEPRIVED—*John Goss Skelton, Jr.* ... 141

PART THREE
THE ADDICTED

8. REHABILITATION OF THE ALCOHOLIC—*George V. Clark* ... 153
9. ALCOHOLISM—*Harry G. Davis and Preston E. Harrison* ... 161
10. THE DRUG ABUSE PROGRAM OF THE TEXAS REHABILITATION COMMISSION—*Larry C. Rhoades* ... 181

xiii

11. THE EFFECTS OF MOOD ALTERING DRUGS: PLEASURES AND
    PITFALLS—*Paul L. Rosenberg* 192
12. CLINICAL AND COUNSELING PROBLEMS IN DRUG DEPENDENCE—
    Charles L. Bowden and James F. Maddux 213

PART FOUR
THE MENTALLY RETARDED

13. REHABILITATION SERVICES TO THE MENTALLY RETARDED—
    Frank B. Perdue 227
14. VOCATIONAL HABILITATION FOR THE MENTALLY RETARDED—
    John W. Gladden 246

PART FIVE
THE VISUALLY DISABLED

15. VOCATIONAL REHABILITATION SERVICES FOR THE BLIND—
    Randolph H. Greene 267
16. PSYCHOLOGICAL IMPLICATIONS OF BLINDNESS—
    James B. Caylor II 277

PART SIX
THE SEVERELY DISABLED

17. THE SEVERELY DISABLED—A REHABILITATION CHALLENGE—
    John A. Fenoglio 299
18. THE PSYCHOLOGY OF PAIN—*Roy C. Grzesiak* 311
19. MOTIVATION: THE GREATEST CHALLENGE TO REHABILITATION—
    G. Frank Lawlis 346

PART SEVEN
THE EMOTIONALLY DISABLED

20. THE MENTALLY AND EMOTIONALLY HANDICAPPED—
    Clifford S. Knape 369

PART EIGHT
THE CANCER CLIENT

21. MEDICAL AND PSYCHOLOGICAL PROBLEMS IN THE REHABILITATION
    OF THE CANCER PATIENT—*A. Beatrix Cobb* 399
Index 433

SPECIAL PROBLEMS IN REHABILITATION

(PART ONE)

THE PUBLIC OFFENDER

Vocational Rehabilitation of the
Public Offender

The Use of Modeling Techniques in
Rehabilitation of the
Public Offender

Survival Camping: A Therapeutic
Technique to Aid the Rehabilitation
of the Youthful Offender

Chapter 1

VOCATIONAL REHABILITATION OF THE PUBLIC OFFENDER

RANDY JENNINGS AND RICHARD RUSSELL

CRIME AND DELINQUENCY are two of the greatest social problems of this age. The crime bill in this country is estimated to be twenty-seven billion dollars a year by the Department of Justice. *The Challenge of Crime in a Free Society* (1967), a report of the President's Commission on Law Enforcement and Administration of Justice, pointedly states:

> There is much crime in America, more than is ever reported, far more than is ever solved, far too much for the health of the nation. Every American is, in a sense, a victim of crime (page 1).

The myths and stereotypes of crime are crumbling. The view of crime as characteristic behavior of a small segment of our population, is a theory losing favor in view of recent research. Crime is not a single phenomenon that can be examined, analyzed and described in one piece. Crime appears to be a multidimensioned problem which invades every level of our society. Its practitioners and victims are people of all ages, incomes and backgrounds. Its trends are difficult to ascertain and its causes legion.

Many claim that the incidence of crime and delinquency is not nearly the problem that our characteristic manner of attending to the criminal or delinquent is—the *correctional* system. The Criminal Justice System is not a system at all, but a conglomeration of a federal system, fifty state systems, and well over three thousand county and municipal systems, having under its authority on any given day perhaps a million and a half people (Report of President's Task Force on Prisoner Rehabilitation, 1970).

In view of the fact that a sizeable percentage of the persons in the system are being *corrected* for a third or fourth time, to say that the system is rehabilitative by nature is too kind a compliment. Thus, it is wrong to assume that the control of crime is solely the task of the police, the courts and correction agencies. In fact, crime cannot be controlled without the interest and participation of schools (university through elementary level), businesses, social agencies, private groups, and individual citizens.

HISTORY OF THE VOCATIONAL REHABILITATION MOVEMENT IN CORRECTIONAL REHABILITATION

During the past decade, there has been a growing momentum for reform in Corrections. With the passage of the Omnibus Safe Streets and Crime Act

5

of 1968 and the Youth Development and Delinquency Act of 1969, alternatives to the incarceration system have been implemented. There has been an emphasis toward the expanding of probation and parole services, utilizing halfway houses. The trend is away from large institutions and toward community based correctional systems. The "national strategy" of the Youth Development and Delinquency Prevention administration has emphasized the need for diverting from the correctional system juveniles who do not exhibit behavior for which they would be prosecuted if they were adults. Work release and innovative institutional treatment and training programs have gained acceptance in recent years.

With the passage of the Vocational Rehabilitation Act of 1965 (Public Law 89-333), public offenders were deemed eligible for vocational rehabilitation services through the definition of the behavioral disorder as a disabling condition. Mary E. Switzer (1967), then Commissioner of Rehabilitation Services Administration, proposed the following challenge:

> Handling of the corrected offender has come a long way from the cat-o-nine-tails and the pillary. Cooperation between corrections and vocational rehabilitation may well make the full planning of this long climb away from barbarism. We are civilized people and, as such, are compelled to seek humane solutions for our social problems. For decades, we have profited from our decision to use the productive capabilities of physically handicapped citizens. The public offender represents the next great source of underdeveloped human potential. No society can long afford to deny full participation to any large number of its members. Vocational rehabilitation can help many offenders become aware of their own value to their country and community as they are assisted in preparing themselves for useful and meaningful living (p. 23).

Rehabilitation of the public offender, which resulted from the "amendments" of the Vocational Rehabilitation Act, has presented the most significant challenge to the vocational rehabilitation administration in its long history of activity. As a result, alliances between agencies have been initiated and will continue to grow in waging the war against crime. Thus, the involvement of Vocational Rehabilitation in Corrections coincided with a gaining national resolve to reform Corrections from simple custody to a concern for the social adjustment of persons in its charge. A constructive member of the community, by definition, is a working member. It is the ultimate objective of Vocational Rehabilitation with each public offender client to prepare him for constructive citizenship via gainful employment.

To test the effectiveness of the vocational rehabilitation counselor's involvement with the public offender, eight Federal Offenders Rehabilitation Projects (FOR) were authorized under grants from the newly created Social and Rehabilitation Services Division of the Department of Health, Education and Welfare. The FOR Project for Texas was located in San Antonio and sponsored by the Vocational Rehabilitation Division of the Texas Education Agency. One of the results of that Project was the finding that traditional rehabilitation techniques of services delivery would have to be altered and refined to meet the needs of the public offender. Many of the findings of that Project gave impetus to a major involvement of Vocational Rehabilitation with public offenders in Texas. In summary, the final FOR report pointed out that not only did vocational rehabilitation have much to offer the public offender but the offender had much to offer vocational rehabilitation in terms of causing vocational rehabilitation to reassess techniques of delivery of services (even as applied to other clients). Correctional rehabilitation may be painful, but it may be good for us.

With the establishment of the Texas Rehabilitation Commission as the approved Vocational Rehabilitation agency in 1969, the administration of the correctional rehabilitation effort consisted of a Special Programs Section, which included adult and juvenile corrections. With administrative guidance, the Correctional Program began to evolve from isolated experimental projects to a uniform statewide program.

STATE PARTNERSHIPS IN CORRECTIONS

Because Corrections in Texas is divided into the Adult Justice System, governed by penal statutes, and the Juvenile Justice Systems, governed by civil statutes, it was necessary to program separately to meet the needs of the public offender clients in the respective systems.

Adult Corrections

Texas was not the first state to become involved in Correctional Rehabilitation following the 1965 Amendments. Prior to entering this field, an extensive study was made of the involvement of other states, such as Oklahoma and Georgia, in Corrections. Very little was known about the correctional system, and it became obvious that the correctional system knew very little about Vocational Rehabilitation.

In 1966, the Division of Vocational Rehabilitation, Texas Education Agency, began serving the public offenders. The agency contracted with and assigned staff to the correctional institutions that were serving the public offenders. The Adult Correctional Rehabilitation program in Texas has thus been greatly influenced by the Texas Department of Corrections and the United States Bureau of Prisons.

Involvement in corrections at the institutional level was expanded through Rehabilitation Services Administration Grants to the Texas Department of Corrections to improve or establish Rehabilitation Facilities. Both the Diagnostic and the Ferguson Units improved their Rehabilitation Services through established grants from Rehabilitation Services Administration.

As a result of this early direction, the Correctional Rehabilitation Program became institutionally oriented. Within a short period of time, the agency became experienced and proficient in working with the public offender. As counselors became more experienced in the field of Correctional Rehabilitation, it became obvious that the goal of rehabilitation could be best achieved if the program was more closely coordinated with community treatment centers, halfway houses, jail projects, and probation and parole agencies. This awakening was encouraged by community correctional agencies that were beginning to realize the benefits that could be received through a close working relationship with Vocational Rehabilitation.

When the Texas Rehabilitation Commission became a reality on September 1, 1969, it became obvious that the new emphasis would be to provide rehabilitation service on the community level rather than limiting involvement to the large correctional institutions. *To accomplish the ultimate goal of reducing crime, it is necessary that the number of people in the criminal justice system be reduced* has become the philosophy in Correctional Rehabilitation. Preventive rehabilitation has become the most productive and effective method in dealing with the mentally handicapped, especially the public offender. Since more than 90 percent of all institutionalized offenders are eventually released from confinement, the ultimate test of any correctional program cannot be made in the institution; it is made on the street.

The shift from an institutionally oriented program to a community oriented program has now been completed. At the present time, 65 percent of the staff in the Adult Correctional Program is assigned to various District Offices in the "free world" while 35 percent of the staff is assigned to correctional institutions. In addition to the original Inter-Agency Contract with the Texas Department of Corrections, Texas Rehabilitation Commission now has working agreements with the Board of Pardons and Paroles, United States Probation and Parole Offices, several large county jail systems and seven large metropolitan Adult Probation Departments.

Since inception of the Adult program in 1966, production has grown steadily. In 1968 for example, the Agency received 4,500 public offender referrals and closed 556 cases as rehabilitated. In fiscal year 1972, the Agency received 8,100 adult referrals and closed 1,650 cases as rehabilitated. In fiscal year 1970, 43 percent of the cases being closed were in a successful status (status "26"). In fiscal year 1972, this percentage rose to 57 percent successfully closed. In 1971, counselors assigned to the Adult Correctional Program averaged thirty-eight successful closures per counselor. In 1972, counselors assigned to this program averaged sixty-three successful closures per counselor.

The Adult Correctional program has undergone the normal "growing pains" that all new programs undergo. Gradually, the program has become refined as the Agency gained experience in this new field of rehabilitation. The Texas Rehabilitation Commission is committed to providing a strong correctional rehabilitation program that will meet the needs of the handicapped public offender.

Juvenile Corrections

From 1966 to 1969, the Juvenile Correctional Program was primarily an institutional one, centered at Gatesville State School for Boys, under an interagency agreement with the Texas Youth Council. Although public offenders do not enjoy a "blanket" disability (automatic eligibility because of incarceration), most juvenile clients served in that three year period were institutionalized before referral for services. In 1970, with the hiring of a program specialist for the Juvenile Program to provide technical assistance, an attempt was made to expand services to meet the needs of the behaviorally disturbed adolescent, regardless of his location or circumstances. As a result, cooperative agreements were established with thirteen county juvenile probation departments to accept referrals and deliver services. In some instances, counselors were actually officed in the probation departments to facilitate the program more readily. As a by-product of this shift of emphasis from the institution to the community, the large majority of referrals to juvenile program counselors were initiated on juveniles in their home community, prior to the need for their being institutionalized.

There has not been a de-emphasis of the Gatesville School for Boys Program and, in fact, it has enjoyed a considerable degree of refinement, resulting in 85 percent of all transferred active cases to field counselors becoming successfully rehabilitated during fiscal years 1971 and 1972.

In 1971, the interagency agreement with the Texas Youth Council was revised to include emphasis on cooperation between parole officers and field counselors. This new agreement has greatly aided in the continuity of Vocational Rehabilitation services from the institution to the field. There are presently twenty counselors assigned to deliver services to the juvenile offender, mostly in the metropolitan areas.

With the understanding that any public offender is eligible who meets the basic criteria of Vocational Rehabilitation, regardless of correctional status, the Texas Rehabilitation Commission attempted to add a preventive dimension to the Juvenile Program. This was accomplished through grant programs which encouraged referrals of predelinquents from school and other social agencies dealing with disturbed youth. A predelinquent is defined as a juvenile in possession of a behavioral disorder who has no correctional status such as probation or parole. With monies granted by the Criminal Justice Council, an agency awarding grants for programs to combat crime and delinquency, the predelinquent projects were begun in several metropolitan areas. In all of the projects, the purpose and intent was the same—to provide a timely service to the disturbed adolescent in the earliest state of his delinquency, and in his home community.

In one sense, this program is not rehabilitative in nature, implying a restoration to a previous condition, but rather habilitative, a timely intervention and delivery of service.

ESSENTIALS OF REHABILITATING THE PUBLIC OFFENDER

The record of man's approach to criminals and criminality can be summarized as a succession of three R's—Revenge, Restraint and Reformation. The fourth R, Rehabilitation, has appeared and is being incorporated and tried throughout the Criminal Justice System. In discussing important essentials in the rehabilitation of the public offender, it is well to give a definition that applies to most individuals that receive services through the Correctional Rehabilitation Program. A public offender is "any juvenile or adult convicted or adjudicated by a court of competent jurisdiction, whether Federal or State" (Crump, 1969, p. 1).

Disability

A behavioral disorder is the predominant disability found in the public offender population. The establishing of a behavioral disorder as a disability has, until recently, been fraught with confusion. This seems to stem from the nomenclature in current use. A behavioral disorder, as defined by the Rehabilitation Services Administration, is the disability for which maladaptive actions or behavior are the predominant symptoms rather than an impairment of contact with reality or emotional distress typically associated with psychosis or neurosis. A behavioral disorder is a *vocational rehabilitation term* which is roughly synonymous with personality disorders or behavior disorders, of various etiology, as described in the *Diagnostic and Statistical Manual of Mental Disorders, Third Edition* (*DSMIII*), 1968, American Psychiatric Association. There are numerous diagnostic labels from the DSM which fall under the *umbrella* use of the term "behavioral disorder." According to the DSM (pp. 9, 10, 121, 41-46, 48), the following are commonly reported diagnoses:

Paranoid Personality
Cyclothymic Personality
Schizoid Personality
Explosive Personality
Obsessive-Compulsive Personality
Hysterical Personality
Asthenic Personality
Antisocial Personality
Passive-Aggressive Personality

Transient Situational Disturbance
  (Adjustment Reaction)
Inadequate Personality
Other Personality Disorders
  of Specified types
  (Immature Personality, Passive
    Dependent Personality, etc.)
Unspecified Personality Disorders
Sexual Deviations

The establishment of a behavioral disorder is a "double-edged sword." It must be done *diagnostically,* by a psychiatrist or psychologist, and through the substantiating of a deviant *pattern* of behavior. This pattern of behavior is often well documented by social histories, school records, court records, and employment history information. It should be made clear that the establishment of a behavioral disorder as a disability is accomplished on the merits of each individual case. The public offender does not enjoy a "blanket" disability because of correctional status, such as probation, parole, or incarceration. Conversely, a behavioral disorder can be established with a client who has no correctional status. This is a point that often eludes those applying the criteria for eligibility to the public offender. Thus, it must be remembered that the term *behavioral disorder* refers to a disability; the term *public offender* is no more than a social characterization.

Diagnostic Evaluation

Diagnostic evaluation to establish disability and to support the counselor's judgment of feasibility of a rehabilitation plan has come under close scrutiny. Some critics are quite pointed in their evaluation of the usefulness of diagnostics:

> *Diagnostics,* the *sine qua non* of those operating within the parameters of the medical model, has come under increasing attack. There is evidence now available to suggest that much of our elaborate diagnostic evaluations (those predicting general personality functioning) have little value for vocational rehabilitation. The traditional diagnostic instruments tend to have low predictive validity for rehabilitation clients. This attack is leveled against the fancy diagnostics. It should not be construed as a criticism of valid psychological tests and inventories; e.g., school tests, tests of general intelligence, interest inventories, objective personality inventories, etc. The general prevocational evaluations are still considered to be the useful (Wolfe, 1967, p. 24).

During the past few years, the Texas Rehabilitation Commission has begun employing psychologists for the primary purpose of providing diagnostic evaluations. It is not unlikely to expect that diagnostic instruments will be refined that yield more validity and reliability to the rehabilitation process. There is already evidence of more reliance on objective measurement of personality, such as the Minnesota Multiphasic Personality Inventory (MMPI), 16 Personality Factor (16PF), and Motivational Analysis Test (MAT).

There has, in the recent past, been evidence of over-diagnosing the behavioral disorder. This can be attributed to a lack of communication with private practitioners contracted with for diagnostic evaluation. It would be questionable, for instance, whether a discussion of a client's "latent manifestations of suppressed conflicts" (quote from a psychological report) would be materially useful for a counselor's judgment of eligibility or realistic vocational planning. There is evidence to support the conclusion that counselors' *use* of diagnostic evaluations is a function of their *usefulness* (Sindberg, Roberts, and Pfeifer, 1968).

By employing staff psychologists, the Commission has been able to develop a diagnostic system that meets the needs of the counselor in terms of providing diagnostic information that can better be used to establish eligibility and at the same time be used by the counselor as a valuable tool in developing a Vocational Rehabilitation Plan. This has also resulted in a diagnostic system that meets the needs of the client, the consumer of vocational rehabilitation services, in that services have now become more immediate and tangible rather than delayed and long-ranged.

With the establishment of the disability, the vocational handicap is often obvious. Many public offenders have a substantial work history; but it is filled with menial employment, instability, and erratic job performance. Often the public offender does not have a work concept, that is a desire to work toward a career or profession. They do not understand what it means to start at the bottom and work up toward an objective. Offenders can usually get a job. Getting the right job, keeping the job, and gaining job satisfaction is usually a major problem that they seldom can solve by themselves.

One of the most important decisions a counselor can make is the "feasibility" of a client to *benefit from* vocational rehabilitation services. This judgment is greatly enhanced and honed by the use of collaborative support of probation and parole officers and other resource persons. In establishing a client's feasibility for vocational rehabilitation services, the counselor must be cautious not to confuse *feasibility* with *client cooperation*. Cooperation can hardly be used to determine acceptability of the behaviorally disabled client. His very disability makes him uncooperative.

Delivery of Vocational Rehabilitation Services—Special Aspects

The nature of the rehabilitation process, as applied to the public offender, is dictated largely by two factors. First, the essential characteristics of this disability group have great bearing on successful rehabilitation. The following is a list of statements applicable to the behavioral disorder group:

1. A history of continued failure and negative reinforcement as a result of temporary or deadened employment and extended unemployment. Lack of vocational skills.
2. Frequent low self-esteem, alienation and easy discouragement.
3. Multiple and complex barriers to employability including inadequate or inferior education (lack of basic skills in reading, math, etc.), chronic health problems, police records, discriminatory hiring practices on the part of employers, lack of transportation to jobs, and for women, often a lack of adequate child-care facilities.
4. Presence of immediate financial crisis.
5. Resistance to and the inappropriateness of many paper and pencil type standardized assessment devices.
6. Wide differences in values and frequent confusion in value systems. Work attitudes and motivation may be very different from those of the dominant society.
7. Low frustration tolerance for perseverance in lengthy developmental programs.
8. Most clients from economically disadvantaged backgrounds or members of minority groups. Families are likely to be large. The proportion of households headed by women is substantial.
9. Resistance to change.
10. Reluctance to take risks (Wolfe, 1967, p. 27).

Second, since the rehabilitation process is assumed to revolve around a one-to-one relationship between counselor and client, the personality of the counselor contributes to or hinders rehabilitation. The successful outcome of this process is often dependent upon the interaction of personal and social characteristics of the client, such as the nature of the disability and psychological variables, and the counselor characteristics, such as experience, understanding and ability to relate to the client. This characteristic interchange is particularly important in correctional rehabilitation because of the psycho-social nature of the disabling condition.

Certain characteristics of the counselor have been observed to expedite the rehabilitation process. Three of these outstanding characteristics which seem essential to successful counseling will be briefly described.

High Tolerance Threshold

Public offenders are commonly manipulative, impulsive, unpredictable and inconsistent in performance. These client traits are very frustrating to the counselor, particularly if he is accustomed to the reward of verbal appreciation and gratitude from his clientele. A high threshold of tolerance is an asset in working with the public offender.

Communication Skills

The ability to communicate, both verbally and non-verbally, is an important ingredient to the rehabilitation process. Public offenders are notoriously non-verbal and non-committal, and place a burden upon the counselor to establish rapport and *honest* communication. The public offender is adept at picking up cues as to the sincerity and acceptance of him by the counselor.

Unselfishness in Rehabilitation

One cardinal rule of rehabilitation with public offenders is not to attempt rehabilitation in a "vacuum." Protectiveness and fostering of dependency in the client can prove to be disastrous. A concerted effort should be made by the counselor to solicit the cooperation and assistance of other agency personnel and community resources. The use of probation officers, parole officers, social agency caseworkers, etc., in the rehabilitation process improves the counselor's judgment and chances of client success. The behaviorally disturbed public offender is often adept at manipulating counselor and probation officers who are not communicating. Interagency cooperative agreements are written largely to foster effective relationships and to minimize triangulation by the client.

Counseling

The role and function of the Vocational Rehabilitation counselor is the efficient delivery of services to adequately prepare the behaviorally handicapped for gainful employment. Obviously, an integral and vital service, underscoring the entire rehabilitation process, is interpersonal counseling. As opposed to other counseling procedures, such as *treatment, therapy,* etc., Vocational Rehabilitation counseling with the public offender is relatively purposeful and specific—i.e., communicative support of the rehabilitation process and objectives. It is a common temptation of Vocational Rehabilitation counselors, because of the psycho-social nature of the disability, to become heavily involved in therapeutic interaction, sometimes to the neglect of Vocational Rehabilitation objectives.

It is not the intention of this chapter to explore the controversy of *coordination versus counseling* as the primary function of the Vocational Rehabilitation counselor. Both are primary functions of the same role, but the nature of the counseling is subject for debate in correctional rehabilitation. The validity of traditional counseling techniques with the public offender is being questioned. The framework of employing the *fifty-minute* hour of verbal interaction *behind the closed door* is particularly questionable with the public offender. Most traditional counseling techniques have not evolved out of experiences of the rehabilitation agency and have been refined and standardized on persons other than Vocational Rehabilitation clients such as middle class college students and neurotics.

The public offender has been deemed an unsuitable candidate for the traditional approach because of an unwillingness to communicate feelings and problems. This is as much an indication of the Criminal Justice System as it is of the disability. If a client has been incarcerated, he has been exposed to the regimented, dehumanizing characteristic often associated with Correctional incarceration. This naturally predisposes him to a non-committal, non-verbal role in counseling based on the medical model.

Experience with the public offender has brought about a reformulation of the disease paradigm, based on the medical model, into problems of learning.

> Experience has shown that it may be enjoyable to probe for deep, underlying pathology; this approach rarely leads to successful outcomes. Rather, success occurs when we view specific behavior as either adaptive or maladaptive. We can identify deficits in adaptive behavior and then attempt to teach the client appropriate behavior. (Wolfe, 1967, pp. 28-29).

Some of the contemporary techniques based on the maladaptive behavior model are "Modeling", utilizing social learning theory (Sarazon and Ganzer, 1971) and "Reality Therapy" (Glasser, 1965) emphasizing the personal responsibility of one's behavior. Survival camping (Collingwood, 1971) is a promising therapeutic mode for behaviorally disturbed adolescents which can be used to supplement the Vocational Rehabilitation process. One such program in Texas, utilized by Vocational Rehabilitation counselors is *Adventure Trails for Girls* in Dallas, Texas.

There are two not very distinct schools of thought in Correctional Rehabilitation on how to best attend to maladaptive behavior of the public offender (Crump, 1969). One approach is to modify small segments of vocationally relevant behavior by reinforcing acceptable responses of the client. The counselor is not concerned with the public offender's basic personality structure as long as the client makes an adequate vocational adjustment. The other approach is based on confronting the client with self-defeating, anti-social behavior and attempting to motivate him to change it. Through directive confrontation, the client is brought to understand the self-defeating aspect of his behavior and positive alternatives are presented. Both approaches are often used in tandem by counselors in the Texas Rehabilitation Commission Correctional Rehabilitation Program.

The best procedure is to consider each individual referral on its merits, making the best judgment possible with the best information at hand.

> The most unfortunate thing a counselor could do in working with the public offender is to fail to recognize the nature of the population with which he is dealing. An attitude of Pollyanna, like naivete would lead to certain frustrations for the counselor and probable failure for the client. The counselors should recognize that many of the offenders will attempt to "con" the counselor and the agency out of everything they can. He should also recognize that with knowledge and discipline, he can bring about the rehabilitation of the public offender. To do so, however, he must approach the task with his mind and his eyes open (Crump, 1969, p. 42).

The counselor working with the public offender can expect to be "conned" more than once; but if he is really providing services to this group, he will accept this possibility as an occupational hazard that can be minimized through experience and knowledge. A rule of thumb to remember is that the public offender that is most verbal in expressing a need or desire for a certain service is usually "hustling" while the public offender that is the least verbal when expressing a need is usually being realistic and will benefit from the services that he desires.

In summary, the characteristics of the public offender and the correctional framework in which the Vocational Rehabilitation process is applied, dictate specialized techniques of counseling. Traditional techniques have limited usefulness, and newer models are evolving which are directly related to the Vocational Rehabilitation process and the public offender client.

Training

Vocational skill training for the public offender is a vital service. After training more than five thousand public offenders, several important considerations have emerged:

1. Many clients trained in state school or prison units do not seek employment commensurate with that training because of the stigma attached.

2. Immediacy is of the essence in deciding upon a training program because of clients' inability to pause and explore possibilities for vocational planning (FOR Project, 1969, p. 45). Consequently, the shorter length of training necessary to achieve the vocational objective, the greater the chance for success. After six months, the mortality rate for dropping out of training increases markedly. The most ideal training program for juveniles would last three to four months. Information obtained on adult public offenders closed as rehabilitated during fiscal year 1972 revealed that the average number of months from acceptance to closure was ten months (Statewide Plan for Juvenile Correctional Program, 1971).

3. There has been a demonstrated need for more on-the-job training

because of the public offender's resistance to the structured aspects of formal training. The client could also benefit from the fringe benefits on-the-job such as compensation for work while training, employer-employee relationships, etc.

Physical Restoration

Physical restoration is a service provided to only a small percentage of public offenders. Orthopedic impairments are often status symbols to public offenders, giving rise to nicknames, and clients don't often refer to these as handicapping conditions. Although physical restoration is a service that is not often considered when evaluating the public offender referral, the following points should be kept in mind:

1. Referrals off the street may have many physical problems such as diabetes, facial disfigurements, or severe problems with dentition, etc. The public offender very often has little concept or concern about personal hygiene.

2. In contrast, the public offender that is being discharged or paroled from an institution will generally be in good health; and in most cases he will be in better health than when he first entered the correctional institution.

Job Placement

Because of the nature of the disability, the public offender has a wider range of occupational choice, not limited by handicap. In a recent survey of successful closures in FY 71 conducted by the Texas Rehabilitation Commission (Whitcraft, Spring 1972, p. 8), it was found that the behavioral disorder disability groups recorded the most clients and the most occupations in which ten or more were closed: 2,151 and 54, respectively. However, job placement is considered by many counselors to be the single most difficult service to render the juvenile client. This difficulty stems from the limitation of employment opportunities because of age and experience. Legal limitations of Workman's Compensation and Child Labor Provisions restrict the labor market available to a juvenile client. It is important to remember that the employment of a juvenile client is often his first job and does not carry with it the finality and stability often associated with older clients. As an introduction to the labor market, a juvenile client's employment is *not* expected to be terminal. It *is* expected that as a client develops a positive work concept, he will seize opportunities for improving his employment.

With the adult client, legal limitations for placement are less restrictive. The ultimate objective in placing the adult client is to assist him in securing employment, consistent with his abilities, that is positively rewarding for him. Quite often, the public offender has little concept about how one goes about finding the right job. He needs assistance in evaluating his own abilities and aptitudes and in many cases will try *any* job rather than looking for *the* job. The client must be made aware of all the methods of finding jobs and should be encouraged to investigate job leads that the counselor provides. To improve the client's interviewing skills, it is sometimes helpful to role play, with the client playing the part of the unemployed seeking a job, and the counselor playing the part of the employer.

FUTURE TRENDS

The Criminal Justice System can be equated with a screening process. It sorts out the *better risks*—the offender at the end of the process, in prison, is likely to be a member of the lowest social and economic groups in America. Most of the incarcerated population are found in city and county jails, not in a prison system. There are 3,000 county and 1,000 city jails with an average daily population of 1,750,000 persons. In many cases, the jails are archaic and outdated. Only a handful of these jails have implemented rehabilitation programs of any sort. Our local jails have been referred to as "revolving doors", a "study in futility." The recidivism rates run as high as 75 and 80 percent.

The Criminal Justice System has finally recognized this glaring weakness in the system. Thus, the trend towards community-based correctional systems has developed. As a support element to the Criminal Justice System, Vocational Rehabilitation has also recognized the need to develop or strengthen cooperative programs with local jails, in an effort to provide timely rehabilitation services, that can be preventive in nature and hopefully break the revolving door syndrome.

In 1971, Statewide Plans, in both the Adult and Juvenile correctional programs, were conducted by the professional staff of the Texas Rehabilitation Commission. After approximately five years of experience in providing services to the public offender, the attempt was made to analyze and evaluate the present programs for future refinement. The following are significant findings of these plans:

1. As in the development of most special programs in Vocational Rehabilitation, correctional rehabilitation began inside of institutions and evolved into the community. Initial entry at the institutional level was due in part to the controlled environment offered at the prison which supposedly would be more conducive to treatment and rehabilitation.

2. Experience revealed that many prisoners upon release reject the possible benefits of prison programs. The stigma attached to institutional training often precludes the client seeking additional training or employment in that area upon release (Bloeser, 1971).

3. An obvious need for specialty counselors, with knowledge and experience in corrections, was identified.

4. Referral sources, such as Juvenile and Adult Probation Departments, were identified as being in need of full-time counselor assignments.

5. The time involved in securing and utilizing diagnostic information for vocational planning is critical. Because of the impulsivity of the public

offender, streamlining of the diagnostic procedure contributes significantly to the ultimate success of a vocational rehabilitation plan of services.

6. To have an impact on the rate and extent of delinquency, there is a need to program for services to the behaviorally disturbed school drop-out. Most delinquents are not handled officially by courts. The school drop-out has a high probability of pursuing a delinquent pattern of behavior. By providing a timely and essential service to the "pre-delinquent", vocational rehabilitation can provide a preventive dimension to their program, with far-reaching consequences.

7. The criteria for closing a case as successfully rehabilitated often has been interpreted with finality. Because of the psychosocial nature of the public offender's disability, this is inadvisable. The public offender is often referred to vocational rehabilitation because of a maladaptive and inconsistent pattern of vocational behavior, which usually has been exhibited over a long period of time. The vocational rehabilitation process can be successful in *readjusting* that pattern into more adaptive and consistent response to employment. It should be recognized that legal, social and familial stress on the client subject him to change beyond his control. Providing follow-up services to reinforce the client's positive adjustment should be recognized as necessary and expected, particularly with juvenile clients.

8. The correctional program of vocational rehabilitation has evolved a newer model or role of the counselor. As opposed to the independent application of vocational rehabilitation services in a one-to-one relationship, the correctional counselor is involved in the teamwork approach to rehabilitation, incorporating probation and parole officers in the process. Vocational rehabilitation is best applied as a complementary program to traditional corrections, rather than a substitute for it.

SUMMARY

Vocational Rehabilitation in Texas has recognized the inherent limitations in traditional methods of delivery of Vocational Rehabilitation services, in programming to meet the needs of the public offender client. The Texas Rehabilitation Commission is committed, on a large scale, to reducing the numbers of persons in the Criminal Justice System by assisting them to achieve satisfactory, independent employment. Although Vocational Rehabilitation is not a panacea for corrections, there is an obvious merge of purpose and program. As traditional corrections change, Vocational Rehabilitation should be in a position to adapt to emerging trends. Hopefully, the *public values* problem of correctional rehabilitation can be mellowed by the involvement of Vocational Rehabilitation as an advocate of the public offender's being worthy of a rehabilitation effort.

REFERENCES

American Psychiatric Association: *Diagnostic and Statistical Manual of Mental Disorders,* 3rd ed., 1968.

Bloeser, Kenneth: Impact of vocational training on young offenders of the Texas Department of Corrections. Unpublished Research Report (No. 1), Institute of Contemporary Corrections and the Behavioral Sciences, Sam Houston State University, Huntsville, Texas, April 1971.

Collingwood, T. R.: *Survival Camping: A Therapeutic Mode for Rehabilitating Problem Youth.* Arkansas Rehabilitation Research and Training Center, Hot Springs, Arkansas, 1971.

Crump, W. A. (Chairman): *Rehabilitation of Individuals with Behavioral Disorders.* Study Group Report of Seventh Institute of Rehabilitation Sources, HEW/SRS, 1969.

Glasser, William: *Reality Therapy.* New York, Harper & Row, 1965.

President's Commission on Law Enforcement and Administration of Justice: A Report: *The Challenge of Crime in a Free Society.* 1967.

President's Task Force on Prisoner Rehabilitation: *The Criminal Offender—What Should Be Done?* April 1970.

Research and Demonstration Project, No. RG-2080-G, SRS/HEW: *Texas Federal Offenders Rehabilitation Project (FOR) Final Report,* March 1969.

Sarason, I. G., and Ganzer, V. J.: *Modeling: An Approach to Rehabilitation of Juvenile Offenders.* Final Report, R & D Grant No. 15-P-55303 SRS/HEW, 1971.

Sindberg, R. M., Roberts, A. F., and Pfeifer, E. J.: The usefulness of psychological evaluations to vocational rehabilitation counselors. *Rehabilitation Literature,* Vol. 29, no. 10, October 1968.

Switzer, Mary E.: Vocational rehabilitation and corrections: A promising partnership. *Federal Probation Quarterly,* September 1967.

Texas Rehabilitation Commission: *Statewide Plan for Adult Correctional Program.* Austin, Texas, 1971a.

Texas Rehabilitation Commission: *Statewide Plan for Juvenile Correctional Program.* Austin, Texas, 1971b.

Whitcraft, C. J.: Disability occupation study. *Research Utilization,* Texas Rehabilitation Commission, Spring 1972.

Wolfe, R. R. (ed.): *Rehabilitation of the Public Offender.* Study Group Report of Fifth Institute of Rehabilitation Sources, HEW/VRA, 1967.

Chapter 2

THE USE OF MODELING TECHNIQUES
IN REHABILITATION OF THE PUBLIC OFFENDER

VICTOR J. GANZER

T HE PURPOSE of this chapter is to describe how the concept of observational learning, or modeling, can be translated into an objective and viable vehicle for teaching various skills to clients who require some kind of social or vocational rehabilitation. Proceeding from a definition of modeling and its place in theories of social learning, this chapter briefly will review research on modeling, describe the development and application of modeling principles in the rehabilitation of male juvenile delinquents, and discuss some potential uses of modeling techniques in other rehabilitation programs.

THE CONCEPT OF MODELING

Modeling, or observational learning, is a central concept in theories of social learning (Bandura, 1969b). Observation of the behavior of others may have three different effects (Bandura and Walters, 1963).

The first is a learning effect. An observer may acquire (learn) a variety of responses simply by observing another person's (the model's) behavior. This is true regardless of whether or not the observer imitates or matches the model's response following its occurrence, and regardless of whether or not reinforcement, either to the observer or model, is contingent upon any aspect of the behavior. There is considerable evidence that the observation and imitation of modeled behavior plays a major role in the acquisition of inappropriate as well as adaptive behavior and that this is true in whatever sociocultural context the learning occurs (Bandura and Walters, 1963; Bandura, 1969a). An enormous diversity of behaviors is learned through the observation of models. These behaviors include vocational skills, various motives and aspirations, sex appropriate roles, and numerous kinds of verbal and nonverbal responses. The category of models includes many types of persons: parents, adults, one's peers, and symbolic and film mediated models such as are observed on television and in motion pictures.

The second effect of observing modeled behaviors derives from the consequences of the model's actions. The inhibitory responses of an observer may be strengthened or weakened depending on whether the model's behavior is rewarded or punished.

The third effect may be termed response facilitation and does not involve new learning or response inhibition. For example, a person may pause to look up into a tree if he observes another engaged in this activity.

Imitation as a concept in social psychological theory may be traced back to the psychologist Lloyd Morgan who, as early as 1896, was concerned with modeling phenomena. Since that time, other writers have considered imitativeness to be an instinctive or constitutional process, a phenomenon derived from Pavlovian classical conditioning principles, and more recently a special subclass of operant responses in which the concept of reinforcement is useful.

Aronfreed's (1969) research on vicarious learning and internalization provides an example of the importance of observational learning and imitation in contemporary social psychological theories. Aronfreed is concerned with the internalization of social role norms in children, which is the process of adopting these norms as one's own. For Aronfreed, observational learning is a mechanism or vehicle by which internalized behavior control is obtained.

A prototype for much current research on modeling was a series of experiments carried out by Bandura (1962) which demonstrated the importance of modeling effects in the transmission of novel responses from adult models to nursery school age children. In these experiments, children were exposed to films of adult models who behaved in different ways toward a large air-inflated plastic doll. One modeling sequence depicted the models behaving very aggressively and abusively toward the doll, while in another condition the adult models exhibited no agression. Children who observed the aggressive behavior subsequently displayed a significantly greater number of imitative aggressive responses than did children in the non-aggressive modeling condition. Children in the latter condition rarely if ever aggressed toward the doll. These studies are especially suggestive in that they indicated that film mediated models also were effective in transmitting various patterns of behavior to the young observers.

Bandura has conducted other studies which have shown that the consequences contingent upon the model's behavior, such as reward or punishment, will produce differential effects on the subsequent behavior of observers (Bandura and Walters, 1963; Bandura, 1965). In this way, principles of reinforcement have been combined with observational learning and imitation to provide very convincing demonstrations of the importance of these concepts for the psychology of learning and behavior modification.

MODELING AND BEHAVIOR MODIFICATION

It was mentioned that theoretical and experimental developments of the concepts of modeling and observational learning are not new. Also not new is the therapeutic application of modeling procedures to the modification of maladaptive behavior. Modeling has been employed as a therapeutic tool within a variety of experimental and clinical settings. One of the earliest applications of modeling principles to behavior modification was undertaken by

Jones (1924) in an effort to modify phobic behavior in children. Her technique for eliminating phobias was to expose a phobic child to other children who behaved in a fearless manner toward the feared object. The observation of children interacting with the object was in most cases sufficient to reduce the phobic observer's anxious and avoidant responses. Conversely, Jones demonstrated that fears rapidly could be acquired through similar observational processes.

Another early modeling study was conducted by Chittenden (1942). Chittenden was interested in measuring and modifying assertive behaviors in young children. Observation of the free play behavior of preschool children identified two types of assertive behavior: dominating (the direct application of force against another child), and cooperating (non-forceful influence) responses. Children who scored high on the dimension of domination participated in a series of play periods in which they observed small dolls enact social roles similar to the ones in which they themselves experienced difficulties. The role modeling situations de-emphasized domination of others as a play technique. The dolls served as symbolic models to facilitate the childrens' understanding of social situations. The experimenter also served as a model and helped the children to understand and select appropriate responses to various situations. Samples of behavior collected subsequent to the training period indicated that actions of children trained in cooperative social techniques were significantly less dominant than those of comparable children who had served as a control (no treatment) group.

A therapeutically useful modeling technique, termed Fixed Role Therapy, has been developed by Kelly (1955) for use with adults who are interested in modifying or strengthening certain personality characteristics. The client first is required to construct a descriptive characterization of himself. The self-descriptions subsequently are studied by a panel of therapists who suggest ways of modifying them to help the client eliminate inappropriate behaviors and maximize the use of positive assets. A new role sketch or self-characterization is then presented to the client, who is given modeled demonstrations of the new role behaviors. Through imitation and practice the new behaviors gradually are assimilated into the client's repertoire and generalized to the extra-therapeutic environment.

Lazarus (1966) developed a behavior modification technique which is similar in some respects to that of Kelly. Lazarus terms his approach Behavior Rehearsal and employs it with patients who are deficient in some type of assertive behavior. Typically, his patients are individuals who are unable to make assertive or aggressive responses in situations where such behavior would be appropriate. In the treatment situation the therapist serves as a model, playing the role of someone toward whom the patient reacts with excessive fear, inhibition, or anxiety. The patient first observes responses that would be appropriate in the situation, then practices responding to the therapist's role behavior in a more uninhibited and aggressive manner. More recently McFall and Lillesand (1971) demonstrated that subjects who lacked assertiveness in refusing reasonable requests could be trained to become more assertive. Subjects first listened to a tape recorded model who refused another's request and subsequently practiced, with coaching from the experimenter, similar refusal behavior.

A final example of the therapeutic application of modeling procedures is the work of Lovaas (1968) on techniques of teaching verbal and non-verbal behaviors to schizophrenic children. Children were exposed to a successive set of discriminations that required them eventually to imitate an adult model's vocalizations. The verbal imitation training phase employed response-contingent positive reinforcement to establish and strengthen matching behavior. An important finding was that imitation eventually became self-reinforcing. Children would imitate words in the absence of external reinforcement. Lovaas devised a similar training program to establish socially appropriate and self-sufficient behaviors in the children. It is of note that Lovaas considered the therapeutic use of modeling and imitation to have been crucial to the success of his program.

Modeling has been used as a vehicle for behavior change in other areas of research. Examples include Poser's (1967) use of modeling procedures to train behavior therapists. Geer and Turteltaub (1967) employed fearless models to reduce the fears of snake phobic female college students. Bandura, Blanchard and Ritter (1969) developed similar methods to modify dog phobic behavior in children. DeWolfe (1967) demonstrated that student nurses became less afraid of contracting tuberculosis as a result of their association with unafraid nurses who served as models with whom the students could identify. Olson (1971) found that preferences for magazines among adult male schizophrenic patients could be modified by exposing the patients to models who expressed different kinds of preferences. In a different context, Sarason, Ganzer and Singer (in press) have shown that *S*s who are defensive about admitting to negative personal characteristics and problems in an interview situation can be influenced to make more problem-oriented statements if they first listened to a tape recorded model who discussed his problems in an open and honest manner. Marlatt (1971) demonstrated similar effects through the use of live models.

The above summary of research on modeling is by no means inclusive. It was meant to serve two purposes: (1) to illustrate the variety of behavior which has been successfully modified through the provision of various kinds of observational learning opportunities, and (2) to provide theoretical and empirical justification for applying observational learning procedures as rehabilitation techniques. We may now describe the development, procedures, and results of a modeling project which was concerned with the rehabilitation of juvenile offenders.*

The Cascadia Project

In different ways psychoanalytic, psychological, and sociological theorists have considered observational learning and the imitation of modeled behavior to be important explanatory concepts in accounting for the development and maintenance of delinquent behavior (Sarason and Ganzer, 1971). Similarly, a guiding principle in the research reported below was that if parents or significant others functioned as models of inadequate or deviant behavior, then impressionable observers such as children might well imitate and acquire various deviant behaviors. Conversely, the provision of adequate and prosocial models for children who have learned to behave maladaptively might be expected to facilitate the learning of new skills and more socially adaptive responses.

This research sought to attain two general objectives: (1) Working from the premise that rehabilitation is facilitated and recidivism is reduced by strengthening the juvenile offenders' social response repertoire, the project sought to teach institutionalized male delinquents more appropriate social skills and ways of coping with problems which they would encounter during their institutional stay and after release. The first objective was to demonstrate that the teaching of appropriate behaviors could be effectively accomplished through the systematic provision of relevant observational learning opportunities. (2) The second objective was to evaluate modeling techniques in terms of how easily they can be learned and applied by persons unfamiliar with behaviorally oriented rehabilitative methods. The urgent need to develop and utilize the potential skills of line personnel is a focal issue in the community mental health movement (Cowen and Zax, 1967). The development of simple, standard procedures for training people in the use of role modeling techniques might represent a significant step toward achieving this goal.

Background

The initial research in which observational learning opportunities were provided in an effort to increase the social-interpersonal skills of institutionalized male juveniles was conducted at Cascadia Juvenile Reception-Diagnostic Center located at Tacoma, Washington.* This institution, which is described

*The modeling research reported in this chapter was supported by grants from the Social and Rehabilitation Service of the Department of Health, Education and Welfare; and from the Law and Justice Planning Office, Planning and Community Affairs Agency, Olympia, Washington. Professor Irwin G. Sarason of the Department of Psychology, University of Washington, was the Project Director. The author served as Associate Project Director.

*Former Superintendent Robert Tropp, Superintendent William Callahan, Assistant Superintendent Keith Gibson, and Cottage Supervisors Lawrence Castleman, James Gibbeson, and John Sanguinetti and their staffs at Cascadia Juvenile Reception-Diagnostic Center contributed importantly to the conduct of the research described in this chapter. Completion of the project would not have been possible without the assistance and cooperation of Cascadia staff psychologists Sarah Sloat, V. M. Tye, and Ralph Sherfey; the Washington Division of Institutions, Juvenile Parole Services, the Office of Research, and the superintendents and staffs of the state's juvenile institutions.

more completely elsewhere (Sarason and Ganzer, 1969, 1971), is a facility of the State's Office of Juvenile Rehabilitation. Cascadia serves as the initial reception, treatment and diagnostic center for all children between the ages of eight and eighteen who are committed as delinquent by the State's Juvenile Courts. It houses approximately two hundred in twelve self-contained residential cottages. The average length of stay for children in the diagnostic program is six weeks.

The ingredients of a "modeling situation" were at this point only generally conceptualized. First, it would be a small group situation, consisting of at least two models or group leaders (in this project, graduate students in clinical psychology training) and four to six boys. Second, the purposes of the group meetings would be to teach the boys some behavior or skill in which they were deficient. Third, the teaching would be carried out by the models who would demonstrate (model) various roles and behaviors while the boys observed. The final step in the learning process would be the boys' imitations of the modeled behaviors which, when accompanied by social reinforcement (e.g., praise), would further the learning process and the development of new skills.

Development of Modeling Procedures

Since information on previous work involving group modeling techniques with institutionalized adolescents was not available, it was necessary to build the procedures virtually from the ground up. The four psychology graduate students who were to serve as the models began preliminary work on the project by meeting informally with small groups of boys in order to better understand the juvenile offender. Some of the purposes of these informal meetings were to develop ideas of what were the boys' problems and major concerns and to determine how the models could best interact with them in order to maximize their influence and desirability as persons with whom they would want to identify. Another purpose was to establish the project in the institution's residential cottages as an accepted part of their day-to-day operation since boys often regard strangers and innovations with suspicion and mistrust. As a further safeguard against arousing boys' antagonism and defensiveness, the project was introduced as being under the auspices of the University of Washington and *not* connected with any aspect of the institution's diagnostic process.

Many informal conversations were conducted and tape recorded over a period of several months. The sessions focused on the boys' problems, their perceptions of the adult and peer worlds, their needs, goals, feelings about themselves, and their identities in general. Informal content analyses were performed on the recorded material, and major problem and interest areas were noted and summarized. Subsequent groups of boys were asked to spontaneously role-play some of the problems. For example, the problems that teenagers have in dealing with authoritarian adults served as one topic around which spontaneous role-playing behavior was elicited. One boy or one of the assistants would play the role of an authoritarian teacher, and another boy would act the role of a teenager who was being disciplined. Or, two boys would role-play a dialogue in which one boy tried to convince the other not to experiment with narcotics. These and many other areas of importance to adolescents were role-played and the performances were tape recorded.

Further study of the boys' spontaneous behavior in these situations resulted in a series of revised and expanded dialogues which were typed in script form. The scripts were similar to those used by actors when learning various parts for plays. Depending upon the content and situations, roles for two to four people were written into the scripts. The sixteen to twenty of these scripts which were developed in this manner may be categorized into three or four general content areas. Some dealt with the problems teenagers often have in coping with authority. For example, one script dealt with how to appropriately interact with police officers; and another focused on appropriate behavior during a job interview. A related content area concerned the importance of planning ahead, which also involved some aspects of impulse control. Other scripts were based on the problem of negative peer pressure: how to recognize it, what it means, and various ways to cope with it. Another general topic concerned ways of making a good impression on others, not in the sense of manipulating somebody, but rather with aspects of dealing with people through acceptable and prosocial means. Most of the materials in some way dealt with the problem of impulsive (primarily aggressive) behaviors and various ways to recognize and appropriately express them.

The models practiced the various roles included in the scripts. These practice efforts were tape recorded, replayed, and the behavior of the models as well as the content of the scripts further were modified. Most of the scripts were tried out in groups with the boys as an audience. Their reactions to and opinions of the material regarding its realism and appropriateness were obtained. In a very real sense, the contents of the modeling procedures were developed largely by the boys themselves; they defined their problems, and the research staff worked with them on possible solutions.

Several common problems which other workers have noted as being particularly characteristic of delinquent youth became apparent during this preliminary work. These problems concerned the boys' motivations to work in groups and their often very short attention span. Learning through observing modeled behavior involves these two important variables. It was initially estimated that the boys' general level of attention could be maintained for approximately twenty minutes to one-half hour. Several techniques were instituted to increase this short and fluctuating attention span. One was the provision of a soft drink for each boy about half way through an hour's session. While initially perceived as a "bribe" by many of the boys, the soft drinks soon were readily accepted as something that the models wanted to share with them. Another, and perhaps the most important, method of maintaining attention is the actual amount of physical activity which the modeling situations require. Models and boys are on their feet and actually moving about the room a great deal during the sessions. This physical activity, combined with the heavy emphasis on affect and non-verbal expressive gestures, did a great deal to facilitate motivation and attention to the content and purpose of the group sessions. Since many delinquent boys are primarily action and movement oriented and rely considerably less on verbal skills, this dimension of the group procedures has proven to be very important. Another method of maintaining interest was the replay of the audio, and later the video, tape recordings after the boys had imitated various roles. This feedback was of considerable interest to the boys since it afforded them the opportunity to correct elements of their own behavior. Another method of maintaining attention was to ask one of the boys to summarize the situation that first had been enacted by the models. Boys did not know beforehand who was going to be asked, so it was necessary for them to be attentive in order to answer the questions satisfactorily. The fact that each boy knew that he would be expected to imitate the model's behavior also promoted increased attentiveness. It was estimated that these procedures were able to hold boys' attention and interest for an hour or more.

The Main Experiment

The subjects were 192 male first offenders between fifteen and eighteen years of age. Half of them were drawn from each of the two cottages in which the research was conducted. Sixty-four boys each participated in modeling groups, guided discussion groups, and the control group. Subjects were comparable in age, intelligence, chronicity of pre-institutional delinquent behavior, and diagnostic classification.

All boys were administered a battery of tests upon admission to the cottages. The tests included self-report trait, attitude, and self-concept measures. A number of dimensions of their behavior were rated by cottage staff on two specially devised behavior rating scales. These instruments are more fully described elsewhere (Sarason and Ganzer, 1971). Boys who arrived at the cottages on nearly the same days were selected in groups of four or five to serve as experimental group subjects. This procedure allowed the group members to participate together for the same number of sessions without having them disrupted by losses or additions of new boys. Additional admissions also were tested and served as a pool from which the control group (i.e., no special treatment) subjects concurrently were drawn.

Boys in the modeling groups participated in sixteen hour-long sessions which were conducted four times a week during a four-week period. Procedures for conducting the groups were very uniform, and the sequences of events which occurred during the sessions were virtually the same. Each session was attended by at least two models and four or five boys. One complete script was used for each meeting. One of the modeling scripts which deals with a home problem situation is presented below as example material.

Home Problem
Scene I

INTRODUCTION: Almost all teenagers differ with their parents on the rules and restrictions that are set down. For example, hair styles and getting hair cuts, clothes, choice of friends, and hours to be home are important sources of conflicts. Most kids get into power struggles with their parents on at least one of these issues with the result that no one usually wins. Kids see parental standards as restrictions on their freedom, and often over-react to this by fighting or simply disobeying. Parents often over-react, too, and today's scene is about a typical family fight, the ways it might start, and some of the ways it might be prevented. There are three parts to this scene: in the first part the situation ends up in a family fight, in the second part a fight is also started but the boy's behavior will probably have more positive results, and in the third scene the fight is averted.

SCENE: *It's Saturday evening and John, a parolee, is home with his mother and father. John's mother is in the kitchen working and his father is in the front room watching television and drinking beer. John comes out of his room with his coat on and is walking toward the kitchen door to leave, as his mother confronts him. Notice how John helps set up a fight between his parents and doesn't get his problem settled.*

(Model Only)

Mother:	"Where do you think you're going?"
John:	"Out."
Mother:	(*angrily*) "What do you mean, 'out'?"
John:	(*also angrily*) "I mean 'out'!"
Mother:	"You're not going anywhere! I'm getting sick and tired of you thinking you can take off anytime you want to. It'll do you good to stay home now and then."
John:	"Man, it's Saturday night—everybody goes out on Saturday night. All you expect me to do is stay home. Who wants to stay home all the time anyway?"
Father:	(*from the other room, looks into the kitchen*) "Shut up out there."
John:	(*walking into the front room*) "Why? Why can't I go out?"
Father:	"You settle that with your mother. I'm trying to watch television."
John:	"You always say that. Why don't you *ever* see my side of something? You always side with her."
Mother:	(*walking into front room*) "You're crazy. He doesn't side with anybody. He just sits in his chair and drinks beer all night."

Father:	"Don't start that crap again. I'm getting sick and tired of your bitching."
Mother:	"Don't you yell at me. You never take any responsibility for that boy."
	(*Parents start fighting between themselves. John leaves the room, runs out the back door, slams the door, and takes off.*)
COMMENT:	John was *set* to react negatively because he *knew* he'd be questioned.

Scene II

SCENE: *The scene is the same as Scene I except that John speaks to his mother first before heading for the door. He still has his coat on.*

(Model)

John:	"Mom, I'm going over to Jerry's for awhile."
Mother:	"What are you going to do at Jerry's?"
John:	"Oh, just mess around."
Mother:	"What do you mean *mess around?* The last time you and Jerry went out and messed around you both got arrested. You stay away from that kid. He's a bad influence."
John:	(*angrily*) "What do you know about it, you don't even know him. I don't tell you how to pick your friends, so don't try to tell me."
Mother:	(*angrily*) "That settles it. You're not going anywhere. All you and Jerry are going to do is go out and get in trouble, and end up in another institution. Haven't you got enough of a record as it is?"
John:	(*trying to control himself*) "Do you have to keep throwing that record bit up to me all of the time? How am I supposed to prove that I can stay out of trouble if all you do is throw that up to me and never give me a break?"
Mother:	"Well, you're *not* going anywhere."
John:	"Man, it's Saturday night—everybody goes out on Saturday night. All you expect me to do is stay home. Who wants to stay home all the time anyway?"
Father:	(*from the other room, looks into the kitchen*) "Shut up out there."
John:	(*walking into the front room*) "Why? Why can't I go out?"
Father:	"You settle that with your mother. I'm trying to watch television."
John:	"You always say that. Why the hell can't you *ever* see my side of something? You always side with her."
Mother:	(*walking into front room*) "You're crazy; he doesn't side with anybody. He just sits in his chair and drinks beer all night."

John:	"Oh, *shit,* here they go again."
Father:	"Don't start that crap again. I'm getting sick and tired of your bitching."
Mother:	"Don't you yell at me. You never take any responsibility for that boy."
John:	(*walks out of room into bedroom*)
COMMENT:	Okay, that's one way to handle a parent problem. Now here's another way.

Scene III

SCENE: *The scene is the same, but John's approach is different than in Scenes I and II, and he doesn't put his coat on first.*

(Model)

John:	"Mom, would you mind if I went over to Jerry's for awhile?"
Mother:	"Well, I don't know. What are you going to do?"
John:	"Well, we'll stay there for awhile, then I guess we'll go downtown and either go to the dance or shoot some pool or something. I'll be home when I'm supposed to."
Mother:	"Well, the last time you and Jerry went out and messed around you both got arrested. You stay away from that kid. He's a bad influence."
John:	"Ah, mom, you don't even know him. (*Laughs*) Besides, do I tell you how to pick your friends?"
Mother:	"That's not the point. You and Jerry *did* get in trouble, and they sent you to that state institution."
John:	(*trying to control himself*) "I know, but I wish you wouldn't keep throwing the record thing up to me all the time. How am I supposed to prove that I can stay out of trouble if all you do is throw that up to me and never give me a break? I'm *not* going to get into any trouble."
Mother:	"Well, I don't know. Go ask your Dad and see what he thinks."
John:	(*walking into the front room*) "Dad, do you mind if I go out for awhile tonight?"
Father:	"What? . . . Well, I don't know. You settle that with your mother. I'm trying to watch TV."
John:	(*starts to get angry, but doesn't say anything, turns around and goes back into the kitchen*) "Well, he doesn't seem to care one way or the other. He said to ask you."
Mother:	"Well, okay, but you'd better be home on time."
John:	"Okay, okay, I will. See you later."

(Imitate II and III)

MAIN DISCUSSION POINTS:

1. How are these three ways of dealing with a family problem different?
2. John's belligerent attitude helped set the family fight up.
3. Notice how easy it is to get a fight "snowballing" when everyone's mad.
4. Discuss possible influence of expectancy effects. John's mother communicated that she *expected* him to get into trouble. Does this have any influence on someone's behavior?
5. Leaving only temporarily solves his problem; both parents will be mad when he returns, for disobeying them. Besides, it's very easy to get into trouble or do something destructive when you take off from home in a bad mood.
6. Again John didn't get anything settled, but he used a little different approach in Scene II.
7. Going to his room and waiting until the fight subsides is a better way of coping with the problem than just taking off and leaving home.
8. Even if waiting and trying again doesn't work for John, it would be a good idea to wait and discuss the problem with the JPC, since continuing to struggle with the parents over matters like this usually doesn't get anywhere.
9. In Scene III John was more honest in details about what he was going to do; he didn't get angry, especially when the question of his record was thrown up to him by his mother. This is a difficult item for most parolees to handle, and it frequently occurs in the family.
10. Trying to be reasonable with parents of course doesn't guarantee that a situation like this will always have a better outcome, but it increases the chances of it.
11. Point out that provoking a fight between the parents is a good way not to get anything solved. Discuss other ways of avoiding three and four way family fights—for example, not going to one parent saying, "(Mom/Dad) said I could go out," when it isn't quite true.

(pp. 1-4 of **Home Problem**, Scene II)

A detailed orientation and modeled example scene was presented to groups during their first meeting. Each subsequent session was conducted in the following sequence: (1) One of the models began the session by introducing and describing the particular scene that would be enacted during the session. The introductions previously had been memorized by the models. They served the purpose of orienting the boys to the group's work for that day and to afford them a rationale for the inclusion of the particular scene in the sequence. (2) The models then role-played the particular scene for the day while the subjects observed. Since the scenes were usually separated into two and three-part sequences because they were often too long to be retained with sufficient recollection for good single imitations, only a first segment initially was modeled. (3) One boy was called upon to summarize and explain the content and outcome of what he had just observed. (4) Models and subjects commented upon and briefly discussed the scene; then an audio or video tape segment of the modeled behavior was replayed. (5) Depending on the number and kind of roles involved, either two or three boys or one boy and one model then imitated the modeled behavior that they had just observed. (6) Following one or two imitations, a short recess was taken while soft drinks were served and one of the previous role imitations was replayed. Participants also used this time to comment upon each other's behavior. (7) After the recess the boys who had not participated then enacted the situations. Insofar as possible, each boy participated in each session. (8) One of these two or three performances was replayed and commented upon. (9) The group's final task involved comments concerning the material, aspects of its importance, and its general applicability in other interpersonal situations.

The efficacy of the modeling procedures was evaluated by comparing the participants' subsequent behavior with that of other boys who were involved in guided discussions of the same content material but without modeling or role-playing. That is, while modeling group boys observed and then imitated appropriate behavior in a family problem or job interview situation, boys in discussion groups would only talk informally about such behavior. Every effort was made to insure that the conduct of the discussion groups was in other respects as similar as possible to that of the modeling condition (e.g., breaks, use of feedback, number of sessions).

Following participation in the experimental sequence, all subjects were readministered the same battery of tests; and their behavior was again rated by cottage counselors. Control group subjects also were retested and rated after a comparable time interval. All boys were discharged from the institution within a week after this second assessment was obtained. Approximately 14 percent of the subjects were paroled back into their communities. The remaining boys were sent to other juvenile institutions, and behavior ratings again were obtained on these boys after a four-month period in residence. A longer term follow-up evaluation provided further data through personal interviews after parole discharge and through records of recidivism. Indices of recidivism were obtained on all subjects at a risk period of at least eighteen months after release to parole.

Evaluation of the Project

The major results of this research are summarized below. Omitted are the numerous statistical analyses that were performed on the more than forty dependent variables which were measured in the study.

1. Boys who participated in both the modeling and guided discussion

treatments showed more positive or favorable changes in their attitudes, self-concepts, and rated overt behaviors than did control group boys.

2. Further analyses of these measures suggested that less socially adequate, more dependent boys who required greater direction and structure, responded most favorably to the modeling procedures.

3. Behavior ratings obtained during the four-month follow-up evaluation were complete on 82 percent of the subjects. Comparison of these ratings with the second Cascadia behavior ratings revealed that most experimental group boys continued to maintain favorable behavior or continued to show improvement. Fewer control boys continued to improve, and more changed in a negative direction.

4. Personal interviews and retesting with a small sample of fifty-three subjects following discharge from parole suggested that more former modeling than discussion group boys remembered and applied the information and concepts that they had learned in the groups. They more frequently expressed favorable or positive attitudes toward their experiences in institutions and on parole than did either discussion or control group subjects.

5. Fewer experimental than control group subjects reported engaging in further delinquent activities while on parole.

6. Data on recidivism were obtained on all subjects. Recidivism was defined as: (a) the return of a boy to a juvenile institution, (b) conviction in superior court resulting in probation as an adult status offender, or (c) confinement in an adult correctional institution. This data indicated that the rate of recidivism for controls was somewhat more than twice as high as that for experimentals. The control group contained twenty-two recidivists whereas there were twelve in the modeling group and nine in the discussion group. The difference in proportion of recidivists among the three groups was significant ($p + .06$, Chi-square test). Both the modeling ($p = .06$) and discussion ($p = .01$) groups had significantly fewer recidivists than had the control group. While recidivism is not an infallible indicator of the success of a rehabilitation program, these data do suggest that the experimental treatments employed in this research did favorably influence the subsequent adjustment of the subjects in the sample.

EXTENSIONS OF THE MODELING PROJECT

One practical yardstick of the value of any rehabilitation program is the extent to which it is applicable in different situations and with different kinds of clients. Perhaps an even more important question is whether a treatment approach can be readily learned and effectively applied by other rehabilitation workers. Could modeling techniques be utilized in institution settings other than Cascadia? How easily could models other than university graduate students be trained to conduct modeling groups? Would other models be as or more effective than had been the graduate students? While the modeling procedures showed several specific advantages over those employed in the discussion groups, modeling was not more effective overall than was guided discussion. Would a new procedure which combined the most therapeutic elements of the modeling and discussion approaches provide an even more efficacious rehabilitation technique? New variations of the original modeling groups were initiated and conducted at three other juvenile institutions in Washington in an effort to answer these questions.*

In addition it was hoped that the new modeling programs would overcome two factors which were viewed as major problems in the Cascadia research. One problem in the Cascadia project was that the graduate student-models were relatively unacquainted with the subjects, interacted with them for only four-week periods, and rotated their participation in different groups on a part-time basis. The unfamiliarity factor would not exist in the new groups because institution staff social workers and counselors would serve as models. The boys would be well acquainted with the models since they had known them for several months prior to participation in modeling sessions. It was expected that familiarity with and trust in the models would enhance the effectiveness of the modeling situations. The second advantage was that modeling groups would be made up of boys for whom parole was an imminent reality (e.g., in 1 to 2 months). The major focus of modeling groups always had been on the development of skills and coping behaviors which would facilitate post-institutional adjustment. In the Cascadia research a problem arose because this emphasis seemed of little relevance to many boys, since for most of them institution release was an event that would not occur for many more months. In view of the limited psychological reality of the future for most delinquent youth, the Cascadia project which was aimed at a period so far ahead often may have appeared irrelevant.

Training New Models

Approximately twenty social workers and staff counselors, both male and female, expressed interest in learning modeling techniques. Some of them were experienced in leading small groups, and some had never participated in group situations. Their educational backgrounds varied from high school graduate to the Master's Degree. However, they all had at least several months' experience in working with adolescents. A training period of four to six two-hour sessions was sufficient preparation time to enable new models to begin conducting their own groups. The training sessions in each institution followed a similar sequence. First was explained the theoretical rationale underlying the techniques. The development of the procedure, content of the sessions, and the role and function of models were discussed in detail. Audio tapes of previous Cascadia modeling groups were played and discussed as example material. Videotapes later were made of two groups, and their sub-

---

*Echo Glen Children's Center, Greenhill School, and Mission Creek Youth Forest Camp were the facilities in which modeling groups were conducted. The support and participation of the administration and staff of these institutions is gratefully acknowledged.

sequent use of teaching aids further facilitated the learning process for new models. The scripts then were used in practice sessions which closely approximated the course of actual modeling groups. Models began to work in informal groups after two or three practice sessions. Research staff participated in some groups and frequently consulted with the models to discuss procedures and any problems that arose. The only apparent difficulty that was noted was an initial tendency of the models to miss various parts in the role imitations where boys needed cues because they had forgotten part of the dialogue. During particularly long imitations, boys often forgot parts of their roles; and models had to be alert to provide cues to enable them to continue their performances. This was never a major problem and was overcome after several group sessions.

Procedure Changes

It was mentioned that the evaluation of the Cascadia project failed to demonstrate that modeling was clearly superior to guided group discussion as a rehabilitative technique. It was for this reason that the most effective elements of both procedures were incorporated into the structure and conduct of new modeling groups. Six major changes briefly may be described: (1) Groups were conducted in a more informal and less highly structured manner. While the sequence of events which occurred during each meeting remained generally the same (i.e., modeling followed by role imitations), both models and boys were permitted more latitude in their adherence to the roles. (2) Considerably more discussion, both structured and informal, accompanied the modeling and role imitations. (3) Role reversals and improvisations more frequently were employed. For example, boys more often were encouraged to take the role of adult authority figures after they had imitated a subordinate role. These three changes were accompanied by more active efforts to involve boys in an ongoing process of critically appraising and modifying modeled roles in an effort to develop the most appropriate and relevant, example behaviors and coping and problem solving techniques. This greater emphasis on making the group sessions more meaningful and relevant appeared to foster more group cohesiveness and provided an additional incentive for active participation among boys. (4) Groups were larger, containing six to nine boys, which required a reduction in the number of imitations during each session. (5) Meetings were longer, often lasting one and one-half or two hours each. Lengthier sessions were necessary because of increased group size, greater emphasis on discussion, and the development of new and longer three- and four-part situations. (6) Although varying among the institutional settings, the number of sessions conducted with each individual group was reduced from sixteen to eight or ten.

Some Results and Effects

At present over thirty diferent modeling groups have been conducted within the revised format outlined above. No formal evaluation has been made of the usefulness or effectiveness of the new procedures and groups. However, a number of subjective impressions were formed based on the observations of the author, the models and boys, and other institution personnel. Several of these observations briefly may be mentioned. Modeling groups contained boys who were accorded both high and low status among their peers. Low status boys frequently were scapegoated on campus and within their respective residential cottages. Group participation facilitated more positive interactions and stronger friendships among status-different boys, with the result that weaker boys gained in status through the protection and encouragement of the stronger boys. In all instances these effects were quite immediate, which result in part attests to the rapid impact that modeling procedures have on group members. It was the feeling of all concerned that group participation had a salutory effect on the ability and willingness of the boys to communicate more openly with adults as well as with peers. It also was noted that boys in the groups formed closer interpersonal relationships among themselves.

A number of the boys experienced situations in which they were able to apply successfully new coping behaviors which they had learned in the groups. One boy with a history of assaultive behavior was one of the best participants. He as well as several staff counselors felt that his aggressiveness had been brought under better control, in large part because of his group experiences. Another impulsive boy employed several self-control techniques, which he had learned in a modeling scene dealing with controlling anger, to avoid becoming belligerent and being isolated by a classroom teacher. A boy who had been on extended leave returned to the institution, sought out his caseworker, and described how the job interview modeling situation had been a key factor in his ability to secure a job which had been promised to him upon release. Another reported how the dealing with authority materials which were used in groups had been a major factor in keeping him out of trouble during a month's leave from the institution. This boy directly stated that he would not have lasted successfully for that month without the benefit of his group experiences.

These reports were offered spontaneously by boys as evidence of the immediate usefulness of the procedures and serve as indications that they have had practical utility for group participants.

CONCLUSIONS

Previously cited research on the therapeutic application of modeling principles has demonstrated that they are useful in individual and group approaches to rehabilitation. They may be employed as either a primary or supplementary means of teaching new skills to clients, of strengthening existing appropriate but weak behaviors, and of modifying maladaptive responses.

Furthermore, both live and filmed or videotaped models have been used to successfully achieve various therapeutic goals.

Modeling techniques are relatively simple, objective, and effective methods of modifying behavior. While the procedures specifically adapted for the present research only have been applied in the rehabilitation of institutionalized adolescent males between the ages of twelve and eighteen, there is no compelling reason to believe that, with certain modifications, they would be any less effective with females of that age or with adults of either sex. The approach has shown favorable results with boys of different ages, of different personality types, and in different institutional settings. In view of these findings, it may be concluded that the first objective of the research was achieved: there is evidence that rehabilitation programs can be strengthened through the use of modeling procedures.

The second objective, the evaluation of how easily the procedures can be learned and applied by institution personnel, also was partly achieved. A number of persons who were totally unfamiliar with modeling techniques, learned them, and became comfortable enough with them that they were able to begin conducting groups after approximately ten hours of training. Training was accomplished through didactic discussion, live and video-taped modeled demonstrations, and rehearsal sessions in which new models practiced and sharpened their newly acquired skills. Modeling procedures are learned equally rapidly by persons with and without previous experience in working with small groups. The experience variable appears primarily important in that models who are familiar with group processes initially are more self confident and skillful in leading discussions of modeled behaviors than are inexperienced models. However, these differences are much less obvious after as little as two or three hours of group participation. Also, effective models need not be persons holding advanced degrees in the behavioral sciences. The importance of this factor to rehabilitation and mental health work may be of considerable importance.

As is true of any technique, the use of modeling and role imitation procedures is not without problems and cautions. Conducting groups is time-consuming. Time means cost to any rehabilitation program. The development of relevant and interesting content for use in groups may take substantial time and energy. At least two and sometimes three models are required to initiate each modeling session, although one model is usually able to conduct a group after the initial phase. Models also usually spend additional time rehearsing their roles prior to each group meeting. However, the cost per group in terms of time seems balanced by the fact that models can be easily and quickly trained. This factor is one of the basic strengths of the application of these procedures in group work.

Other potential problems involve the specificity of modeled behavior. Models perform a specific sequence of observable verbal, affective and motor behaviors. Care must be taken to select and develop the most appropriate example behaviors to illustrate the purposes of the modeled situation. The examples should have some relevance for each client in the group, and ingenuity often is required to come up with situations which meet this requirement. The specific nature of modeled behaviors also demands that generalization be provided for at some point during the group session. Clients probably will never engage in situations where they confront a problem or are required to exhibit a behavior exactly as it was illustrated in a modeling session. It is therefore necessary to provide for adequate generalization to insure that learned behaviors will be applied in a variety of similar settings. Both group discussion and the modeling of several similar but not identical situations may be used to facilitate generalization.

Role modeling techniques appear to work, but what are the important ingredients which make them successful? As is true of other approaches to therapy and rehabilitation, there seem to be a number of factors which contribute to the success of the procedures. Modeling is a method or vehicle for presenting information to clients. It also serves as a potent stimulator for group discussion. Discussions help assure that the purposes of the modeling are understood. The practice afforded by role imitations serves to sharpen observers' skills as well as to promote better retention of what is learned. Modeling always focuses and holds the attention and interest of group participants, in part because it is an action-oriented as well as a verbal procedure in which clients learn by observing and by doing. Beginning a group by modeling a sequence of behavior immediately focuses on relevant aspects of the material. Because of this feature, groups start off rapidly, and there is little groping or searching for topics to discuss. Modeling has the advantages of role playing in that participants can feel safe being in the role of another person, yet they are free to express their own characteristic attitudes and behavior. Modeling permits but does not require self-exploration, discussion of personal problems, or the achievement of insight. In this respect it has some of the advantages of traditional group therapy.

Finally, participation in modeling groups is fun, and this factor may be of particular importance for adolescents. Almost all group participants, models and boys alike, at various times indicated that they enjoyed the sessions. While most people learn and work more effectively if they are enjoying themselves, this may be particularly important for adolescents because many of them lack the self-discipline to persist at something they dislike. While modeling procedures continue to develop and evolve, they may be considered effective as methods of modifying behavior, both with respect to their impact upon the clients with whom they had been used as well as the ease with which they can be learned and applied by group workers.

REFERENCES

Aronfreed, J.: The concept of internalization. In D. Goslin and D. Glass (Eds.),

Handbook of Socialization Theory and Research. Chicago, Rand McNally, 1969.

Bandura, A.: Behavioral modification through modeling procedures. In L. Krasner and L. P. Ullmann (Eds.), *Research in Behavior Modification: New Developments and Implications.* New York, Holt, Rinehart and Winston, pp. 310-340, 1965.

Bandura, A.: The influence of punishing consequences to the model on the acquisition and performance of imitative responses. Unpublished manuscript, Stanford University, 1962.

Bandura, A.: *Principles of Behavior Modification.* New York, Holt, Rinehart and Winston, 1969 (a).

Bandura, A.: Social learning theory of identificatory processes. In D. Goslin and D. Glass (Eds.), *Handbook of Socialization Theory and Research.* Chicago, Rand McNally, 1969 (b).

Bandura, A., Blanchard, E. B. and Ritter, B. J.: Relative efficacy of desensitization and modeling approaches for inducing behavioral, affective, and attitudinal changes. *Journal of Personality and Social Psychology, 13*:173-199, 1969.

Bandura, A. and Walters, R. H.: *Social Learning and Personality Development.* New York, Holt, Rinehart and Winston, 1963.

Chittenden, G.: An experimental study in measuring and modifying assertive behavior in young children. *Monograph of Social Research and Child Development,* Vol. 7, no. 1, 1942.

Cowen, E. L. and Zax, M.: The mental health field today: Issues and problems. In E. M. Cowen, E. A. Gardner and M. Zax (Eds.), *Emergent Approaches to Mental Health Problems.* New York, Appleton-Century-Crofts, pp. 3-29, 1967.

DeWolfe, A.: Identification and fear decrease. *Journal of Consulting Psychology, 31*:259-263, 1967.

Geer, J. and Turteltaub, A.: Fear reduction following observation of a model. *Journal of Personality and Social Psychology, 6*:327-331, 1967.

Jones, M. C.: The elimination of children's fears. *Journal of Experimental Psychology, 7*:383-390, 1924.

Kelly, G. A.: *The Psychology of Personal Constructs: A Theory of Personality.* New York, Norton, 1955.

Lazarus, A.: Behavior rehearsal versus non-directive therapy versus advice in effecting behavior change. *Behaviour Research and Therapy, 4*:209-212, 1966.

Lovaas, O. I.: Some studies on the treatment of childhood schizophrenia. In J. Schlein (Ed.), *Research in Psychotherapy.* Washington, D. C., American Psychological Association, 1968.

Marlatt, G. A.: Exposure to a model and task ambiguity as determinants of verbal behavior in an interview. *Journal of Consulting and Clinical Psychology, 36*: 268-276, 1971.

McFall, R. M. and Lillesand, D. B.: Behavior rehearsal with modeling and coaching in assertion training. *Journal of Abnormal Psychology, 77*:313-323, 1971.

Olson, R.: Effects of modeling and reinforcement on adult chronic schizophrenics. *Journal of Consulting and Clinical Psychology, 36*:126-132, 1971.

Poser, E. G.: Training behavior therapists. *Behavior Research and Therapy, 5*:37-41, 1967.

Sarason, I. G. and Ganzer, V. J.: Developing appropriate social behaviors of juvenile delinquents. In J. D. Krumboltz and C. E. Thoreson (Eds.), *Behavioral Counseling: Cases and Techniques.* New York, Holt, Rinehart and Winston, 1969.

Sarason, I. G. and Ganzer, V. J.: Modeling: An approach to the rehabilitation of juvenile offenders. Final report to the Social and Rehabilitation Service. University of Washington, June 1971.

Sarason, I. G., Ganzer, V. J. and Singer, M.: The effects of modeled self-disclosure on the verbal behavior of persons differing in defensiveness. *Journal of Consulting and Clinical Psychology,* (in press).

Chapter 3

SURVIVAL CAMPING: A THERAPEUTIC TECHNIQUE TO AID THE REHABILITATION OF THE YOUTHFUL OFFENDER

Thomas R. Collingwood

THE CRISIS in our youth is becoming more and more pronounced. Among them are problem youth (the drug abuser, the delinquent and the drop-out) and potential problem youth (the disadvantaged, the turned off) who are not able to successfully progress or develop within society. At the same time, the scope of rehabilitation services to serve the public offender is expanding. With this expansion there is a search for effective programs to facilitate the rehabilitation, avocationally as well as vocationally, of delinquent or problem youth.

The key questions confronting rehabilitation are how to prevent potential problem youth from becoming marginal adults and how to rehabilitate those who are delinquent already. In relation to this challenge, there is an increasing awareness of the totality of effort demanded to deal with the whole person that is oftentimes needed for successful outcome with this group. There is a realization that physical, intellectual and emotional needs of delinquents, as well as their vocational-educational needs, must be dealt with if successful rehabilitation is to occur. In a very real sense, prevention and rehabilitation can be concretized into one basic question as to how to facilitate the development of effective and fully functioning youths into effective and fully functioning adults.

The total development of youth to live effective instead of ineffective lives, can be viewed on three levels (the physical, the intellectual and the emotional-interpersonal) within a Human Resource Development Model (Carkhuff, 1971). The majority of rehabilitation programs for delinquents have usually been oriented toward just the intellectual (educational and vocational evaluation and training) or just the emotional (counseling and guidance), with little emphasis placed upon the physical or upon an integrated "total" program that will affect all three life spheres. This, unfortunately, leaves a gap in the scope of necessary rehabilitation services. There is a critical need to develop and implement more "total" rehabilitation services to serve the young offender.

While educational and vocational rehabilitation services do meet many of the needs of the youthful offender, the outcome data tell us that in actuality these services are often not enough. Many writers (Erickson, 1956; Jesness, 1967) have emphasized the importance of providing therapeutic experiences to affect the delinquent's negative self-concept, even his lack of personal identity, lack of effective behavior, and his resultant recourse to antisocial behavior. In turn, the dearth of successful outcomes with delinquents may be directly related to a failure to provide the type of experiences or services that facilitate positive change in those dimensions. By the same token, the delinquent has a high preference for action for solutions to conflicts and tensions, for action as a style of life. In fact, traditional cognitive approaches (counseling psychotherapy, guidance) employed to modify the undesirable behavior of delinquents have had rather tenuous results.

For many delinquents, existing services may not be enough to meet their needs. Although needs of the young offender in many respects are developmentally the same as for all youth, only magnified in intensity, he *needs* to learn appropriate, functional, and more purposeful behavior, to develop his own identity and increase interpersonal effectiveness. He *needs* to undergo rewarding success experiences to develop a more positive self-concept and to learn the most important survival skill—discipline. At the same time he prefers action, such as results from meeting concrete challenges. The fundamental question keeps coming back: *how* can we meet these needs?

The basic conclusions from the field all point to the desirability of developing and utilizing new and more total therapeutic techniques in order to "turn around" many delinquents. Oftentimes extra effort, extra service, or extra techniques may be required to meet the needs of the young offender. One such technique or mode is survival or rugged camping with a strong physical base.

SURVIVAL CAMPING AS A SERVICE TO DELINQUENTS

Some of the major delinquent needs which existing services do not always meet are those pertaining to the delinquent's preference for action and his need for constructive challenges and appropriate behavioral change. Over the years, camping programs have been developed to provide for problem youth, challenging, action-oriented experiences which are meant to serve as constructive learning experiences for the participants, both personally and socially.

The effective camping programs for male and female delinquents (see experiences cited in Kelly and Baer, 1968; Loughmiller, 1965; and Weber, 1969) are rugged in nature with an emphasis on wilderness survival, are systematic and functional in operation, and are integrated within a total treatment or rehabilitation program. On the other hand, the less effective programs tend to be neither systematic nor rugged (recreation in nature), and to be neither very challenging, nor integrated into a delinquent's total rehabilitation program.

The basic premise underlying most camping programs for delinquents is that, inherent within the camping and outdoor experience, are tremendous therapeutic benefits. However, the therapeutic potential in a rugged camping situation must systematically be capitalized on to be functionally relevant for changing problem youth. Without this, the program could be nothing more than a two-or-three-week vacation for a youth.

The sources of gain from rugged survival camping experiences are derived from a unique process. We have already seen that the camping process itself provides a therapeutic and total context. On a physical level, experience cannot be made more real or undistorted. A physically based process provides a very concrete and honest experience with immediate feedback which cannot be rationalized away. As such, it has tremendous potential as a learning process. The twenty-four hour challenge of individual and group survival in the camping process, lends itself as a potent learning vehicle as well. Having to undergo physical hardships such as procuring one's own water and food facilitates responsibility rather quickly. In short, the context of a survival camping experience provides basic challenges so that the learning of more effective physical, intellectual and emotional-interpersonal behaviors, self-discipline, self-responsibility, and self-respect can be greatly enhanced. By affecting those particular factors, a rugged camp program can meet the needs of delinquents and directly facilitate their rehabilitation.

The words "rugged" and "survival" are emphasized in describing the concept and utilization of effective camping programs to differentiate them from the more recreational types of programs and to demonstrate the physically challenging ingredients of the process of a good camping program are the ones which offer the basic therapeutic potentials for client change. In certain respects the delinquent is "delinquent" because he is not able to survive functionally within society. Consequently, the young offender can benefit from a program that gets down to basic survival. Hopefully, by being able to survive successfully at that level, he can evolve to the point whereby he can get *turned on* to himself and his own development and can more effectively survive once he is back home. The very basic physical demands of such a camping process can enable the problem youth to develop and become aware of strengths and potentials. He can experience a very intense, concrete, and *earned* success experience. In turn, the realization of seeing change and growth can serve as a springboard for him to view himself in a more realistic, a more functional and a more confident perspective.

Generally, survival camping can be regarded as a type of therapeutic vehicle to aid a young offender's rehabilitation. As a client service, a survival camp program should be developed and/or utilized to meet certain client goals whether they be physical, psychological or social. Of utmost importance is the use of such camping programs to meet *behavioral change* goals. To get a more complete picture of the development, utilization, role and effects of a survival camping program as a client service for delinquents, the following report of a unique camp project is presented.

CAMP CHALLENGE*

The need for a total approach to serving delinquents in Arkansas led to a cooperative effort between the Arkansas Rehabilitation Service, Aldersgate Methodist Camp of Little Rock and the Arkansas Rehabilitation Research and Training Center to develop an innovative client service camping program that had the potential to positively affect the *total* person. The end result was the development and implementation of "Camp Challenge," a rugged three-week camping program designed as both a client service and as a demonstration project for male problem youth in Arkansas.

The general aim of the "Camp Challenge" project was to develop and implement a challenging survival camping program, capitalizing upon the therapeutic potentials within the camping process, which would serve as a functional program for the rehabilitation of delinquents. The program was developed and structured to function as follows:

1. *An integrated program* within the youth's total rehabilitation program; the camp program was not an isolated experience for the participants. From the very beginning the youth, his rehabilitation counselor and the project director defined and organizationally structured the program as a major client service program within the total rehabilitation plan. The camper's performance in the camp project affected further rehabilitation plans, etc. The camp was to function as a first step program prior to vocational and/or educational training.

2. *A systematic program* which demanded increasing levels of performance from the participants. The youths were taught the necessary camp and survival skills starting with the least hardest skills to the most difficult skills. Performance demands were from least hardest to hardest as well. In a sense, systematic success experiences were built in.

3. *A functional program* in which the experiences, demands and reinforcements placed upon the youths were very relevant to their day to day survival. There was a functional purpose and a functional reward for the various program aspects the youths went through.

4. *A challenging program* which presented new and confronting experiences for the youth where they could learn and utilize more effective physical, intellectual and emotional-interpersonal behaviors. The program provided the youth a chance to test themselves.

5. *A consolidated program* whereby the youth looked at themselves (their strengths and weaknesses) and where they are going in their lives to develop some direction.

6. *A therapeutic program* in the sense that the youths learned effective physical, intellectual and emotional-interpersonal behaviors and underwent an intensive success experience. Self-enhancement and self-worth emerged from the experience that, in turn, can serve as a springboard for success in all areas of their lives.

7. *An inexpensive program* that elicited cooperation from existing functional professionals as project staff members. The only way that a camping program such as this could be implemented in a practical and efficient manner was to secure cooperative efforts from community resources.

*Reprinted in part from *Survival Camping: A Therapeutic Mode for Rehabilitating Problem Youth* by the author. Monograph Series. Arkansas Rehabilitation Research and Training Center, 1972.

8. *A demonstration program* to assess the effectiveness of the camping program as a vehicle to affect positive change in problem youth and in an inexpensive fashion. Assessment of the program's effect on behavioral and psychological dimensions relevant to rehabilitation outcome, as well as outcome assessment, should demonstrate the feasibility of employing such a camp program on a larger basis.

In short, this camping program could be viewed as an initial therapeutic client service to help prepare the youth and get them *in shape* for the vocational rehabilitation process in terms of more effective and positive behaviors and attitudes.

Participants:

Nineteen boys between the ages of 15-18 started and completed the program. Three of the boys were from one of the training schools in Arkansas, ten were from the Arkansas Rehabilitation Service First Offender Program (most were charged with drug abuse) and six were from a large rehabilitation facility (all were categorized as behavioral problems). All nineteen boys were rehabilitation agency clients and were volunteers.

PROGRAM DEVELOPMENT

The development of any effective program must account for three major areas: (1) the effectiveness of the staff implementing the program in terms of the functionally relevant skills they have, (2) the effectiveness of the program in terms of its being developed in a systematic manner to accomplish its goals, and (3) the effectiveness of the organizational process in terms of the structures and procedures that integrate the staff with the program for optimum helpee gain.

The development of the camp project can be delineated according to those three areas.

STAFF CONSIDERATIONS:

Staff Selection:

The key to staff selection is to select those who have the functional skills needed to implement the program. Aldersgate Methodist Camp had a pool of camp leaders of which four were selected. The basis of the selection was in their having the campcraft and survival skills and experience necessary to function effectively in the program. All four leaders had been camp leaders for two years and had previously participated in rugged camping. The Project Director, besides having experience and skill in the survival camping area as well, also had skills in the interpersonal/counseling skills area, physical fitness and program development area as they relate to helping processes.

The four camp leaders were not selected on other relevant dimensions such as interpersonal skills, program development and physical fitness which have been demonstrated to be key variables in effective helpers (Carkhuff, 1971). Future programs such as this, however, need to select staff on these dimensions as well.

Staff Training:

All staff received a week long campcraft and first aid course as part of the Aldersgate Camp pre-camp training. The four leaders also received approximately ten hours of interpersonal skill training and orientation/familiarization to the clients with the rehabilitation counselors. Reading materials relevant to the program were assigned. Many hours were also spent in reviewing several skills such as map reading, etc., and acquiring any new skills that were needed.

As the time for the camp program approached, all five staff members developed a program outline for the three weeks. Potential backpacking and camping areas were reconnoitered and a tentative route was planned.

Staff Conclusions:

1. Staff selection needs to be based upon relevant physical, intellectual, emotional-interpersonal, and specialty skills, such as: (a) fitness level—physical, (b) program development skills—intellectual, (c) interpersonal skills—emotional, and (d) campcraft and survival skills—specialty. This involves getting the highest functioning helpers for the program.

2. Plenty of staff training time needs to be allocated with a focus upon the same skills you select staff on. The most critical skills are the campcraft and survival (hygiene, fire building, food and water procurement, cooking, shelter making, hiking and backpacking, orienteering and first-aid) and fitness.

3. Staff need a good orientation to the clients with whom they will be working and living.

4. Staff pre-training especially in physical areas insured their readiness for the program.

5. Staff need to know the big picture. They need to have all the information relevant to the camp's purpose and goals . . . specifically as it functions as a rehabilitative tool for the individual client. They need to know where they are contributing.

6. Staff need to be more directive than is usually the case with camp counselors.

PROGRAM CONSIDERATIONS:

Pre-Camp Orientation:

All clients were interviewed by the project director or counselor. A brief description of the program and its goals was presented to the individual client, emphasizing the challenging aspects of the program. Communication was set up so that he would explore what he would like to get from participation as well. It was detailed out what he could expect from the staff and the program and what the staff expected of him. Following a commitment to the program, the necessary legal, parental, medical and counselor approval was obtained. In some cases an orientation also had to be given to parents and training school authorities where appropriate.

Camp Stages:

The total camp program lasted approximately three weeks. There were four basic stages to the program: (1) basic training, (2) backpacking expedition, (3) counseling, and (4) follow-through. Out of twenty-one clients, nineteen started and completed the program. Campers and staff were broken down into functional units of six men (one leader and five youths) for a total of four groups.

The participants spent the first eight days at the resident camp learning to work together as a team, learning the basic camping and survival skills and getting into physical shape. The physical training consisted of running, calisthenics and hiking, with the skill training in outdoor living consisting of the following areas: personal and camp hygiene, axmanship, fire building, food and water procurement, hiking and backpacking, trail discipline, cooking, shelter making, orienteering (map reading, compass and star reading), first-aid, snake identification and general campcraft. The majority of skill acquisition sessions were done within the small functional unit or with two units together (twelve persons). Toward the end of the basic training week they participated in several backpacking hikes and one overnight to practice tearing down and building a camp site properly.

Following the basic training portion of the program the participants went on a nine-day backpacking expedition through the Ozark mountains. Everything they needed to survive they carried on their backs. A portion of their food had to be secured from the land (snakes, polk salad, fish, crayfish, burdock plants, wild berries, sassafras roots and water). Toward the end of the nine days, pairs of participants went on a twenty-four hour survival by themselves, whereby they had to secure their own shelter, food and fire while alone.

After returning to the resident camp the participants spent two days of group counseling, recreation and equipment clean up. Besides the group session, there were individual consultations between the individual participant and his leader and with the project director. The thrust of the discussions focused around exploring the gains the participants made in successfully completing the program and the implications for them in acting successfully in other areas of their lives. Specific content also focused upon had to do with future plans vocationally and avocationally.

The participants reported back to their rehabilitation counselor after leaving the camp program. A concrete rehabilitation plan was then developed with the aid of the camp staff reports and personal consultations. Three month follow-up reports were obtained and personal consultations have been initiated as needed between project director and counselor and, on a few occasions, directly with the client. Personal letters of encouragement have also been communicatd to all clients.

Camp Process:

The entire program was devised to proceed in a rather systematic fashion. It was attempted to build-in success at every step of the entire process.

During the basic training portions, skills were taught at a group and individual level so that competency could be obtained regardless of initial level. Skills and physical tasks were taught and attempted from the least difficult to most difficult. From the basic training to the end of the backpacking phases, the participants earned increasing responsibility and decision-making functions. Every day, especially during the basic training phase, certain tasks and goals had to be met. Self-discipline was striven for. Rewards such as coke breaks, smoke breaks and free time were employed or withdrawn to increase skill acquisition and cooperative work effort. However, the key reinforcement that aided the program to proceed systematically was the functionality of the situations into which the participants were placed.

At all stages of the program, the demands placed upon the participants were functional. From the very beginning, in resident camp, they had to build their own shelter, cook their own food and function as a unit. This placed a very real demand on them to learn the skills and to cooperate with each other in order to meet day-to-day necessity needs. Functionality was most pronounced during the backpacking phase whereby the meeting of everyday needs and day-to-day survival was dependent upon individual and group performance. How well an individual got into shape during the basic training phase affected his backpacking pace and, in turn, his group's pace. How well an individual learned to read the stars, compass and maps could determine whether he or his group got lost. How well an individual learned to find food and water directly affected his own and his group's survival. Cooperation, responsibility, leadership and followership were functionally demanded twenty-four hours a day or else one went without shelter, fire, food and water. Every participant had functional responsibilities to meet for himself and his group.

The intensity of the functional aspect of the program, especially during the backpacking phase, was made known in that the participants had to learn to perform while fatigued, lonely, scared and at times uncertain as to what was going to happen. There were many functional challenges to meet every day, such as finding food and water, climbing mountains and orienteering (not getting lost). By the same token, there were some dangerous challenges as well. Encounters with poisonous snakes were a daily experience and there were black bears in the area. All the preceding, coupled with the new and unfamiliar surroundings, served to make the process functionally confronting for the participants.

At one level, the basic program process, skills learned and participant gains from the program could be interpreted in terms of physical, intellectual and emotional-interpersonal functioning. Physically, they had to learn fitness, hiking and many outdoor skills. Intellectually, they had to learn many new facts and how to use them in outdoor living. Emotionally-interpersonally, they had to learn to deal and cooperate with each other, to trust themselves and to gain self-confidence. These gains, though functionally tied to the survival camping process, are transferable to other situations and underscore the total therapeutic potentials of the program.

Program Conclusions:

1. Systematic contact and orientation for the clients is a necessity so that they are better prepared for the program. A pre-training client program emphasizing fitness is important.
2. The camp process needs to be as systematic and as structured as possible to insure progressive gains.
3. The development of physical fitness needs to be emphasized during the basic training.
4. Specific program goals need to be operationalized in as concrete a manner as possible.
5. Alternative plans need to be developed fully, especially during the backpacking phase in case a program change is necessitated.

ORGANIZATIONAL CONSIDERATIONS:

From the standpoint of rehabilitation agency functioning, the camp functioned as a referral client service. Since this was a demonstration project, there was no cost for the service. The details of the program were presented to those rehabilitation counselors and supervisors who worked with delinquents and they, in turn, made a list of potential participants from their caseloads. The criteria employed for inclusion on the list was (1) the client could benefit from the program, and (2) the client was physically able to undergo the physical activity.

Potential participants were interviewed by the project director and asked to volunteer for the program. Their counselors strongly recommended that they participate. Once clients were selected for the project, the program was written into their rehabilitation plans as a specific client service.

Close contact was maintained between the client's rehabilitation counselor and the project director. Each participant who successfully completed the program got a positive progress report sent to the appropriate legal authorities. The counselor received a personal evaluation report of a client's reaction and progress in the program from all project staff. Personal consultation was initiated between the project director and a client's counselor in regard to the client's vocational and rehabilitation plans in light of the new learnings about him from camp program participation. There was a strong emphasis placed on following through on rehabilitation plans immediately after returning from camp. Follow-up contact was maintained between project director, counselor and client for consultive purposes as needed.

In short, the camp program was developed, from the very beginning, to serve as an integrated and basic client service to function as a springboard for the client rehabilitation program and not as an isolated incident. By working it as an integrated program, the gains from the camp experience could be optimally capitalized upon.

Community Resources:

Aldersgate Methodist Camp was a resident camp which could provide basic training facilities and staff for the program. The expense of the program was 3500 dollars payable to Aldersgate for equipment, food, staff salaries, insurance and rent of facilities. If the program was procured on an individual client basis, it would run around 175 dollars an individual.

Aldersgate Camp was selected as a key resource of the program because (1) there were functionally effective staff, (2) there were appropriate facilities, (3) it was organized in a fashion that could accommodate the clientele without any difficulties, and (4) it had a director who supported the program and was willing to facilitate such a venture.

Other community resources which were elicited included borrowing equipment from the local national guard (at no cost). This included canteens, belts, ponchos and shelter halves. Also, a rehabilitation agency supervisor lent the use of his deer camp in the Ozarks as a base camp during the survival portion of the program.

All of the physical necessities (equipment, supplies, etc.) as well as the majority of staff for the project were elicited or procured from existing community resources.

Organizational Conclusions:

1. A good orientation program needs to be provided for agency and community personnel who will be involved.
2. Steps for the implementation of an integrated program need to be defined within the organizational structure and responsibilities assigned.
3. Feedback channels need to be developed between program, agency, and community resources.
4. Follow-up and follow-through need to be coordinated and adhered to.
5. All possible avenues for discovering and implementing functional resources to build a better program need to be developed.
6. The more isolated the camp setting can be (for all stages), the better the learning conditions.

PROGRAM ASSESSMENT

In viewing the participants' progress through the entire program, there appeared to be two basic types of boys. The majority of the participants appeared at the start to have many inadequacies and little strengths. It seemed that they turned to drugs or antisocial behavior as a self defeating means to overcome these inadequacies and belong to a group. The camping program served as an intense success experience for these boys "filling" them up with adequacies, more effective behaviors and accomplishments that increased their self-confidence and self-esteem. There were a few boys who had many adequacies and strengths, but they would use their resources for whatever end they wanted to achieve and would tend to make a game out of everything. These boys learned to cooperate and act more responsibly as time went on, especially in the Ozarks. Some demonstrated some constructive leadership. The program had the effect, hopefully, of offering them an alternative direction to use their resources for.

Generally, the camping experience facilitated positive change in all the participants. The depth and breadth of change will vary by individual. For some of the participants the program appeared as a real critical experience in their lives to serve as a springboard to develop competencies and live a productive life.

Results:

Several different approaches to statistically assess the effect of the program upon the participants were employed. Participant, rehabilitation counselor, and parent evaluation of the program's effect and behavioral ratings assessing physical, intellectual, and emotional-interpersonal functioning were employed to assess the program's direct effect. Participant follow-up was also recorded.

Physical fitness, body attitude, self-concept, and internal attitude measures were also employed to assess the hypothesis that a healthy attitude toward oneself progresses through the physical sphere. Specifically, it is felt that a key source of gain for the participants from successfully completing the program was an increase in physical fitness which facilitated an increase in positive body attitude which resulted in an increase in general self-concept and internal control.

The participants were administered the several fitness tests, Body Attitude Scale, Bills Self-Concept questionnaire and the Internal-External Scale before and after the three week program. Pre and post "t" tests on mean differences were performed and significance tested for.

The physical fitness testing consisted of four basic measures: (1) Cardiovascular functioning as measured by resting pulse rate following the step test; (2) Power as measured by time to run the fifty yard dash; (3) Dynamic strength as measured by number of situps and pushups; and (4) Overall fitness as measured by the Kraus-Weber series. Following the camping program the participants demonstrated significant decreases in resting pulse rate ($p=.005$), time for the fifty yard dash ($p=.001$) and significant increases in pushups ($p=.05$), situps ($p=.005$) and performance on the Kraus-Weber series ($p=.05$).

A shortened form of the Body Attitude Scale, a form of the Semantic Differential developed by Osgood, Suci and Tannebaum (1957) was administered the participants in which they rated bipolar adjectives on a seven point scale for several body parts on three dimensions: (1) Evaluative (good or bad), Potency (strong or weak), and Active (active or passive). The participants demonstrated significant increases on the evaluative ($p=.05$) and potency dimension ($p=.05$) and an non-significant increase on the active dimension. Bills Index of Adjustment and Values (I.A.V.) developed by Bills, Vance and McLean (1951) was given the participants as the self-concept measure. The I.A.V. contains adjectives which are rated by the individual on a five point scale to yield the following: (1) present self-concept score; (2) self-acceptance score; and (3) ideal-self score. The participants demonstrated a significant increase on the present self-concept dimension ($p=.005$) and nonsignificant increases on the other two dimensions. The Internal-External Scale developed by Rotter (1966) was also administered the participants before and after the camp program. The participants' ratings of internal control significantly increased ($p=.05$) following the camp experience while their ratings of external control demonstrated a significant decrease ($p=.05$).

Rehabilitation counselors and parents of the participants rated their behavior before and after the program using the Behavior Rating Inventory and Quay's Behavioral Problem Checklist (Quay and Peterson, 1967). The two scales together contain over seventy-five items for which individual ratings must be made. These items, in turn, were categorized according to whether they focused on physical, intellectual or emotional-interpersonal behavior.

The Behavior Rating Inventory is a seven point scale in which level 1 means that a particular behavior is never emitted to level 7 where the behavior is extremely frequent. According to the scale ratings, the participants demonstrated an increase of positive physical functioning from 3.25 to 5.00, an increase in positive intellectual functioning from 3.12 to 3.61 and an increase in positive emotional-interpersonal functioning from 3.21 to 4.11.

Quay's Behavioral Problem Checklist is a three point scale in which each behavioral item is rated a *0* if it is not a problem, *1* if it is a mild problem and *2* if it is a severe problem. According to the ratings, the participants demonstrated a reduction in behavioral problems in terms of quantity and severity. In terms of physical behaviors, there was a 14 percent increase in the no problem category, a 10 percent decrease in the mild problem category, and a 4 percent decrease in the severe problem category. In terms of intellectual functioning, the percentages were a 13 percent increase in the first category and decreases of 5 percent in the mild category and 7 percent in the severe category. The percentages for emotional-interpersonal functioning were a 9 percent increase in the no problem category, 4 percent decrease in the mild category and a 5 percent decrease in the severe category.

The subjective evaluations of both the participants and their rehabilitation counselors bear out the preceding data results. Both sets of evaluations were consistent in rating the camp program as having a positive effect on such dimensions as physical, intellectual and emotional-interpersonal functioning, potential to deal with problems, rehabilitation outcome, preparation to do better in school or training, desire to be more effective and effort put forth in counseling relationships. Some of the most underscored notes were that the camping program increased the participants's overall self-confidence, self-discipline, and ability to deal with people.

The participants' status six months following the camping program also bears out the program's positive effect. Prior to the camping program, three of the boys were in vocational training, one was in school, none had a job, three were in the training school, and twelve were on probation doing nothing. Six months following the camping program, eight of the boys are in vocational training, seven are in school, two are on jobs, none are in the training school and two are unaccounted for.

Discussion:

The various assessment data all point to the positive effects the camp program had upon the participants. The results also note that although the camp process was basically a physical process, there were many therapeutic benefits of a total nature. The changes in fitness could have facilitated a more positive attitude toward their bodies and, more globally, toward their total selves as well. The more positive attitude toward one's self and one's body were an outgrowth and consolidation of actual behavioral accomplishments (i.e., they became more fit, they learned physical skills and successfully met many physical challenges). The more positive feelings of potency and effectiveness, in turn, led to their believing they had more personal control over their own lives. In short, they proved something to themselves.

The camping process served to facilitate positive behavioral and attitudinal changes in the participants relevant to their rehabilitation and development as fully functioning individuals. On a general level, the participants experienced a very intense, concrete and earned success experience in that the program presented challenges and confrontations for the participants to function more effectively and change, especially on a physical level, which they were able to meet. Consequently, the realization of seeing change and growth could serve as a springboard for the participants to confidently try to succeed in their life situations back home.   (pp. 2-36)

The project reported was a therapeutic camp, implemented to help delinquents and designed to provide an intense experience whereby challenging demands were placed upon the participants. In turn, they were taught the skills to meet these demands, they were confronted with them and expected to meet them successfully. The sources of gain for the participants were derived from the functional and systematic process. At one level, the survival camping process functioned as a vehicle to provide a learning and therapeutic success experience. The participants were able to leave the program not only with a sense of accomplishment, but hopefully with more effective behavior and with attitudes more relevant to their rehabilitation.

The sources of gain from participation in that project were not so much from the global principle that "camping is good for delinquents" as from the fact that a systematic, functional and challenging process was instituted. The physical nature of the process brought things down to a very basic level for the boys. Part of the reason they were delinquent was that they were *turned off* to themselves (their potentials) and to society. They were not able to functionally survive. The camping process, especially the survival portions, put them in touch with some very basic needs and feelings. They were forced to attend to and act on their own needs and the needs of the group. As a consequence, they became more attuned to themselves and to reaching goals while experiencing growth at many levels. The results that the project facilitated illustrate the tremendous therapeutic potentials that survival and rugged camping programs can provide for the young offender.

THE ROLE OF SURVIVAL CAMPING
WITHIN THE REHABILITATION PROCESS

Few experiences can provide the intense physical, emotional, and social challenges that delinquents need as fully as survival camping will. As a therapeutic vehicle to facilitate client change, the rugged camping process capitalizes upon the youths' preference for physical action. At that level, the camping process provides a training modality to which the young offender can readily respond and from which he can readily learn. It can provide a milieu or setting for client gains which may offer greater potential for constructive behavioral change than the classroom or counseling office. For this reason, survival camping warrants consideration as *a key therapeutic program,* to be emphasized as *an integrated portion of a total rehabilitation experience for delinquents.*

Participation in a systematic survival camping program can serve to prepare the youthful offender physically and psychosocially for the rehabilitation process. In a conventional sense, it could be viewed as a very intense and challenging personal-adjustment program. Just as a delinquent client may be referred to group counseling or psychiatric treatment for psychosocial adjustment or behavioral change, so might he be referred to a survival camping program. Survival and/or rugged camping experiences can definitely be viewed as preferred modes of treatment for the youthful offender.

Survival and rugged camping programs have been utilized and can be further employed within the continuum of rehabilitation services for delinquents either as a specific service area provided by a rehabilitation agency, correctional agency, or facility, or as a program service to be obtained and used from the community (YMCA, Boys' Club, Boy Scouts) or private concerns. For example, in many rehabilitation agencies, there is a special program for the youthful offender in which camping may be an important cohesive component. By the same token, a camping program can be a key adjunct to a training school's total program. In all of these examples, the survival camping experience is but one therapeutic element in a more total, more completely integrated rehabilitation design.

Whether viewed as an intervention strategy, a preferred mode of treatment, or as a major therapeutic technique, a survival camping program can be realistically feasible in terms of practical considerations such as money, time and resource. Some rehabilitation and correctional agencies have developed or are developing their own programs. Cooperative efforts such as the project presented have also been developed. There are many private and community agency programs which are also available as program services. Practical and functional programs can and have been developed on a short term basis utilizing weekends or longer periods (up to four weeks).

In summary, the general role of a survival camp program can be viewed as a basic therapeutic mode to facilitate physical and psychosocial behavioral change in delinquents. It can serve many separate roles in terms of the specific needs of individual clients, and, as a program, survival camping can be viewed as a means to reach goals—client goals—to aid them in becoming successfully rehabilitated avocationally and vocationally.

SURVIVAL CAMPING FROM A PRACTITIONER PERSPECTIVE

A concerned practitioner (whether counselor, evaluator, supervisor, etc.) should be open to all possible avenues and approaches that offer the promise of facilitating a client's rehabilitation. Survival and/or rugged camping has been presented here as a therapeutic approach or mode to help facilitate relevant psychosocial and behavioral change in the youthful offender. As such, it can be viewed as one type of program or method that can be employed within a given client's total rehabilitation plan.

Most practitioners function on two levels—as a direct service provider or as a service arranger. On the direct level, a practitioner can work to develop and implement a survival camping program for delinquent clientele. Working through rehabilitation agencies, grant opportunities, or through cooperative efforts, he can set up or crystallize a direct service program. On a smaller scale, short term (weekend) survival camping experiences can be arranged between an individual practitioner and his clients. One important side benefit of this type of endeavor is the facilitating effect such a camping experience can have on the helper-client relationship.

The arrangement and procurement of specific services is often a time consuming yet important function. If a rugged camping program appears justifiable to meet the needs of a young offender and there are no existing agency or correctional programs, then potential community and private resources can be canvassed. Existing programs through YMCA's Boy Scouts, farm organizations, etc. can be utilized and procured as a client service or, with a little cooperative effort, restructured to meet rehabilitation needs.

Whether one is directly involved in developing, implementing, utilizing or procuring a survival camp program or not, there are some basic conclusions from past programs relevant to helping the delinquent which perhaps offer some general implications toward their rehabilitation. The young offender makes discriminations and responds more readily to an action-oriented, more physical approach. In other words, he or she can accept functional challenges, physical and otherwise. When both the helper and the client know where the other stands (what the functional and reciprocal demands are), there is more of a chance for a positive and working relationship. In short, many of the underlying dynamics of the survival camping process (as described in the Camp Challenge example) can be appropriate for any helping approach to assist the young offender to "survive" (become rehabilitated). A systematic, functional, active and goal-oriented approach to serving the young offender holds more promise than an unsystematic, non-functional, passive, diffuse process.

Even though survival camping is but one approach or one type of client service program that can be available to the practitioner, competent programs have demonstrated the effectiveness and potentials of the camping process as a therapeutic mode for helping the young offender. All in all, survival camping deserves attention as a valid, integral approach in planning for deliquent services or in planning *one* individual client's total rehabilitation program.

SUMMARY

Camping programs for delinquents are not new ideas. Over the years many camping experiences (long and short term, resident and day camping, work camps, recreational and educational camps) have been provided young offenders for therapeutic purposes. However, the utilization and demonstration of systematic survival or rugged camping programs have not been as fully provided or made known to the field.

Survival camping as a therapeutic process is one vehicle that can aid delinquent rehabilitation. The systematic functional and goal-directed process can facilitate relevant behavioral and attitudinal changes through the physical, action-oriented, challenging nature of the camping process. In short, survival camp programs, as innovative approaches, offer unique therapeutic potentials.

The Human Resource Development Model outlined by Carkhuff (1971) contends that to aid fully in the development of human resources or in individual rehabilitation, all avenues need to be investigated. Functional programs developed and run by functional helpers insure a greater probability of success. A functional survival camp program is one potential, physically based avenue that can provide an integrated rehabilitation approach to the young offender.

REFERENCES

Bills, R. E., Vance, E. L., and McLean, O. S.: An index of adjustment and values. *J of Consult Clin Psychol, 15*:257-261, 1951.

Boy Scouts of America: *Fieldbook for Boys and Men.* New Brunswick, N. J., 1967.

Carkhuff, R. R.: *The Development of Human Resources,* New York, Holt, Rinehart and Winston, 1971.

Collingwood, T. R.: *Survival Camping: A Therapeutic Mode for Rehabilitating Problem Youth.* Monograph Series, Arkansas Rehabilitation Research and Training Center, 1972.

Department of the Air Force: *Survival—Training Edition,* AF Manual 64-3, Washington, D.C., 1969.

Erickson, E.: *New Perspectives for Research in Juvenile Delinquency.* Children's Bureau Publication No. 356, Washington, D.C., 1956.

Jesness, C. F.: *The Jesness Personality Inventory,* Palo Alto, Calif., Consulting Psychologists Press, 1967.

Kelly, F., and Baer, D.: *Outward Bound Schools as an Alternative to Institutionalization for Adolescent Delinquent Boys.* Boston, Fondel Press, 1968.

Loughmiller, C.: *Wilderness Road.* Austin, Texas, Hogg Foundation for Mental Health, 1965.

O'Brien, T.: Forestry camps praised. *Challenge, 12*(5):15-17, 1969.

Osgood, L., Suci, G., and Tannenbaum, P.: *The Measurement of Meaning.* Urbana, U. of Illinois Press, 1957.

Quay, H. C., and Peterson, L.: *The Behavioral Problem Checklist.* Morgantown, W. Va., R. F. Kennedy Youth Center, 1967.

Rotter, J. B.: Generalized expectancies for internal versus external control of reinforcement. *Psychological Monographs, 80,* No. 1, 1966.

Weber, S.: Six camps for delinquent boys. In R. Cowan, *Readings in Juvenile Delinquency,* New York, J. B. Lippincott, 1969.

(PART TWO)

THE DISABLED DISADVANTAGED

VOCATIONAL REHABILITATION OF THE
DISABLED DISADVANTAGED

THE DISABLED DISADVANTAGED

ROLE INDUCTION FOR PSYCHOTHERAPY:
A PROMISING TECHNIQUE FOR THE
REHABILITATION CLIENT

MOTIVATING THE CULTURALLY
DISADVANTAGED

Chapter 4

VOCATIONAL REHABILITATION OF THE DISABLED DISADVANTAGED

DALE H. PLACE

THIS CHAPTER will provide information on the philosophy and procedures utilized in a State-Federal rehabilitation agency to provide vocational rehabilitation services to the disabled disadvantaged client. Specifically, it will focus on the Texas Rehabilitation Commission program and its concerted work with other agencies (local, state and federal) in attempting to meet the needs of disabled disadvantaged clients. Observations of other state rehabilitation agency programs designed for the disabled disadvantaged will also be reported. A great deal of emphasis will be given to the agency's work with disabled recipients of public welfare. The history of the movement, and agency operations with this client population, will be examined in detail.

Legal Background and History of the Vocational Rehabilitation Movement in Serving the Disabled Disadvantaged

The Vocational Rehabilitation Movement has served the disabled disadvantaged client since its inception as a program. As E. B. Whitten (1969), Executive Director of the National Rehabilitation Association, suggests:

> Physically and mentally handicapped individuals are, of course, disadvantaged individuals in every sense of the word. As a rule, they are also poor people; over one-half of those who come to the agencies (VR) have no income at all when they apply for services, and 90 percent have incomes at time of referral below what is commonly referred to as a poverty level (p. 1).

The Vocational Rehabilitation Movement began on June 2, 1920, when President Woodrow Wilson signed into law the Vocational Rehabilitation Bill (Obermann, 1965). For the first time the United States had provided national funds for the disabled citizen to rise above his disabilities. The program was limited to the physically disabled, and provisions were not made for physical restoration services to remove or reduce the disability or to pay the living costs of the handicapped client while he was being rehabilitated.

In 1934 and 1935, a special appropriation of 70,000 dollars monthly was provided for vocational rehabilitation services to public assistance cases only. The money was obtained through a transfer of funds from the Federal

Emergency Relief Administration (Obermann, 1965). Although a substantial percentage of the Vocational Rehabilitation caseload were poor people, this is the first mention of earmarking of funds specifically for the poor (*50 Years of Vocational Rehabilitation in the United States, 1920-1970*).

In 1935, the Public Welfare program was created through the Social Security Act. The purpose of this program was to provide economic relief to disabled and dependent citizens in the United States. The aged, blind and children only were included in this program. Welfare case workers carried caseloads of four to five hundred and their main charge was to provide the correct amount of aid. When clients needed social services, they were referred to community agencies such as the vocational rehabilitation agency for *free* help.

In the 1943 amendments to the Vocational Rehabilitation Act, services were broadened to include: surgery, hospitalization, transportation, licenses, tools and equipment, prosthetic devices, maintenance, books and training materials while undergoing training. "These services were offered to disabled individuals found to require financial assistance . . . ." (Obermann, 1965). The mentally ill and retarded could also now be accepted as rehabilitation clients as well as the physically disabled.

A concerted effort was begun in America in 1965 with the creation of Public Law 88-452, the Economic Opportunity Act. At all levels of both public and private sectors of the establishment, people began looking for ways to involve themselves in this massive effort to insure a better life for every American. This prompted Mary E. Switzer, Commissioner of the Vocational Rehabilitation Administration, to write the following words relative to the role the Vocational Rehabilitation program would play in the poverty program:

> It is appropriate that there should be an alignment between the poverty program and vocational rehabilitation. The philosophy, methods and techniques that have been successful in rehabilitation have value for the socially disabled. The need is to evolve the most creative and meaningful ways to fulfill the potentials of vocational rehabilitation in this rapidly expanding area.
>
> The massive problems that the poverty programs are considering will not be solved by conventional means. If this battle to break the barriers between affluence and poverty is to be won, new ways must be found to do it, and success will not be achieved if the same paths that have been used for past decades are still followed. If the Great Society's program to up-grade the poverty stricken is to be effective, it will be necessary to undergo radical shifts and changes in views, methods and organization.
>
> To underline the relationship between poverty and rehabilitation, the poor person who is disabled is eligible to receive rehabilitative services. With increases in funding for both programs, there will be a tremendous growth of new resources in the community. In addition, comprehensive workshop improvement and development programs are going to become more and more important in the community approach to work training and work evaluation. These factors will influence the success of some of the more extensive efforts of the poverty program in urban areas.
>
> The counselor has always been the anchor man in vocational rehabilitation.

As these programs expand, the counselor has to work with more clients, and learn to handle their problems more expeditiously. Therefore, techniques and new organizational patterns must be devloped for delivering service. Underlying this are the basic elements that go into counseling and the personal aspects of the counselor-client relationship. How the counselor's talents are multiplied and how agencies will function with a minimum of counselors and a maximum of people for them to serve is one of the great challenges. The idea of assisting an individual to help him redirect his life, no matter what the causes for his dislocation and dependency may be, is inherent in rehabilitation counseling and the broad spectrum of rehabilitation services.

The professions and programs require ideas, a clarification of problems and the establishment of guidelines both for training and its practical application. This ultimately should assist impoverished and dependent people to bring themselves to an optimum level of self-sufficiency and productivity. It is apparent that the needs are not going to be met by master's degree level personnel only. They are needed, but also required is something dramatically different to supplement this basic group of professional workers in terms of training techniques, service and staffing patterns.

Some experimental approaches are necessary to recruit young people who want to serve within these kinds of programs. New efforts at pre-service and in-service training must be attempted to bring this potential reservoir of young workers to a sufficiently high level of functioning so that they can provide service to clients sooner and more efficiently than under existing programs.

Through planning and a unification of resources, philosophy and purposes, the debilitating effects of poverty can be eliminated. The Vocational Rehabilitation Administration is most anxious to participate in this effort and to assume a responsibility for stimulation and leadership in this direction (Cohen, 1966, p. vii).

The need to closely align the State Vocational Rehabilitation agencies and the Public Welfare departments was felt earlier than 1965. In 1962, with the passage of Public Law 87-543, amendments to the Public Welfare Law, the Bureau of Family Services of the Welfare Administration and Vocational Rehabilitation intensified efforts in coordinating their respective services. A special committee on Public Welfare worked with the Council of State Directors of Vocational Rehabilitation to review joint action plans and recruit the full cooperation of vocational rehabilitation agencies (Hansen, In Press). One of the direct results of this collaborative effort was the development of twenty-six Research and Demonstration projects in the United States. Several of these projects are worthy of mention, as a historical base for the State Vocational Rehabilitation agency programs now serving the disabled disadvantaged client.

Pruitt-Igoe Project*

The location of this project was the Pruitt-Igoe public housing complex in St. Louis, Missouri. This was a five-year (1963-1968) experimental project designed to test the feasibility of offering vocational rehabilitation services to the severely culturally, educationally, and economically disadvantaged. A total of 344 cases were accepted, and of this number 257 were closed rehabili-

*See Houston and Finley, 1969.

tated, and 87 were closed not rehabilitated. A high proportion of the group was female; single, divorced, or separated; on welfare; responsible for dependents; limited educationally; low IQ scores; and limited work experience. Hansen clearly summarizes the significant findings of the project:

> The ability of a culturally disadvantaged person to be rehabilitated was clearly demonstrated and was one of the brightest points of the project. Clients who are culturally disadvantaged have identifiable characteristics which pose as much a barrier to employment as do physical handicaps. The counselors learned that immediate help is essential in disadvantaged cases and the assistance must be tangible to be of any value. Also, counselors learned that short-term goals are most effective but must be followed by later counseling or pre-vocational training (Hansen, In Press).

San Antonio Rehabilitation-Welfare Project**

This project was located in San Antonio, Texas. Office space was provided by Victoria Courts, a public housing project, and the project ran three years. Joint office space for Vocational Rehabilitation counselors and Welfare (DPW) caseworkers was provided and caseloads were limited to sixty cases. Applicants and recipients of AFDC, under sixty years of age, comprised the target group in this project and included a large number of Latin Americans and migrant workers.

Developed in this project and the Houston Project (*Houston Rehabilitation-Welfare Project Report,* 1967), was a pre-vocational evaluation-adjustment program (The San Antonio Rehabilitation-Welfare Report on Curriculum Developed for Pre-Vocational Evaluation-Adjustment Classes, 1967). The San Antonio Pre-Vocational program consisted of a sixty-day pre-vocational adjustment program for all project clients. Seven primary points received attention in these classes:

1. Understanding the world, utilizing current events on a base beyond the client's narrow scope of information.
2. Utilizing information sources such as newspapers, radios, telephone, magazines, etc. to secure employment.
3. Civic participation geared at greater understanding of the local, state and federal government; voting, police, community service agencies, and social security.
4. Budgeting for home and money management.
5. Developing an adequate self-concept.
6. Tutoring in basic English, spelling, reading and arithmetic skills.
7. Completing job applications and preparing for job interviews.

The San Antonio Project rehabilitated 70 percent of all accepted cases and 38 percent of all cases referred to the project, with a mean cost of 560 dollars per successful case.

**Research and Demonstration Grant Number 1513, 1967.

Wood County Project*

In 1963 the State of Wisconsin Division of Vocational Rehabilitation, directed by Adrian Towne, and the University of Wisconsin Regional Rehabilitation Research Institute, directed by Dr. George N. Wright, proposed the nation's first broadscale project to demonstrate the effectiveness of rehabilitation methods in meeting the needs of all handicapped persons, including the culturally disadvantaged. Wisconsin DVR and the University of Wisconsin, Madison collaborated in one of the largest research and demonstration projects yet sponsored by the Vocational Rehabilitation Administration, now the Rehabilitation Services Administration (RSA).

The million-dollar five-year grant called for a model rehabilitation agency to operate with redefined eligibility criteria, and it provided funds and staff to meet the broadened objectives. The definition of *handicap* was extended to include any physical, mental, educational, or socio-economic deficit or inadequacy which made it difficult for a person to secure or maintain employment commensurate with his capacities.

Total rehabilitation meant saturation coverage in order to make services available to virtually every handicapped person in Wood County. The experimental agency extended services horizontally to medically disabled persons who, though legally entitled, had not been served because of budget and staff inadequacies. It extended services vertically to the culturally handicapped, for the first time entitling them to vocational rehabilitation.

Researchers tested four major hypotheses of total rehabilitation during the five-year study:

1. That the intensive Vocational Rehabilitation program will increase the number of successful rehabilitations of the physically and mentally handicapped.

2. That the project's rehabilitation experience with the culturally handicapped will be as effective as with the physically and mentally impaired.

3. That the project will result in economic benefits to the county by increasing employment and reducing welfare costs.

4. That the project will improve public attitudes toward and increase public knowledge of vocational rehabilitation.

These assumptions proved correct in the most ambitious effort toward total rehabilitation yet attempted.

Findings of the Wood County Project point to the need for continued expansion in vocational rehabilitation well beyond the limits still narrowly defined by law. Rehabilitation's brief career has been marked by sub-total programs.

Although these programs have done much to assist the nation's handicapped, the Wisconsin experiment shows that vocational rehabilitation has

---

*See G. N. Wright *et al.*, 1969.

done little more than scratch the surface. Many medically handicapped persons and virtually all of the non-medically handicapped remain cut off from one of the best tools yet to combat poverty: Vocational Rehabilitation. The Wood County Project embodies the philosophy that vocational rehabilitation programs cannot remain static. They must be flexible and geared to human need. A sub-total vocational rehabilitation program, no matter how well done, still answers the need of but a small percentage of the handicapped.

In the future Vocational Rehabilitation policies and procedures should reflect considered professional advice and the results of tested research. The Wood County Project may well influence such policies and procedures in the direction of total rehabilitation.

Early Referral

California (Merrill, 1967) and Washington, D.C. (O'Neill, 1968) studies demonstrated the importance of early referral. Both projects assigned Vocational Rehabilitation counselors and welfare caseworkers to joint caseloads. Referrals were made to these teams when the public assistance application was granted. A higher number of successful cases resulted after early referral techniques were developed in these projects.

Hansen (from Grigg, 1969) aptly summarizes the findings of fourteen Research and Demonstration projects involving 7,694 clients:

1. Of 7,694 applicants in the 14 projects, 2,786 (36 percent) were accepted for services, and complete data was available on 2,614 of the applicants.
2. 1,146 (44 percent) of the 2,614 cases were closed as rehabilitated and another 879 clients (34 percent), some of whom would become rehabilitated, were still being served.
3. Only 6 percent of the 1,146 clients who were closed as rehabilitated indicated they were unemployed after their case was closed; compared with 78 percent before services. Of those clients rehabilitated, 68 percent were working in the competitive labor market, and 78 percent were working full-time (some in sheltered settings), compared with only 5 percent when referred.
4. With all other factors constant, the cost-benefit ratio for Negroes was lower than for Whites and Latin Americans, due largely to the higher expected cost of services. In this regard, the difference between Negroes and Latin Americans was especially noteworthy, and prevailed also with respect to the percentage still being served in the projects: 58 percent of Latin Americans versus 20 percent of Negroes.
5. Of the 2,614 clients for whom data was analyzed, 56 percent were men, 44 percent women; 62 percent were White, 26 percent Negro, and 11 percent Latin American. Their ages ranged from under 20 to over 60, with 90 percent of the clients' ages spread rather evenly between 20 and 60.
   42 percent of the clients had less than 8 years of schooling; only 17 percent of the clients had 12 years of school or more.
   Prior work experience of the clients had been mostly in service, semi-skilled, and housewife areas, 46 percent having such work backgrounds.
   77 percent of the clients were on AFDC. In all, about 72 percent were receiving some form of public assistance, but 28 percent were getting no aid when referred.
   79 percent of the clients had not been referred for services to the State Di-

visions of Vocational Rehabilitation during the 4 years prior to acceptance into these projects.

6. All of the clients accepted were disabled in addition to being economically dependent. The most frequent primary impairments were amputation and orthopedic or bodily deformities (28 percent), psychiatric and behavior disorders (14 percent), and cardiac problems (6 percent). A full range of impairments was present in the total group, and at least one-half of the clients suffered also from secondary disabilities.

7. In brief, the majority of those clients served were functioning only marginally in our society, as shown by their low educational attainment, skimpy work histories, and economic dependency.

8. Major reasons for nonacceptance into projects were little or no functional work capacity, "declined services," no substantial disability, and combination of disability, illiteracy, and lack of skill.

9. Of 11 social services rendered to project clients, health care was used most often, followed by vocational and financial and self-support help.

10. The AFDC groups, which received more public welfare services under matching funds than other public assistance categories, had a better rehabilitation rate than any other public assistance group. The study data does not, however, tell us whether or in what manner welfare services affect rehabilitation outcome.

11. The most frequently used of 10 rehabilitation services were diagnosis, maintenance and transportation, surgery and related treatment, training and training materials, prosthetic appliances and hospitalization. Those clients who were rehabilitated received more of these services than those clients who were not rehabilitated.

12. Needs and types of service varied by race and ethnic group. Whites needed more major medical attention and Negroes needed more job training or retraining. Negroes received relatively more maintenance and transportation, but their urgent training needs were not met.

13. Those clients who were rehabilitated had an average treatment cost of 561 dollars, compared to 502 dollars for those not rehabilitated.

14. The average increase in weekly earnings after successful rehabilitation was 46 dollars, with men and those with higher educational attainment gaining the most.

15. Expenditures were greater for men than for women, and greater for those clients with higher levels of education (pp. xiii-xvi).

The period from 1963 to 1969 was a fruitful period for research and demonstration of ways and means of providing Vocational Rehabilitation services to the disabled disadvantaged client. During this same period of time, there were some major revisions to the Vocational Rehabilitation Act which had relevance to the disabled disadvantaged client population.

In 1965, the definition of disability was broadened to include the behaviorally disabled (Public Law 89-333). Physical or mental disability was defined as:

> . . . a physical or mental condition which materially limits, contributes to limiting, or if not corrected, will probably result in limiting an individual's activities or functioning. It includes behavioral disorders characterized by a pattern of deviant social behavior or impaired ability to carry out normal relationships with family and community which may result from vocational, educational, cultural, social, environmental, or other factors (p. 136).

Lamborn, writing in the *Rehabilitation Record,* publication of the Rehabilitation Services Administration, stated: "No longer can (the applicant) be excluded because the cause of the disability is rooted in poverty or cultural deprivation rather than in disease, or accident, or a congenital defect" (Lamborn, 1969).

One other new provision of the 1965 Vocational Rehabilitation Act Amendments was the revised definition of "substantial handicap to employment," the second of three Vocational Rehabilitation eligibility criteria.:

> "Substantial handicap to employment" means that a physical or mental disability (in the light of attendant medical, psychological, vocational, educational, cultural, social, or environmental factors) impedes an individual's occupational performance, by preventing his obtaining, retaining, or preparing for a gainful occupation consistent with his capabilities or aptitudes (RSA Regulations 401.1).

Previously, it had been required that there be demonstrated a direct causal relationship between the disability and the handicap to employment. The new regulation recognized that limited educational, medical, social, or other factors provided fewer resources for coping with the effects of a disabling condition without the disabling condition's directly affecting the occupational performance (*Rehabilitation of Individuals with Behavioral Disorders*, 1969).

The Council of State Administrators of Vocational Rehabilitation issued the following statement:

> The current definition of disability in the regulations governing the administration of the Vocational Rehabilitation Act results in millions of handicapped people who are "eligible" for vocational rehabilitation services. In addition to individuals whose disabilities are the result of medically definable physical or mental impairments (the traditional sources of agency clientele), there are added millions whose disabilities consist of behavioral disorders characterized by deviant social behavior or impaired ability to carry out normal relationships with family and community, which may result from vocational, educational, cultural, social, environmental, or other factors. Eligibility for vocational rehabilitation services under such a definition may include the public offender, the alcoholic, the drug addict, and the socially and culturally deprived, provided these people are truly "handicapped" in finding and holding suitable employment. In considering the relationship of disability to handicap, one considers all of the factors—environmental, educational, and social—which will impede a person's performance and intensify the vocational handicap.
> This broader definition of disability is intended to free State vocational rehabilitation agencies from the restrictions imposed by previous definitions of disability and its relation to handicap, and to enable them to use their services and skills freely to serve handicapped people who obviously can profit from vocational rehabilitation services, but who might have been excluded from such services because they did not appear to be "disabled" under traditional interpretations of the meaning of disability (p. 10).

The Vocational Rehabilitation Act was amended again in 1968 when Section 15, the Work Evaluation and Work Adjustment provisions were added. Although it has never been funded by the Congress, the two services referred to—work evaluation and work adjustment training—could be provided to disadvantaged individuals as a community service. Public Law 90-391 (Section 15) defines disadvantaged individuals as:

Individuals disadvantaged by reason of their youth or advanced age, low educational attainments, ethnic or cultural factors, prison or delinquency records, or other conditions which constitute a barrier to employment (p. 14).

Services to the disabled disadvantaged were identified as a top priority in the Rehabilitation Service Administration of the Social and Rehabilitation Service in 1970 (Edward Newman, Commissioner's Letter 70-27, February 18, 1970).

On August 19, 1971 Congress appropriated 26.6 million dollars in expansion grant funds to the states, earmarked for use only to expand the number of disabled public assistance recipients rehabilitated. The Texas Rehabilitation Commission was able to expand the number of joint rehabilitation-welfare projects from seven to sixteen. These funds will enable the Commission to serve an additional 3,000 disabled public assistance recipients annually. A majority of the states applied for these expansion grant funds to serve additional disabled public assistance recipients.

Through earmarking of funds, expansion projects, Research and Demonstration projects with public assistance recipients, outreach efforts, and amendments to the Vocational Rehabilitation Act, the State Vocational Rehabilitation Agency has provided Vocational Rehabilitation services to the disabled disadvantaged client since the inception of the Vocational Rehabilitation Movement. This client population is a top priority with SRS and RSA and will remain as a top priority for many years to come, since the reduction of dependency and poverty is a national goal and will be for many years to come.

Joint Rehabilitation-Welfare Project Description

In the sixteen joint rehabilitation-welfare projects in Texas, the Texas Department of Public Welfare (DPW) and the Texas Rehabilitation Commission (VR) have staff jointly housed and carrying the same caseload. Comprehensive services are provided in the project with close supervision of case flow. In most projects a Pre-Vocational Evaluation-Adjustment training service is available.

Philosophy of Joint Project Operation

Emphasis is placed on early referral of the disabled public assistance recipient, along with the provision of immediate or "sudden" services. Coordination of VR and DPW services and community involvement of as many local private and public agencies in the provision of services is important. The joint project staffs reach out to the community to purchase or arrange for services needed by the client but unavailable in the project.

An atmosphere of goal-oriented team action is present in the projects. Services needed by clients are planned by the project team (including the client). Staff opinion conflicts are settled in favor of what will be best for the client. Constant communication between staff members through staff meetings and informal staffings keeps conflicts at a minimum. Deep involvement of agency supervisory staff is a key to maintenance of a low number of staff conflicts. Open sharing of client information is also a key to preventing staff opinion conflicts.

A social and rehabilitation approach is taken with each client with emphasis on the whole person. All facets of the client's life and environment are considered in planning project services.

The following summary of findings in the New Haven Special Project for vocational rehabilitation of the socioculturally disadvantaged poor is also applicable to the Texas joint projects' philosophy (Goldin, George J., *et al.,* 1970).

1. The concept of enablement is paramount in the vocational rehabilitation of the ghetto poor. By enablement is meant the provision of an accepting non-defensive psychosocial climate in the service delivering organization within which the client can explore his capacities and pursue meaningful goals. Enablement does not mean doing for the client nor does it mean the imposition of norms and values of a culture alien to his own. It means, rather, providing him with an opportunity structure within which he can grow and develop as well as helping him with the motivation and wherewithal to overcome social and psychological barriers to maximum use of opportunities for training and vocational growth.

2. The concerting of services by involved agencies is a procedure which is beneficial to the rehabilitation of the poverty bound client in rehabilitation. The attainment of a true concerted services approach is exceedingly difficult because each agency or organization approaches the resolution of the client's problems in terms of its own philosophy and value structure. The area in which to work, therefore, is the integration of philosophical differences among the concerting agencies. Once this is achieved, agencies can easily work together in role allocation in behalf of the client.

3. Not all problems of the poverty bound client in rehabilitation are sociocultural. Very frequently this point of view is overstressed. Psychodynamic or intrapsychic forces stemming from family relationships and other psychobiological developmental forces play an important part in the adaptive patterning of the poor as they do in the middle class. The intrapsychic forces of the poor are different, but they can be understood in dynamic psychological terms.

4. During the process of rehabilitating the socioculturally and economically disadvantaged client, staff members of the rehabilitating agency must be prepared to accept and absorb massive amounts of hostility and alienated behavior. The client because of his long period of deprivation and social rejection comes to the agency with anger and demands which appear to middle class oriented staff as irrational and ungrateful. Staff must be helped to understand such behavior in the light of its social origin.

5. Indigenous community workers are of much value in the process of vocational rehabilitation of the ghetto poor. However, it is of vital importance that they maintain their identification with the group that they are serving. The training and supervision of the community worker should be performed by individuals thoroughly familiar with the culture of poverty in the ghetto.

6. The personality structure and area of commitment of personnel is of great importance in influencing the functioning of the organization for rehabilitation of the poor.

7. In many instances jobs for the poor must be developed, modified and tailored

to meet the needs of the particular client. The use of the role of job developer as experimented with in this project proved valuable in aiding the rehabilitation of the poverty client.

8. Communication with the poor must take place on an emotional as well as a semantic level. Such communication can take place when the rehabilitation worker makes an honest attempt to learn their language. When the professional worker makes an attempt to understand and communicate with the culturally different poor in their own language, the poor respond reciprocally and attempt to understand the language and value structure of the middle class.

9. Although self-determination is a prized concept in dealing with the ghetto poor, completely nondirective techniques can be anxiety provoking for some clients. There are instances in which the expertise and authority of the professional are of value in helping the client to come to a decision and motivating him to action.

10. In many instances confrontation between counselor and client is of value in clearing the air and establishing a climate of honesty between counselor and client. This is a valuable technique since the disadvantaged client of the ghetto has a basic mistrust of the professional whom he perceives as representing the establishment.

11. Social disability is no mere academic concept. It is a condition which exists and is characterized by the inability of the poverty client to enter into negotiations with social institutions in the community to have his social, emotional and concrete needs satisfied. Such social disability stems from lack of opportunity for experience in social skills, a lack of information about the greater culture, and the anxiety which stems from these conditions.

12. Intensive follow-up utilizing supportive counseling is of crucial importance following vocational placement of disabled poor. The individual who is socio-economically disadvantaged is particularly susceptible to stress and sensitive to problems which mobilize his feelings of inadequacy and powerlessness. It is, therefore, important to manipulate the environment around him so that negative comments and behavior around him are mitigated until he gradually can be helped to deal with them and absorb them (pp. 103-105).

Staffing Patterns of Joint Projects

All joint projects in Texas have a full-or-part-time supervisor from VR and DPW, responsible for administration of staff and for case management. A VR counselor and DPW Social Service worker on a full-time basis make up the crux of the team. In larger metropolitan areas several teams of VR counselors and DPW social workers work in the joint projects. Social and rehabilitation services are coordinated by these staff members.

Pre-Vocational Evaluation-Adjustment Training is provided by a full-time joint project Instructor-Evaluator. In the larger metropolitan areas a joint project may have two or more full-time Instructor-Evaluators.

In most of the joint projects, one-half or full-time psychologists are employed to provide client psychological evaluation for the determination of disability and information for the joint project team to better plan services with the client. Psychologists are being added in each of the joint projects as funding and manpower are available.

Job Development and Placement Specialists are being added to the joint project teams. Although only one joint project has this staff member available, plans are to add these positions as funding and manpower is available.

Community Service Aide, Social Service Aide, and Rehabilitation Technician positions are available in some of the joint projects. Usually these are former clients and/or personnel *indigenous* to the project locale. These staff members do outreach work and help bring clients into the projects. These staff members are available in helping the professional to communicate with the client.

Eligibility of Disabled Disadvantaged for VR Services

Jennings and Russell in a discussion of eligibility of the Public Offender client for VR services cover the above topic very thoroughly as do various Government publications listed at the end of this chapter.

Special Groups of Disabled Disadvantaged Clients Served by VR

A very adequate description of some special groups of disabled disadvantaged clients is found in the following remarks (Kunce *et al.*, 1969).

There are certain groups of the disadvantaged that have all of the previously noted characteristics to a greater or lesser degree, yet are identifiable through additional special characteristics. Some of these groups are (1) migrant workers, (2) mentally handicapped, (3) physically handicapped, and (4) racially handicapped.

MIGRANT WORKERS: Domestic migratory workers number almost 500,000. Although large numbers of individuals leave the migratory force each year, it is replenished by ". . . displaced tenant farmers, hired farm workers displaced by mechanization, an inflow of . . . Puerto Ricans, and some unskilled jobless workers from the city (U.S. Department of Labor, p. 74, 1966a.

Three-fourths of the 1964 population of migratory workers were men, with 60 percent less than 35 years old and 25 percent non-white. Their annual average income was 1,016 dollars with two-thirds earning less than 1,000 dollars. Lenore Epstein has summed up the flow of migrant labor as follows:

"There are three major migrant streams for domestic migrants. The largest, followed by about 250,000 workers, is the mid-continent movement made up largely of Texas-Mexicans, with home bases in south Texas. About 100,000 workers follow the western states migrant stream, which moves from southern California northward through the Pacific Coast states. The East Coast migrant stream attracts almost 100,000 workers—southeastern Negroes, Puerto Ricans, and some Texans. This stream moves north from Florida to North Carolina to New York State and then back to Florida.

"These people are caught in a number of economic squeezes. Their work is hard and irregular, pay is low, and mechanization is displacing them. Also, they are excluded from the protection of the Federal Minimum Wage Law (U.S. Department of Labor, 1965). Failure to meet state residence requirements usually rules out eligibility for any type of welfare."

MENTALLY HANDICAPPED: A second special poverty group includes the mentally and emotionally disabled. From a report by the U.S. Department of Labor (1966a) the following information was gleaned. The mentally handicapped of working age in the United States number approximately 3.5 million. Many of the retarded, particularly those with mild intellectual defects, are members of an ethnic minority, live under substandard conditions, and lack proper educational and cultural opportunities. The prevalence of psychological, environmental, or genetic mental retardation is not of itself evidence that brain damage is greater in lower socioeconomic groups. Nevertheless, impoverishment may be a factor in retardation. For example, one significant factor linked to the cause of mental retardation is premature birth, which may be caused by poor nutrition and/or inadequate prenatal care—situations that, in turn, are likely to be intensified by low income. Mental or emotional disorders may affect the ability of an individual to obtain and hold a job and to support one's dependents; and these frustrations may contribute to the onset and recurrence of such disorders, thus creating a vicious cycle.

PHYSICALLY HANDICAPPED: Five million U.S. citizens are classified as physically disabled individuals. An additional 1.4 million males and 1.6 million females are handicapped in terms of employment because of chronic health conditions (U.S. Department of Labor, 1967). Chronic illness, low income, and unemployment were found by the National Health Survey to be interrelated and mutually sustaining factors (U.S. Department of Labor, 1966a). To summarize the employment situation of the physically handicapped:

The blind: 450,000 are of working age, but only 50,000 are employed.

Paraplegics: 60,000 are of working age, of whom 10 percent are veterans. Only 39 percent of the veterans and 47 percent of the nonveterans are employed.

Epileptic: Of the 2 million epileptics in the United States, 400,000 are of working age. Their employment rate is estimated to be from 15 to 25 percent.

Cerebral Palsy: An estimated 200,000 are of working age, and yet relatively few are at work. The United Cerebral Palsy Association strives for 10 percent rate of employment.

. . . The number of such persons rehabilitated under federal-state programs has been rising: 1,900 epileptics rehabilitated in 1961, 3,282 in 1966; 4,500 blind in 1961 and almost 6,000 in 1966; 1,500 deaf in 1961 and over 2,700 in 1966. Other groups also have been rehabilitated in increasing numbers.

The presence of physical disability without appropriate financial and personal resources may lead to chronic unemployment and dependency upon others and may result in conditions of poverty. It is not surprising to find a high incidence of disability and chronic illness among the disadvantaged.

RACIALLY HANDICAPPED: Of all the special groups of disadvantaged in the United States, none is more significant than that portion of our population designated as "non-white". The geographical distributions of American poverty are strikingly similar to those of the non-white elements of our society. This is especially true of the Negroes (or blacks) who account for about 90 percent of all non-white Americans. There are other non-white Americans such as Indians, Mexicans, and Asians. With few exceptions, all that can be said of the Negro applies as well to these other smaller, non-white segments of the community (pp. 11-13).

Pre-Vocational Evaluation-Adjustment

An integral part of the joint project is a program designed to provide the client needing behavior modification with some enrichment in survival skills as a prerequisite to job placement. In the Pre-Vocational Evaluation-Adjustment program the client is removed from an environment in which it is acceptable to have excuses for not being productive, to one in which he is rewarded for having positive attitudes toward himself as a productive and responsible member of society.

Based on a covert academic vehicle, the program provides the client information and experience of successful mastery in areas where those experienced with the disabled disadvantaged population find deficiencies. A set of values wherein self-help, self-worth, cooperation with families, among coworkers are valued above martyrdom to disability, insufficiency, and dependency (*The San Antonio Rehabilitation-Welfare Report on Curriculum*

Developed for Pre-Vocational Evaluation-Adjustment, 1967).

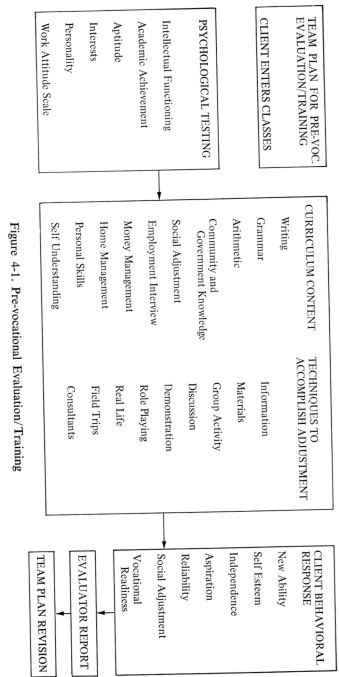

Figure 4-1. Pre-vocational Evaluation/Training

In the projects, clients spend approximately sixty days in these classes, five days per week, six hours per day. An Instructor-Evaluator conducts the program. In all projects the classroom space for this program is located under the same roof with the other project staff. This close proximity allows intensive counseling sessions to occur with the client in addition to the Pre-Vocational Evaluation-Adjustment program services. This program has proven to be very beneficial to clients and has been made an integral part of the VR Project program.

Report on a Non-Project Pre-Vocational Evaluation-Adjustment Class

A Pre-Vocational Evaluation-Adjustment Training Program has been utilized with success in a rural area (Wadsworth, 1972). A rehabilitation counselor carrying a general caseload recognized the need for such a program when faced with several individuals referred by the Public Welfare. The individuals were primarily Mexican-American and Negro-American and had been *hired hands* for ranchers in West Texas. They were poorly educated, culturally deprived, had many dependent children, and had been disabled by a physical or mental disability. All of these prospective clients were unskilled and many of them could not speak the English language. All of these people lived in or near three small West Texas towns with populations not exceeding 2,000. Many rehabilitation counselors would have closed these peoples' cases as *not feasible* for services. This rehabilitation counselor did not feel such action would be necessary if a program could be arranged to ameliorate the many handicaps present in these rural people. The counselor retained, with case service funds, the services of a woman who had taught Spanish at the high school level, kindergarten, and first grade. This lady was also of Mexican descent. He arranged with the local high school to use a classroom three evenings weekly for three hours nightly. The high school Principal also allowed use of the school library.

Classes met from September to June. The objective of the program was to help these disabled disadvantaged individuals to make personal and social adjustment, learn to read and write, and do arithmetic.

Sixteen clients were served the first year of operation. These clients had a broad range of physical and mental disabilities. Their stay in the class ranged from two to nine months with a mean stay of seven months. Ten clients or 62.5 percent were employed or advanced to Vocational training; two clients were *undecided* or *incomplete;* and four clients received little benefit or were unsuccessful. A review of all of the cases indicates that fifteen clients were male and eight were female. Their ages ranged from eighteen to fifty-four years with a mean age of thirty-five.

In the second year of classes nineteen clients were enrolled. It is too early at this time to gauge any results from this class, but the counselor estimates that 75 percent of these clients will be successful. Surely this is a very promising program for the rural disabled disadvantaged client (Wadsworth, 1972).

Joint VR-DPW Project Operating Procedure*

Certification of AFDC, APTD and OAA Recipients

Certain recipients in AFDC, APTD and OAA public assistance cases are eligible to be considered for referral for Joint Project-VR-DPW services. Disabled family heads and disabled youth over sixteen years of age in AFDC families are eligible for referral, as well as disabled OAA and APTD recipients. All recipients with a primary visual impairment are referred to the Commission for the Blind (CB).

Selection of Recipient for Referral to Project

The primary source of referral for joint projects is the AFDC, APTD and OAA case records of the Department of Public Welfare (DPW). Other sources of referral include non-project VR caseloads and public or private agencies; however, it is mandatory that DPW certification be established prior to acceptance for joint project services. The first line member of the team effort is the DPW field social service worker who may refer cases on an assumed or apparent disability. This referral is the result of a review of DPW case records or a personal contact with the client. Readiness factors considered are age, limitations of the disability, availability of child care, and client interest and motivation. When the referring field social service worker identifies a potential Project client, he initiates the joint referral form and/or routes the case folder to the Project DPW supervisor or a designated representative. Screening activity does not preclude services nor is it the basis for the denial of services, but it serves to provide more timely introduction to appropriate services.

Screening for Project Participation

Upon receipt of the referral and the financial and social service case folders, the Project DPW supervisor and the Project VR supervisor or their designated representatives conduct further preliminary screening of the case. If all factors for client participation appear positive, the case is assigned to a team comprised of a project Social Service Worker and a VR counselor.

Intake Activity

DPW INTAKE: Upon receipt of the case folders, the Social Service worker assigned to the project again reviews the case information in order to make his determination of case readiness and case approach before scheduling the initial interview with the client. The caseworker makes prompt contact with the client, preferably in a home visit, and reviews the full scope of Project

---
*This writer shares credit for the development of this project procedure with his colleague in the Texas Public Welfare Department, Mrs. June Oliver, Consultant for Social Services, with Mrs. Adelle Casseb, Texas Public Welfare Department Supervisor, and Mr. H. L. McLerran, Texas Rehabilitation Commission Program Specialist.

Services with him. He explains the team concept and relevant Project policies and procedures. During this contact, he arranges a meeting between the client and the assigned VR Counselor. He shares with the counselor all positive and negative aspects of client potential that may have been uncovered in the initial contact. He accompanies the client to the initial counselor-client meeting, and introduces the client to the counselor and remains long enough to lay the groundwork for fruitful VR intake. It is at this point that the stage is set for all future teamwork activity.

VR INTAKE: In the initial VR intake meeting with the client, application for services is completed, and counseling and guidance are provided regarding services that may be available. The VR counselor makes preliminary educational and vocational assessment and initiates general medical examination and other specialist examinations necessary for eligibility determination and plan development.

DPW ASSESSMENT PROCEDURE: The primary responsibility of the Project Social Service worker is the family unit. For example, during the initial interview for a particular case, the Social Service worker learns of existing family problems and begins at once to assess the abilities and disabilities, the assets and liabilities of the various members of family. In his close association with them, he continues to assess strengths, weaknesses and environmental obstacles. He considers child care, family relationships, transportation, clothing needs, budget management, health and family planning in his work toward the development of a long-range social and economic plan. The plan is designed to resolve the immediate problems which pose a threat to Project participation, as well as the continuing problems encountered by welfare clients. He develops with the client a long-range goal affording the client maximum opportunity for vocational success, emotional and economic stability, and reduction of dependency upon public financial support. Family problems are identified, and an appropriate plan of services, formulated to overcome these problems. At all times the Project Social Service worker shares with his counterpart, the VR counselor, all aspects of client and family potential that he has discovered. While the Project Social Service worker is engaged in this diagnostic procedure, the VR counselor is making *his* diagnostic plan for services.

VR DIAGNOSTIC PROCEDURE: The primary responsibility of the VR counselor is the disabled client. He identifies and assesses the client's desires and goals, his abilities and his limitations. He gathers pertinent medical, vocational and educational information, as well as hospital records, in his effort to begin comprehensive vocational planning. He makes arrangements and appointments for the medical and other evaluations necessary for establishment of eligibility. Upon determination of eligibility status, he arranges a convenient date for the approaching joint staff-client conference.

Joint Staff-Client Conference

After completion of the diagnostic studies, the project team (including the client) meets in a joint conference to consider the following:

1. Acceptance for full project services.
2. Determination of client ineligibility for full project services resulting in referral to other appropriate community resources.
3. Identification of social service needs.
4. Budgetary and economic considerations.
5. Completion of the vocational and social plans by the team and the client—the type and length of the plans, goal of the plans, and the kinds of supportive services are identified.
6. Formulation of pre-vocational training plan complete with entry date and identification of team services.
7. Option to by-pass pre-voc in favor of other VR services—e.g., vocational training, physical restoration or job placement. The criteria for pre-voc by-pass will be based upon recency of employment, client need, length of eligibility, client interest and motivation, and academic level.

Criteria for By-Passing Pre-Vocational Evaluation-Adjustment Training by the Client

The client's realistic desire for and ability to gain immediate employment or to benefit from vocational training are dependent upon the following criteria:

1. Recency of work history (during last six months).
2. Recency of dependency on welfare (less than six months).
3. Educational attainment or functional level of twelve years or equivalency (based on vocational objective).
4. Mutual agreement by Counselor/Social Service Worker/Client team to by-pass pre-voc evaluation-adjustment training.
5. Absence of negative personal and social problems which could defeat the attainment of the vocational objective.
6. Availability of training or employment.

First Formal Staffing and Screening Conference

Following the joint staff-client conference, a written, formal staffing review will be completed documenting decisions made at that conference. This staffing serves to reflect the current status of the client, services rendered to date, and necessary services anticipated by both agencies. The Staffing Review Record indicates the team decision either to accept or screen-out. Screen-out may result from one or more factors: it may occur because of unwillingness to attend pre-voc training (in those cases where pre-voc is indicated and prescribed), confirmation of medical ineligibility to participate in Project services, a request for withdrawal from the program, inability to obtain child care, severe family problems that preclude participation, and any other conditions which indicate poor prognosis for rehabilitation. All clients thus screened-out are assured that future requests for service will be considered, and they must be given the opportunity for referral to other appropriate services in the community.

Pre-Vocational Evaluation-Adjustment Training

The client enters Pre-Vocational Evaluation-Adjustment Training according to plans developed in the joint staff-client conference. This plan is completed before the beginning of pre-voc activity. Both team members review and fully discuss the pre-voc activity with the client so that the client is emotionally prepared for exposure to a new, sometimes threatening, sometimes overwhelming group experience. One member of the team, usually the VR counselor, accompanies the client to the classroom for the introduction to the Instructor-Evaluator and to the classroom environment. The Instructor-Evaluator, for a period of time, supervises client academic effort, psychological testing, achievement endeavor, and general pre-voc activity.

When need indicates, the Instructor-Evaluator provides team members with reports of client performance, attendance, attitude, cooperation, motivation, and general academic achievement. Frequency of these reports is determined by agreement of the project staff. Team members carry joint responsibility for resolving problems affecting client progress. This information is utilized by team members in their formulation of plans with the client.

VR Formulation of Vocational Plan

During pre-voc activity the VR counselor summarizes his client evaluations and assessment. Pre-Voc records, client attitude, interests and past vocational experience are factors to be considered in the crystallization of the VR plan. The plan may take the direction of training employment or physical restoration, based upon type and extent of disability. The vocational plan reflects the counselor's best efforts toward the improvement of client productivity and attainment of a realistic vocational goal.

The VR counselor remains alert to DPW eligibility factors in male incapacity cases (AFDC) and cooperates with the Social Service worker in the exchange of medical information which is important in the DPW medical eligibility extension for this group of clients. A copy of all vocational plans is provided to the DPW project Social Service folder. In all medical incapacity cases this information is submitted to the project Social Service worker for forwarding to DPW Financial Service worker for appropriate action in consideration of the DPW medical eligibility extension.

It is the responsibility of the VR counselor to schedule the next joint staff-client conference. This conference may include any other appropriate individuals who have concern with the case.

DPW Provision of Support for Vocational Plan

As a long-range vocational plan is being formulated, DPW provides active support of this VR activity. On the basis of the original and ongoing assessment made of the recipient and his family, services are given as needed to ensure that the recipient is able to participate fully in the pre-vocational program and to follow through with any specific procedures necessary to the program. The services may be as specific as helping the recipient arrange for child care or daily transportation to and from training, or they may be supportive such as providing counseling with the recipient regarding guilt feelings he or she may have about leaving her pre-school child in a day care center; or it may offer counseling with a teenage daughter about the new responsibilities that the vocational rehabilitation program has thrust upon the entire family.

Alert to a new problem-risk level created by the recipient's participation in VR, the Social Service worker makes himself available to the recipient for immediate assistance. The model followed in this provision of services is crisis intervention. Problems are resolved quickly and soundly in order to maintain in the recipient a high level of confidence and hope about his participation in the new venture and his ultimate achievement of self support.

Areas of special concern are child care and protection of the recipient's assistance grant during the period of pre-vocational or vocational training. All social services are closely coordinated with DPW financial service for continuation of eligibility in those cases where eligibility may expire due to medical determination. Examples of high risk cases are those wherein a male head of household is disabled and his medical eligibility may be influenced by a Financial Service worker's verification of continued need due to his participation in a VR program.

Joint Staff-Client Conference

A mutual team decision establishes the joint staff-client conference which will cover the following items:
   1. Revised vocational plan.
   2. Revision of the plan for supportive services when indicated.
   3. Budgetary considerations, including training-related expenses (when indicated) and public assistance grant.
The client emerges from this conference with a clear understanding of his role and a definite sense of vocational direction.

DPW Continues Provision of Support for Vocational Plan

The Project Social Service worker remains in contact with the client throughout the training program or in the first weeks of employment, whichever the VR plan indicates. Regular client contacts are made for purposes of support, reinforcement, encouragement, and resolution of family problems. In some situations in which demands are placed upon the client that are out of the realm of his usual experience, the need for counseling may be extensive. The Social Service worker is alert to the need for what could be called emergency intensive encouragement and support, and remains in close contact with the client in order to maintain the rapport that is established. In addition to the new training or employment experience, family relationship problems, intercurrent illnesses, unexpected events, and motivation let-downs are among the many problems the Social Service worker watches for and resolves.

VR Implementation and Evaluation of Vocational Plan

The VR counselor maintains close contact with the client whether the latter is in employment, training, or engaged in a physical restoration program. The counselor is responsible for the provision of appropriate vocational supportive services, which might include intensive counseling and guidance, the procurement of prostheses, orthotic devices, or tools, perhaps additional training, and placement assistance. The VR counselor remains sensitive to threatening circumstances which may alter or disrupt the VR plan. Motivational let-down, intercurrent illness, resistance to employment, resistance to DPW approaching denial (where need or incapacity no longer exists) are problems for the VR counselor to detect and resolve.

Revision of Plan, If Indicated

The revision of the vocational and social plans is necessary when unexpected factors influence them. The decision to revise the vocational plan is a mutual, coordinated team agreement which is accomplished and implemented with the same care as that exercised in the original plan. The team continues to work closely with client and the family to secure maximum participation and supportive effort.

Employment

The client arrives at employment through direct placement (by-pass of pre-voc) or after the completion of pre-voc or a training program. Both the VR counselor and the Project Social worker have had a part, along with the client, in the selection of an employment goal in the placement after training. Staff of both agencies make a combined effort to provide encouragement, support and counseling in this critical stage of the client's vocational activity. The client has arrived at the crossroad: forfeiture of a certain and predictable financial resource as opposed to an independent effort toward unguaranteed economic independence. Since any client receiving VR services has a disability, his fears of denial and rejection are real and legitimate. The first areas of competition in the economic arena include those of physical and mental ability, vocational prowess and staying power. Surely sustained efforts in counseling, guidance, encouragement and assurance are necessary from both team members at this crucial stage in the program.

DPW Monitors for Economic/Emotional Stability

While the client is in employment, he is assisted into a recognition of the positive values of self-determination and financial independence. It is the responsibility of the Project Social Service worker to make every effort to assure that the client's budgetary needs are met by communicating them to the DPW Financial Service worker. If need still exists, after earnings have been netted, the client is assured of continued State earnings on a reduced scale. If the client's employment earnings dictate denial (or if denial is imminent in medical incapacity cases), the client is prepared for the cessation of State assistance and reassured as to his ability to become self-sustaining. The Project Social Service worker may continue to provide social services to denied clients for ninety days following denial, and reassures the denied client that should circumstances demand, he may re-apply for financial assistance. Also, the Social Service worker will acquaint the client with his right to appeal a denial of a grant or an adverse grant decision. The Social Service worker relates to the VR counselor any changes in the financial grant.

VR Monitors for Employment Stability

The VR counselor remains in contact with the client for a minimum of thirty days of employment prior to case closure and continues to respond to client needs for an appropriate period of time beyond closure. He makes every effort to insure that the client is engaged in compatible employment, that the client is receiving adequate compensation for his employment, and that the client is not being exploited. He remains in close contact with the Project Social Service worker so that he may be aware of any forthcoming changes in the client's financial condition, and so that the worker can act on the closure.

Final Form Staffing and Closure

When the client has functioned successfully in employment for thirty days and related conditions are assessed to be satisfactory, the case is ready for a final staffing and closure. The conditions of employment, home and family relations, and client vocational stability are reviewed for advisability of closure, accompanied by DPW denial or transfer of case for continuance in the usual DPW capacity. Where family size and netted earnings leave an unmet need, DPW financial assistance is retained in the grant to supplement the earnings and the case is transferred to other DPW units for continuance of services.

In the event that the vocational effort has not been successful and there is no reasonable expectation that a revised plan will succeed, the VR counselor closes the case as unsuccessful and the DPW case is transferred for continuance.

Every effort is made by the team to work in close cooperation toward the final objective of successful closure. Formal closure and denial of the public assistance grant do not always occur simultaneously. In cases where financial assistance must be denied prior to VR closure, the VR counselor continues to provide VR services until the case is closed. The Project Social Service worker may continue social services for ninety days following denial of the financial grant. Decision of the team to close the case is shared with the client. The final Staff Review Record is completed by each team member indicating the team decision, services provided, and the results of the services. Copies of the Staff Review Record are placed in both agency folders and a copy is used as a Project accounting record.

Follow-Up

Follow-up action by the VR counselor is determined by the need of the client. In cases where denial of DPW financial assistance occurs, social services may be given for ninety days following denial. Where DPW financial assistance is continued, the DPW case is transferred to other DPW units for continuance of Social Service. Social Services will be continued by another DPW Social Service unit if desired by the client, and the financial case will be handled routinely by another financial service unit.

REFERENCES

Beck, R. B., Pierce-Jones, J., Lamonte, A., McWhorter, C. C.: *The San Antonio Rehabilitation-Welfare Report, Final Report,* RD1513, Texas Rehabilitation Commission, U.S. Department of Health, Education and Welfare, SRS, 1967.

Cohen, Julius S., et al.: *Vocational Rehabilitation and the Socially Disabled.* School of Education, Syracuse University, 1966.

Goldin, George J., Margolin, Reuben J., Stotsky, Bernard A., Marci, Joseph N.: *Psychodynamics and Enablement in the Rehabilitation of the Poverty Bound Client.* Lexington, Mass., Heath Lexington Books, 1970.

Grigg, Charles M., Holtman, Alphonse G., and Martin, Patricia Y.: *Vocational Rehabilitation of Disabled Public Assistance Clients: An Evaluation of Fourteen Research and Demonstration Projects.* Institute for Social Research, Florida State University, No. 8, 1969.

Hansen, Carl E.: Research findings in the rehabilitation of the public welfare recipient. In Hardy, Richard E., and Cull, John (Eds.), *Rehabilitation of the Public Welfare Recipient.* Springfield, Thomas, In Press.

Houston, David G. and Finley, Jerry: *Rehabilitation Versus Poverty, Final Report,* Project 1250-64-5, Missouri State Department of Education, Jefferson City, 1969.

Kunce, Joseph T. and Cope, Corrine S. (Eds.): *Rehabilitation and Culturally Disadvantaged.* Columbia, University of Missouri, Regional Rehabilitation Research Institute, Research Series No. 1, 1969.

Lamborn, J. S.: *Issues Relating to Rehabilitation of Individuals with Behavioral Disorders.* Seventh Institute on Rehabilitation Services, U.S. Department of Health, Education and Welfare, Social and Rehabilitation Service, 1969.

Merrill, S. M.: *Early Referral: A Demonstration of Early Evaluation of Rehabilitation Potential of Public Assistance Recipients,* Final Report, RD-1119, California Department of Rehabilitation, U.S. Department of Health, Education, and Welfare, SRS, 1967.

Obermann, C. Esco: *A History of Vocational Rehabilitation in America.* Minneapolis, T. S. Denison and Company, Inc., 1965.

O'Neill, R.: *Vocational Rehabilitation of Disabled Persons Receiving Public*

Assistance Grants. Final Report, RD-1639, Washington, D.C., Department of VR, U.S. Department of Health, Education, and Welfare, SRS, 1968.

Seventh Institute of Rehabilitation Services: *Rehabilitation of Individuals with Behavioral Disorders.* Washington, D.C., U.S. Department of Health, Education, and Welfare, SRS, RSA, 1969.

Texas Education Agency, Vocational Rehabilitation Division: *The Houston Rehabilitation-Welfare Project Report,* RD-1334-D-63, Austin, Texas, May, 1967.

Texas Education Agency, Vocational Rehabilitation Division: *The San Antonio Rehabilitation-Welfare on Curriculum Developed for Pre-Vocational Evaluation-Adjustment Classes,* RD1513, Austin, Texas, 1967.

U.S. Department of Health, Education, and Welfare: *50 Years of Vocational Rehabilitation in the United States, 1920-1970.* Washington, D.C., 1970.

Wadsworth, O.D.: Pre-vocational training for the disabled/disadvantaged in non-urban areas. Unpublished paper, 1972.

Whitten, E. B.: Disadvantaged individuals and rehabilitation. *Journal of Rehabilitation, 35*(1), January-February, 1969.

Wright, G. N., Reagles, K. W., Butler, A. J.: *The Wood County Project,* Final Report, RD-1629. The University of Wisconsin, Regional Rehabilitation Research Institute, U.S. Department of Health, Education, and Welfare, SRS, 1969.

Chapter 5

THE DISABLED DISADVANTAGED*

KENNETH KRAUSE

THIS CHAPTER will provide a conceptual framework for understanding and working with the disabled disadvantaged. It will attempt to integrate psychological, sociological, and treatment theories to provide a rationale and guide for rehabilitation practice. This approach will be based on the assumption that the disabled poor are, in most ways, like all other people and, in some ways, unique because of their economic and physical status. Specifically, the following discussion will focus on the physically disabled adult with few financial resources living in an economically depressed area. This chapter will first consider some psychological characteristics of normal adults, then some psychological conditions associated with poverty, and last, some psychological needs of the disabled. Based on these considerations, certain goals for rehabilitation counseling will be identified and a model for practice presented.

PSYCHOLOGICAL CHARACTERISTICS OF NORMAL ADULTS

In his discussion of normal adult psychological functioning, Erik Erickson (1964) identified a schedule of virtues, or qualities of strength, which he postulates develop from healthy past life experiences. These virtues are hope, will, purpose, competence, fidelity, love, care, and wisdom. These characteristics will be briefly discussed below. It is an assumption of this paper that the disabled disadvantaged will need to achieve these virtues if they are going to enjoy the benefits and responsibilities of adulthood in modern society.

Hope

Hope is the earliest and the most indispensable virtue inherent in the state of being alive. It enables people to believe and trust in themselves, in others, and in the future. It enables people to face their present situation with confidence and optimism as they feel that their wishes and goals can be attained. In spite of limitations and set-backs it enables people to face life with the

---

*Portions of this paper were presented at a conference sponsored by Medical Rehabilitation Research and Training Center Number Twenty, Northwestern University and the University of Chicago Center for the Study of Welfare Policy, April 15, 1971.

belief that things *can* change. Hope is an essential virtue of adulthood and an adult without hope will not survive.

Will

To will is to gain the power of increased judgment in the pursuit of life goals. A healthy adult is able to will, or determine by choice, decisions that affect his own situation and that of others. Will, therefore, is the determination to exercise free choice as well as self-restraint in making decisions. An adult must learn to will what can be and to renounce as not worth willing, what cannot be. As man must have hope, so must he have will in order to live.

Purpose

To have purpose is to have an aim in life. A psychologically healthy adult will have purpose and will use it as a blueprint to give direction to his internal strivings and his external activities. Purpose is the courage to pursue valued goals. Purpose must be realistic and related to what can be achieved and what cannot be achieved. An adult must have purpose to give meaning to his life.

Competence

To be competent is to be qualified and capable of contributing to society. Competence is related to workmanship and the ability of an adult to perform necessary life tasks. Competence is the free exercise of dexterity and intelligence in the completion of tasks which are needed by society. Man develops the rudiments of competence in his early schooling in the form of language skills, grammar, mathematics, mechanics, and the ability to think. These tools enable the adult to develop competence and without them he would be unable to contribute to his society. Man might be able to survive without competence, but he would be of little value to his fellow man.

Fidelity

Fidelity is the ability to freely enter into and to sustain pledged loyalties in relationships with other people. This virtue implies such characteristics as truthfulness, sincerity, devotion, fairness, trust, integrity, and a high sense of duty. The adult needs the fidelity of others, such as family members, co-workers, and friends; and they need *his* fidelity. Society, too, needs the fidelity of its members and their potential power of solidarity. Man and society without fidelity would both be weakened in their pursuit of common goals.

Love

Love is the greatest of all human virtues and the dominant virtue of the universe. Adult love is the mutuality of mates and partners in a shared identity, through an experience of finding oneself, as one loses oneself, in another. Adult love is actively chosen and entered into freely by both partners. Families are created and children are born, educated and socialized to take their place in society. Man has the need and the capacity to love and to be loved, and fulfillment of this drive will mutually benefit man and society.

Care

Care is the quality of extending solicitude and concern to other persons. It is the shifting of preoccupation with oneself to the needs of others. Man, by his nature, has a need to teach and to care for his fellow man in order to perpetuate mankind. Teaching and caring benefit both the giver and the receiver as well as society. In order to meet this challenge we need to utilize the ingenuity of workers and thinkers of many kinds. Adults have the need and the capacity to meet this challenge and, in so doing, benefit themselves, other people and society itself.

Wisdom

Wisdom is the ability to view mankind and life itself in some perspective. It is the capacity to become detached from day-to-day activities and concerns and to consider the long-range needs and problems of society and all of mankind. The adult who has wisdom can share his heritage with others and yet remain aware of the relativity of all knowledge. A society that fails to utilize this adult virtue may lack the vision and the capacity to provide for future generations.

The above virtues, according to Erickson, are characteristic of healthy adults in all societies. Through exercise of these virtues, man can utilize his potential to the fullest extent possible with mutual benefit to himself and society. But without these virtues man and society will fail.

In our society, the disabled poor, in many cases, have not developed these adult virtues just listed. They have, instead, developed psychological characteristics that discourage self-fulfillment and human potential.

PSYCHOLOGICAL CHARACTERISTICS OF THE POOR

Before discussing psychological characteristics of the poor, it might be important to note some environmental conditions of poverty. These include such things as overcrowded living conditions, poor housing, limited public services, fatherless families and broken homes, large families, unsanitary health conditions, poor schools, low income level, low educational attainment and aspiration, limited and impersonal medical services, more sickness and disability, more unemployment, high crime, low community organization, and limited mobility. It is well known that these environmental conditions contribute greatly to the intellectual and psychological functioning of persons living in them (Hurley, 1969). This chapter will not dwell on these conditions, but it does acknowledge the part they play in personality development and response to life of persons who are both disabled and poor. It will focus in particular on five psychological characteristics generally associated with poverty. These are helplessness, emotional isolation, low achievement motivation, present-time focus, and poor health orientation.*

Helplessness

This psychological condition involves a person's ability to control his environment to help himself and others. Hurley suggests that a person's ability to control his own fate is an indispensable ingredient in maintaining a positive self-image and psychological health (1969). He further notes that the poor have attitudes of fatalism, dependency, helplessness, and inferiority. Seeman describes the poor as being alienated from society and feeling powerless, meaningless, normless, value isolated, and self-estranged (1970). Roth associates poverty with lack of self-respect (1969). Irelan adds that the poor feel life is uncontrollable (1967).

The poor have become isolated from society as they have been unable to contribute to it and benefit from it. They have rejected the norms and values of major society as being unattainable or incompatible with their life style. The poor have been unable to realize the potential in themselves and in society, and society has been unable to realize the potential of the poor. This psychological condition of helplessness affects the behavior of the poor and their aspirations, values, relationships, use of society and their commitment to life itself.

Emotional Isolation

Emotional isolation is the psychological condition of being alone and without meaningful personal relationships. It is the condition of not being loved by anyone and not loving. There are several environmental characteristics of poverty that contribute to this phenomenon. In their child rearing practices the poor emphasize discipline and control and not psychological development. There are more single-parent families among the poor, more fatherless families, and more broken homes. Poor families have larger families, resulting in limited opportunities for parental involvement in socialization of children. These factors, and others, contribute to a condition of social and psychological distance in family relationships. As a result, family members cling less to each other for close emotional support.

As the poor become isolated emotionally from other people, they become unable to meet their own psychological needs or to meet the needs of others. This lack of emotional interdependence may be especially devastating to the poor in times of crisis. For example, the importance of interpersonal relation-

---

*It might be important to note, however, that many persons living in poverty do not hold these attitudes but, instead, possess the attitudes identified by Erickson. How some persons have been able to break from the bonds of poverty (and disability) may be an important area for further study.

ships was noted by Sussman in his work with discharged mental patients. He found that those patients who held membership in a family, were active in work, had a social group identification, and led active social lives were most likely to be successful vocationally and economically while family isolates had poor rehabilitation records (Sussman, 1969).

Low Achievement Motivation

This psychological condition relates to the degree of motivation a person has to achieve success educationally, socially, economically, and occupationally. The poor child is limited from birth. Larger families mean lower I.Q's due to socialization factors (Hurley, 1969). Parents lack education and have lower achievement aspirations for their children. Parents are unable to provide the time, ability, space, and stimulation to help their children achieve in school. The children of the poor have limited life experiences and understimulation of their tactile senses. The poor take few trips to the country, buy few educational toys, have few books, attend few cultural activities, and have little concern for national and world events. Further, as Seeman points out, learning depends on the expectation that behavior will lead to successful outcome and the value of that outcome (Seeman, 1970). The prospect of a college degree, or even a high school diploma, for the poor youth is dim and its value doubtful. The difference between aspirations and real opportunity for the poor is illustrated in an interview reported by Henderson in his work with black ghetto youth (1966, p. 41).

Int. What would you like to be when you grow up?
Boy A school teacher.
Int. Why would you want to be a school teacher?
Boy Because I think I'd like to teach and I think I'd be good at it.
Int. What do you think you *will* be?
Boy A pimp.
Int. Why do you think you will be a pimp when you want to be a school teacher?
Boy Because I'd never be able to afford to go to college but I can be a pimp and make plenty of money.

What may look like lack of ability among the poor could be a result of physical and emotional environmental circumstances. The condition of low achievement motivation and the lack of opportunity prevent the utilization of the poor and result in a loss of benefits for society and the individual.

Present-Time Focus

This psychological condition relates to the time focus of the poor. Simply stated, the poor are more concerned with staying alive today than being alive next year.

They are more concerned with food, bus fare, rent, and utility bills than they are with the rewards of a lengthy education, the future of the economy, or city politics. Because of this present-time focus, the poor have little disposition to postpone gratification. If they do have extra money, it is more likely to be spent for today's pleasures than saved for tomorrow or invested in an educational program. This psychological condition limits the poor from anticipating future needs and from transforming human potential into vocational and educational skills. This condition distorts the vision of the poor so that they are unable to discern what could be from what is. Further, they are unable to identify what knowledge and values are important to pass on to their children to insure personal and societal fulfillment.

Poor Health Orientation

Before discussing this psychological condition it might be important to mention several factual connections between poverty and poor health. There is generally a higher rate of disease among the poor (Irelan, 1967). There is the highest concentration of maladjusted individuals and the highest concentration of persons suffering from schizophrenia among persons from the lowest social stratum (Roman and Trice, 1967). The poor are hospitalized for illness later, and they stay longer, resulting in a piling up of people from lower classes in some hospitals (Myers and Bean, 1968). Lower classes have a lower age at death and a higher death rate than the general population (Myers and Bean, 1968). There is 300 percent more disability among the very poor than among the general population (Sussman, 1969). Persons from the lowest income group have more than twice as many of the job disability days per year than do persons from the highest income group (Hurley, 1969). The poor know less about health care and health programs (Irelan, 1967). The poor do not spend money on medical care, and good health occupies a low place on their value hierarchy. The poor are more likely to obtain medical services in a clinic where they receive impersonal and partialized treatment than from a family physician who would coordinate all of their medical needs. Hurley (1969) illustrates the fatalism in the cyclical relationship between poverty and poor health by suggesting, "A man becomes sick . . . he loses a steady job . . . he becomes poorer . . . sicker . . . and he dies."

As a psychological condition, a poor health orientation commits the poor to a frame of mind that is destructive and prevents utilization of existing knowledge and resources. As a consequence, the poor tend to accept physical discomfort and physical limitations as inevitable, a way of life. They turn to their friends for medical advice, diagnose and treat their own illness, and make frequent use of patent medicines (Irelan, 1967). They fail to take advantage of what medical services are available and often do not follow through on the medical advice that is given (Roth, 1969). The result is an under-utilization of scientific and human potential and a mutual loss to both the individual and society.

PSYCHOLOGICAL NEEDS OF THE DISABLED

A physical disability is a reality, and it defines certain boundaries on activities of disabled persons. Further, a physical disability causes, with variations, behavior and attitudinal reactions from other people towards disabled persons. These factors are important and must be considered in the rehabilitation process. Yuker notes that there are psychological characteristics associated with all physical disabilities and that understanding of them may be as important, or more important, in the rehabilitation process than the extent or nature of the disability (Yuker, 1966). In these pages we will focus on five psychological needs of disabled persons. These are need for security, need to be the same, need to be interdependent, need to be an individual, and need for life goals and self-determination.

Need for Security

The disabled person often has attained a level of adjustment which provides some level of psychological security. Economically, he may be receiving rehabilitation payments that provide a marginal level of existence (Turney, 1964). Interpersonally, he may be receiving attention and acceptance from family and friends because of his disability (Siller, 1969). Socially, he may have an acceptable reason for withdrawal from the problems and demands of life (Burke, 1968). Though not completely satisfactory, this level of adjustment is known and may provide a degree of psychological security.

The disabled person may not want to risk what is known for what is unknown. He may be reluctant to risk leaving welfare because, if he has to, he may have trouble getting back on. He may be unwilling to experiment with new family relationships because they may be more demanding and less satisfying than his present relationships. He may be reluctant to get a job because of his fear of failure.

The recently disabled person has different problems as he exchanges the security he has known for a new security he has not yet found. This person may have to deal with the reality of such things as the loss of a job, loss of money, limitation of activities, limitation of physical ability, different family roles and responsibilities, and new social relationships. The need for psychological security is important, and it may enhance or impede the rehabilitation of disabled persons.

Need to Be the Same

The disabled are different from other people; they may look dissimilar and act differently. Disabled persons may associate these differences with deficiency and see themselves as impotent, a burden, unproductive, and undesirable. This may be a result of how others see the disabled, or others may see the disabled as they see themselves (Barron, 1967). These differences and feelings may be accentuated and confirmed by life experiences and lead to a self-fulfilling prophecy of failure.

The disabled are also the same as other people because they are human. They have the same need and ability as other people to give and receive love, solve problems, develop human potential, and the same natural strivings for growth, productivity, and interpersonal relationships. The disabled have the same capacity to develop the adult virtues discussed by Erickson as all other people. These similarities may be accentuated and confirmed by life experiences and may lead to a self-fulfilling prophecy of success.

The psychological need on the part of the disabled to be the same as other people can be utilized in the pursuit of life goals. Disabled persons can choose to be like other people and build on their strengths and deal with their limits in a realistic way; or they can focus on their differences and resign themselves to a life with limited promise. Actually, there is no alternative, and, as Braceland noted, "the disabled person must act as though he were going to live forever" (Braceland, 1966).

Need to Be Interdependent

The disabled, like all people, are social by nature and have the capacity for reciprocity in interpersonal relationships. However, disabled persons often become preoccupied with their disability, and with related problems, and view other people and society in terms of their own needs while losing sight of what they have to contribute to others (Cohen, 1962). This position limits the contribution of the disabled to others and the benefits to the disabled in terms of life purpose and self-worth. The disabled are often seen as dependent persons, and the goal in working with them is to develop independence. While this approach is valid, a goal of interdependence is more consistent with the nature and ability of man.

In their work with the deaf, Hurwitz and DiFrancisca (1968) noted that it was impaired social functioning and not functional capacities that limited persons in relation to employment. The same might be true for other disabled persons, and the inability to discuss mutual interests, share common concerns, comment on current events, express anger, and show friendship might prevent them from becoming successful in their social and vocational aspirations.

There is, moreover, a tendency on the part of the disabled to congregate and socialize among their own kind (Burke, 1968). Thus the disabled serve as their own reference group for gauging normal behavior (Thorsen, 1968). While this may have value in terms of the social and emotional needs of the disabled, it may limit adjustment in the larger community, as normal behavior among the disabled might not be normal behavior in the community.

Need to Be an Individual

Obvious as it may sound, there is a need on the part of disabled persons to be treated as distinct individuals. Yuker (1966) described the situation at a university that modified its facilities to accommodate disabled persons. Soon, large numbers of disabled persons were enrolled on campus and their presence raised questions such as whether they should be allowed to join fraternities. A spokesman for the disabled argued against any blanket policy on acceptance or rejection of disabled persons to fraternities but urged that they be considered for membership as individuals on their own merits and on the basis of fraternity membership criteria the same as anyone else.

In an inspired article, Prudence Sutherland, a severely handicapped college student, described how she treasured being treated as a human being and as an individual. She related the pleasure she found in being listened to, understood, respected, involved, and liked for what she was, and how her friends helped her to become honest and unashamed in all aspects of being human (Sutherland, 1968).

There are both a reciprocity and a self-perpetuating aspect in mutual relationships. How one views oneself is related to how one is viewed by others and how one views oneself is related to how one approaches life. The disabled person who sees himself as incapable will probably respond differently to life and the rehabilitation process than the disabled person who sees himself as worthwhile. MacGuffie and Janzen (1969) administered self-concept tests to persons applying for rehabilitation services and found that those who scored high on the test tended to follow through on services and were rehabilitated and those who scored low tended to drop out. Similarly, Yuker (1966) found that disabled persons who accepted themselves and their disabilities were relatively well adjusted.

Need for Life Goals and Self-Determination

Disabled persons, like all people, need to have life goals that are rewarding and attainable. Such goals may be influenced by the nature of the disability, family status, intellectual and vocational skills, interests, and social, cultural, and economic factors. Not all goals, of course, are equally valid for all disabled. It is important, however, for all disabled to have some life goals which are identifiable and feasible, and mutually beneficial to the person and society. Further, it is necessary that the disabled person have a part in identifying and attaining goals which are important to him. It is through this process that he can learn that he, like all men, has the ability to be aware of his own behavior and change it (Nadolsky, 1966).

REHABILITATION GOALS FOR THE DISABLED POOR

Thus far this chapter has considered some psychological characteristics of normal adults, the poor, and the disabled. These characteristics are related and a framework for understanding the disabled disadvantaged embraces all of them. The disabled disadvantaged, like all men, have the need and capacity to develop the virtues identified by Erickson: hope, will, purpose, competence, fidelity, love, care, and wisdom. Also, like all men, they have the capacity for reciprocity in human relationships and the right and ability for self-determination. The disabled poor are limited in attaining these goals, however, by an environment which creates feelings of helplessness and emotional isolation.

A present-time focus, low achievement motivation, and a poor health orientation further limit the disabled poor in setting and achieving short and long term goals. In addition, the disabled poor have to deal with feelings of being different from other people, physically limited, and sometimes stereotyped. These considerations suggest some general goals for work with the disabled poor.*

1. **Partialization of Objectives.** The disabled poor have a multitude of problems, and it is important to identify *specific* and *attainable* objectives that can be pursued jointly by the worker and the disabled person. These objectives may be related to physical, personal, social, vocational, and material concerns which prevent full functioning. They may include such things as obtaining vocational training, participating in a workshop, obtaining medical care, continuing welfare benefits, receiving personal and family counseling, obtaining and holding a job, receiving dental care, and, often on a very basic level, maintaining adequate food, clothing, and housing for a minimum subsistence. The important consideration is that these objectives be clearly defined and explicit so they can serve as a focus for mutual activity on the part of the worker and the client in the counseling process.

2. **Utilization of Resources.** The disabled poor often find it difficult to take advantage of specific opportunities and services available to them in the community for a variety of physical, personal, and societal reasons. The rehabilitation counselor, because of his knowledge, community perspective, and work connections, can help make available such things as training workshops, medical services and supplies, transportation money, welfare benefits, psychological testing, psychiatric services, and educational opportunities. Further, the worker may, at times, serve as the client's advocate in such things as obtaining needed services, finding and holding a job, obtaining a scholarship, or handling a problem with an unresponsive individual or organization (Ad Hoc Committee on Advocacy, 1969).

3. **Developing Strengths.** The disabled poor are often not accustomed to building on their own strengths because of their preoccupation with their limits. They are motivated to growth, however, and have ability, creativity, personal and interpersonal skills that can be freed for satisfying and productive experiences. The rehabilitation worker can help identify these strengths, encourage their development, and help find outlets for them in family, community, and work relationships.

4. **Developing Self-Acceptance and Self-Determination.** The disabled disadvantaged must find satisfaction with themselves as human beings and see themselves as valuable and productive members of society. They must be able to accept themselves as they are and gain some measure of acceptance

*The writer would like to express deep appreciation to Shirley Treger, Division of Vocational Rehabilitation, State of Illinois, for her help in supplying case material used in developing ideas presented in this paper.

from others. The disabled person must develop faith and confidence in his ability to identify and solve his own problems, make decisions, and control his own destiny. The rehabilitation worker can encourage these processes through his complete acceptance of the disabled client as a person who is capable of becoming more self-fulfilling as a result of utilizing his own resources.

5. **Developing Faith in Other People.** The disabled poor often have little faith in society and their fellow man. They have all too often been limited in their opportunities, viewed as incapable and a burden on society, and, frequently, underutilized. The rehabilitation worker is in a unique position to change this perspective through his personal involvement in the counseling relationship. The worker can, through a trusting and helpful relationship, enable a client to gain a new view of others and himself. Later, these views may be transferred outside of the counseling relationship and result in new satisfaction.

6. **Developing Perspective on Life.** The disabled poor may be able to benefit from a perspective on life that enables them to look beyond their immediate problems with hope and enthusiasm. This perspective, if present, may help them see their own usefulness, their opportunities, their relationships to others, and the possibility of enjoying life without fear of the future. The rehabilitation worker can, whenever possible, share his perspective on life, his hope and belief that life can be enjoyable and fulfilling for all people, including the disabled poor.

AN APPROACH FOR REHABILITATION PRACTICE

The remainder of this study will be devoted to outlining an approach for practice with the disabled poor. This approach is based on a social work practice model developed by William Schwartz (1961). It considers the psychological concepts discussed earlier in relation to the normal adult, the poor, and the disabled, and the goals for rehabilitation mentioned above.

Assumptions About Man and Society

This model assumes that the relationship between man and society is symbiotic with each needing the other for its life and growth, and each reaching out to the other for self-fulfillment. Society and man, and man and his fellow man, are interdependent and both give and receive in their interactions with each other in pursuit of common goals. Together, man and society will prosper; separate, neither will survive.

This model assumes that man, by his nature, is growth-oriented, positively motivated, and capable of taking responsibility for his own behavior. Man has a fundamental impetus towards other people and a capacity to act in his own self interest and in the interest of others. Man is viewed as a valuable human resource that has the capacity for self-fulfillment and high productivity.

This model notes that in a complex society a variety of things interfere with the ability of man and society to fulfill mutual goals. The impetus of man and society towards each other is often blocked by a symbiotic diffusion, or lack of common goal clarity, and by obstacles which prevent each from using the other. For example, in the case of the disabled poor, obstacles such as personal problems, cultural conditions, limited job skills, physical limitations, and lack of knowledge about community opportunities prevent self-fulfillment and result in a mutual loss to individuals and society.

This paper assumes that the disabled poor need society and society needs the disabled poor and that each has the basic motivation and the resources for interdependent and productive activity. This approach views the disability, and the poverty, as obstacles which can be identified and overcome.

Role of the Agency and Worker

The role of the agency, and specifically the rehabilitation agency, is to help persons and society achieve mutually beneficial goals—or, as Schwartz states, ". . . to mediate the process through which the individual and his society reach out for each other through a mutual need" (Schwartz, 1961). By helping persons become more productive and self-fulfilling, the agency is carrying out a joint commitment to society and the disabled poor, in the end meeting the mutual needs and interests of both. In this way, the goals of client, agency, and worker are the same. The worker carries out the agency function and attempts to bring together individual and societal needs that facilitate or impede symbiotic strivings. With the disabled, focus might be on goals noted earlier, such as improving medical knowledge, utilizing community services, increasing job skills, improving self-concept, developing social skills and social awareness, and changing attitudes.

Tasks of the Worker

Schwartz (1961) identifies the activities of the worker in terms of five tasks, which are searching out a common ground, identifying obstacles, contributing data, lending a vision, and defining limits.

1. **Searching out a common ground.** The first task of the worker is to seek out a common ground between a client's perception of his own need and aspects of social demand with which he is faced. In other words, a common ground involves mutually held goals and needs between the individual and society. More specifically, there may be a common ground between a person and any other person, group of persons, or organization. There may be a common ground between an individual and his family, his friends, his employer, his church, his community, and his government. A common ground between a disabled person and his family might be the mutual goal of keeping the family together, maintaining the best possible health, or having enough money to survive. A common ground between a disabled person and his employer may be good job performance. The first task of the rehabilitation worker is to search out a common ground with the disabled person, and

translate it into specific, realistic, and attainable objectives which can serve as a focus during the rehabilitation process.

2. **Identifying obstacles.** The second task of the worker is to identify obstacles preventing the disabled person from achieving what he wants to achieve. For example, lack of knowledge might prevent the disabled person from utilizing medical services, lack of a job might strain family relationships, lack of social or vocational skills may prevent obtaining or holding a job, and lack of trust may prevent using rehabilitation services. Identification of obstacles by the disabled person himself is often difficult because of their subjective and diffuse nature. The rehabilitation worker can bring objectivity to this process of identifying obstacles and removing them. Once identified, obstacles can serve as a focus for the worker and his client in the rehabilitation process.

3. **Contributing Data.** The third task of the worker is to contribute data in the form of ideas, facts, insights, values, knowledge, and opinions to the counseling process. The worker has knowledge of community and agency resources, insights into human behavior, ideas about solving problems, and a perspective on life that is not available to the disabled client. These data are to be contributed freely, honestly, and openly by the worker as, in that way, the client is encouraged to contribute in a like manner. In this approach, both the worker and the client are actively engaged with each other and both have something to contribute to the rehabilitation process.

4. **Lending a Vision.** The worker has a faith in people and a perspective on life that is often not held by persons who are disabled and poor. He knows, for example, as the client does not, that the rehabilitation process *can* work and the end results are worthwhile. The worker can lend his perspective, his vision, his faith in life, and his hopefulness in his contacts with his clients. The worker can convey to the disabled person that he is worthwhile and that he can use his own ability and the resources of his community to achieve his desired life goals.

5. **Defining Limits.** The final task of the worker is to define the limits and boundaries of the rehabilitation situation. These limits are determined primarily by the rehabilitation task as it was originally set down in the search for a common ground. Once the common ground has been identified, limits on subject content and behavior may be imposed if they are not consistent with it. It is important to note, however, that if limits are imposed, they are determined by the rehabilitation task and not by the authority inherent in the worker or the client. As the worker and the client become more aware of the task that faces them, they will come to see more clearly the behavior appropriate to it.

In general, this model suggests a positive, growth-oriented approach to working with the disabled disadvantaged. It assumes that people can and will strive to improve themselves if given the help and the opportunity to do so. It suggests to rehabilitation workers, a humanistic and goal directed approach in work with clients. For the rehabilitation agency, it defines a mission that serves both society and the individual. This model has been useful to social workers as a framework for practice in a wide variety of settings with different kinds of clients, and it is hoped that it will be useful in work with the disabled poor.

SUMMARY

This chapter has attempted to integrate psychological, sociological, and treatment theories to provide a framework for understanding and working with the disabled disadvantaged. Characteristics of normal adults, the poor, and the disabled were discussed; general goals for rehabilitation practice were identified; and a model for practice was presented. It is expected that this framework, or portions of it, will be useful and serve as a positive guide for rehabilitation workers in their work with persons who are both disabled and poor.

REFERENCES

Ad Hoc Committee on Advocacy: The social worker as advocate: Champion of social victims. *Social Work, 14,* 1969.

Barron, D.: Coping with the stereotype of the handicapped. *Journal of Rehabilitation, 33*:16, 1967.

Braceland, F.: Psychiatric aspects. *Journal of Rehabilitation, 32*:53, 1966.

Burke, D.: Vocational rehabilitation and emerging mental health service needs of the deaf. In Altshuler, K., and Rainer, J., (Eds.), *Mental Health and the Deaf.* National Conference on Mental Health Service for Deaf People, p. 33, 1968.

Cohen, Albert: Personality aspects of multiple sclerosis. *Journal of Rehabilitation, 28*:20, 1962.

Erickson, E.: Human strength and the cycle of generations. *Insight and Responsibility.* New York, W. W. Norton and Co., p. 111, 1964.

Henderson, G.: Occupational aspirations of poverty stricken Negro students. *Vocational Guidance Quarterly, 15*:41, 1966.

Hurley, Roger: *Poverty and Mental Retardation: A Causal Relationship.* New York, Vintage Books, 1969.

Hurwitz, S., and DiFrancisca, S.: Behavior modification of the emotionally disturbed and retarded deaf. *Rehabilitation Literature, 29*:258, 1968.

Irelan, L.: *Low Income Life Styles.* Washington, D.C., Department of Health, Education and Welfare, p. 3, 1967.

MacGuffie, R., and Janzen, R.: Self-concept and ideal-self in assessing the rehabilitation applicant. *Counseling Psychology, 16*:157, 1969.

Myers, J., and Bean, L.: *A Decade Later: A Follow-up of Social Class and Mental Illness.* New York, John Wiley and Sons, p. 61, 1968.

Nadolsky, J.: Diagnosis in rehabilitation counseling: An existential approach. *Rehabilitation Literature, 27*:66, 1966.

Roman, P., and Trice, H.: *Schizophrenia and the Poor.* Ithaca, N.Y., Cayuga Press, 1967.

Roth, J.: The treatment of the sick. In Kosa, J., Antonovsky, A., and Zola, I., (Eds.), *Poverty and Health: A Sociological Analysis.* Cambridge, Harvard University Press, 1969.

Schwartz, W.: The social worker in the group. *Social Welfare Forum*, p. 146, 1961.

Seeman, M.: Behavioral Consequences of Alienation. Mental Health Program Reports—4. Chevy Chase, Maryland, National Institute of Mental Health, p. 127, 1970.

Siller, J.: Psychological situation of the disabled with spinal cord injuries. *Rehabilitation Literature, 30*:290, 1969.

Sussman, M.: Readjustment and rehabilitation of patients. In Kosa, J., Antonovsky, A., and Zola, I. (Eds.), *Poverty and Health: A Sociological Analysis*. Cambridge, Harvard University Press, p. 249, 1969.

Sutherland, P.: On the need of the severely handicapped to feel that they are human. *Journal of Rehabilitation, 34*:28, 1968.

Thorsen, R.: Disability viewed in its cultural context. *Journal of Rehabilitation, 34*:12, 1968.

Turney, W.: Working with the socially handicapped. *Journal of Rehabilitation, 30*:29, 1964.

Yuker, H.: Attitudes as determinants of behavior. *Journal of Rehabilitation, 30*:15, 1966.

Chapter 6

ROLE INDUCTION FOR PSYCHOTHERAPY: A PROMISING TECHNIQUE FOR THE REHABILITATION CLIENT*

HANS H. STRUPP AND ANNE L. BLOXOM

D ESPITE THE FACT that psychotherapy has been a part of Western civiliza-
tion for three-quarters of a century, it continues to fascinate, and often
mystify, people as much as ever.

BACKGROUND

To be sure, the basic concepts of psychotherapy have been very popular
in our modern world, and a vast literature has sprung up. Nevertheless, the
goals and mode of operation of this intriguing treatment remain poorly
understood and shrouded in half-truths. Contrary to contemporary cartoons,
it is very serious business; it is exceedingly hard work for patient and therapist; and it is anything but *fun*. It cannot offer quick or painless solutions to
complex problems—a lure to which contemporary American society seems
particularly prone.

What Is Psychotherapy and Who Can Benefit From It?

Deep-seated prejudice is one of the obstacles to a clearer understanding of
psychotherapy. Others are the multiple meanings of the term "psychotherapy"
and the multiple forms of therapy currently available. And perhaps most formidable of all is the uncertainty, misconception, and lack of definition surrounding the nature of the problems for which one seeks psychotherapy. We
have grouped these problems under the label "neurosis," but this tells us
little of their specific nature, form, or cause.

Perhaps one reason that neurotic symptoms are so hard to define is that
they are constantly changing. These symptoms are partly a reflection of conflicts and struggles prevailing in the culture (or sub-culture or class) in which
the individual must make his adjustment. Despite the many and varied forms

*This investigation was supported by Research and Demonstration Grant No. 15-P-55164 from the
Division of Research and Demonstration Grants, Social and Rehabilitation Service, Department
of Health, Education, and Welfare, Washington, D.C. 20201.

98

of his complaints, we do know that the modern patient, like those before him, suffers and is unhappy. Typically he is anxious, depressed, and discouraged; he may be chronically fatigued or he may have a psychosomatic ailment; he has problems in interpersonal relations; he may be an alcoholic; he may be promiscuous or a homosexual; and he may have other symptoms that stamp him "neurotic." Since he hurts, he wants to be helped. He wants the expert to make him feel better, to do something that changes his current feeling state. Even highly intelligent and sophisticated people have only vague notions about the nature of his help, and, as is true of anyone in distress, they often cling to magical expectations of an omnipotent healer. Modern man in distress is no different, in this way, from the aborigine who looks to the witch doctor for powerful magic. What the candidate for psychotherapy particularly fails to realize is that he himself is contributing materially to his suffering and that in a very real sense *he* is responsible for his troubles. Consequently, one of the hardest lessons for the patient to learn is that *he* must change.

This point of view—that man is largely responsible for his own neurotic suffering—has important implications for the understanding and practice of psychotherapy, including its goals as well as its philosophical underpinnings. First, it means that the model of the medical patient as the passive recipient of an expert's ministrations is grossly inappropriate; thus, the patient must be taught *from the very beginning* that his active participation in the treatment is crucially important. Second, if the patient is so locked into a family structure or circumstances that he cannot, in that situation, possibly be changed, therapy is greatly hampered. This issue becomes particularly salient in dealing with the economically and culturally deprived client. The patient must have the opportunity to make changes within himself, but he must also have the leverage of changing his style of life and external arrangements when this seems necessary. In a real sense, a patient is neurotic to the extent that he fails to take effective action where he can and should, and he fails wildly at self-created obstacles. So long as he pursues contradictory goals, he continues to suffer. The patient must learn which problems are due to himself and which to circumstances, which he can change and which he must learn to accept.

How can the patient be made to realize that in order to *get well* he needs to change, and how can therapeutic change be brought about? That change partly occurs when the patient becomes convinced (persuaded, taught) that change is in his own best interest. This realization is usually painful because the patient is confronted with the necessity of giving up fantasies, beliefs, and ways of relating to others which, while they are shown to be self-defeating and infantile, still involve a certain amount of masochistic pleasure. To illustrate: If, as a result of early life experience, a person has been programmed to feel that sooner or later a significant person (wife, boss, etc.) will exploit him and do him in, and if he is thus driven to fight the oppressor, the resulting feeling of revenge is pleasurable regardless of other consequences. On the other hand, the realization that he is the one who arranges circumstances such that others will exploit and abuse him is difficult to drive home, and when it does take hold, it inevitably results in a sense of lost power and an injury to one's narcissism.

Therapy is an educational enterprise pure and simple. However, it is education of a unique sort: it trains the patient to be more self-aware and more honest with himself; to achieve more adequate control over his primitive impulses and strivings; to be freer in expressing his feelings; to manage his relations with others so that they become more satisfying to himself and more effective in achieving his own realistic goals; to become more tolerant of the human lot, including limitations and shortcomings in himself and others; and to develop an ability to postpone, modify and even forego gratifications whose demands previously seemed imperious. Freud once described the goal of therapy as transforming neurotic misery into ordinary human suffering. We cannot eliminate suffering, but we can teach a person to deal with it more effectively.

Indeed, a primary goal of all therapy is to teach man to take an *active* part in mastering his fate. The task of the therapist, therefore, is not to modify a symptom, or to change a specific external circumstance, or to cure an illness, but to help the patient build the kind of inner support structure which will enable him to face the vicissitudes of life with greater strength and equanimity. The real goal for man is *to stand alone,* which becomes possible when he has obtained insight into the motives for his entanglements with others and has learned new methods of coping with them more effectively and productively.

Psychotherapy and the Lower-Class Patient: A Poor Match

Of the large number of emotionally troubled persons who are referred for help to outpatient clinics, community mental health centers, or similar agencies, only a very small percentage receive psychotherapy for any substantial period of time. A large proportion of applicants never get to see a therapist, and the relatively small number of those who do, frequently stay for only a few sessions. The problem involves selection on the part of the potential patient as well as of the clinic. Services are not offered to many people who seek help, but when they are, there are still quite a few people who do not take advantage of them. The reasons for rejecting an offer of psychotherapy are difficult to assess. Some people obviously are not serious about entering psychotherapy; some have erroneous notions about it and reject it when they become aware of the need for their active participation; some become discouraged by the reception accorded them by the agency to which they apply; some find the prospect of self-examination extremely threatening; and, for others, coming regularly to a clinic entails too many sacrifices.

Many persons in our culture still have a considerable number of inhibitions and reservations about consulting a psychotherapist, and the wish, both conscious and unconscious, to view unhappiness and emotional suffering as a physical ailment is widespread. There is no stigma attached to consulting a physician, and it is not surprising that people most readily turn for help to a general practitioner or internist. They find the pronouncement that they are suffering from a vitamin deficiency, an allergy, or even a heart condition easier to accept than that their difficulties are symptoms of disturbed interpersonal relations, such as excessive dependency on a spouse, seething hatred of a parent, and the like. The fear of being labeled *crazy, a mental case, homosexual,* etc., is far from extinct despite the influence of books, magazines, motion pictures, and television. To be *in psychotherapy* or, preferably, *in psychoanalysis,* is acceptable—even a sign of status and prestige—among many intellectuals in the larger urban centers, but is virtually unknown elsewhere.

It is relatively uncommon for a person to become clearly aware that he is in need of psychotherapy and to come to a therapist on his own. He is more likely to turn to other professionals in the community, for example, a physician or a clergyman. Persons in these professions with an eye for emotional factors in illness or incapacitation are still not numerous, although their number is steadily increasing, and they most often attempt to offer help solely through reassurance and understanding. They make referrals to a mental health clinic only as a last resort.

In view of the massive attempts which are being made to educate the public about the nature of emotional problems in living, we may question whether the information which is being dispensed by the mass media is as useful as it might be. Since the beginning of the modern mental health movement, efforts have been made to remove the stigma of emotional problems by defining their onset as an *illness* (Szasz, 1961). It is hardly surprising, then, that emotional problems have come to be seen in terms of a disease, an attitude encouraged by the use of such terms as *patient, diagnosis, treatment, cure, etc.* The psychotherapist, on the other hand, attempts to make his patients see neurosis as a problem of maladaptation, faulty learning, and the like. The patient comes to realize that he is not the victim of a disease visited upon him by mysterious forces, and that he must take active part in his own treatment. Only in recent years has neurosis come to be viewed as a problem in living and adaptation; consequently, psychotherapy is not a technique for "treating" or "curing" a patient, but rather for increasing his ability to cope adequately with the everyday problems in living.

Very few people have a clear understanding of the processes and goals of psychotherapy, or of the role the patient is expected to play, let alone the kinds of expectations he might reasonably entertain. This problem of inadequate information and lack of understanding is especially acute among the lower socio-economic classes. The Joint Commission on Mental Illness and Health in its final report, *Action for Mental Health,* concluded that the way Americans view their mental health and the professional treatment opportunities available, is very much conditioned by the extent of their education and the amount of money they earn (these two factors being the basic determiners of social class in our society). In interviews of a representative sample of the American population, it was found that one out of four persons reported having experienced a problem for which professional help would have been useful. In defining the nature of their problem, the better educated tended to be more introspective and self-critical, and to take into account their own personality characteristics in connection with their current problems. They typically reacted to stress with predominantly psychological symptoms. People with less education, on the other hand, tended to think more in terms of the external world as the basic cause of their troubles and reacted to their problems with predominantly physical symptoms.

Only one out of seven persons interviewed reported having actually sought some form of professional help. It was those who tended to define their problems in psychological terms (the more educated), who sought a psychological form of treatment. People who saw their problems as arising from sources *outside* themselves were less likely to consult psychotherapists. Only a small percentage of those who sought assistance (of any form) traced their problems back to their own inadequacies with any clarity. "Most were looking for support and advice. Few were prepared to be told that they must accept at least a share of the responsibility for their problems and that they must change themselves accordingly." That may be why so many reported choosing the support of a clergyman or of a physician over the more searching, difficult, and often prolonged therapy offered by the psychiatrist. Yet, in terms of feeling, they had benefited from the professional assistance sought, those who saw their troubles as arising from sources outside the individual fared worse. People who defined their problem in terms of personal adjustment most often reported that the assistance they received had been of value to them.

Approximately 40 percent of people reporting problems for which professional help was needed failed to make any active effort to seek such assistance. They attributed this lack of action primarily to a sense of shame, a fear of stigma, or to inadequate knowledge of where to go. The more poorly educated and lower income groups were least likely to seek professional help. It is important to note that there were no striking differences in the kinds of problems they reported, only in the way they interpreted these problems. Similar patterns of action were reported for day-to-day worries and unhappiness not seen as requiring professional help. Again, the less educated, lower income group reported passive reactions of doing nothing, forgetting the difficulty, letting it run its course, or relying on prayer. In contrast, the more educated, higher income group exhibited more active reactions of self-help or turning to family or friends. Thus, "the people who seek professional help when confronted with major personal problems, the better educated people with higher incomes, also take more initiative in trying to cope with less serious life problems."

Brill and Storrow (1960) point out that it is this type of initiative, coupled with the relationship between education, sophistication, and alertness to psychological resources—more than a social class or economic bias per se—which determines the type of psychiatric treatment given to a patient. Often middle and upper class clients seek and are accepted for therapy on the grounds that they are most able to benefit from this type of treatment. The lower class client is seen as less intelligent and less educated, as defining his present problems as physical rather than emotional, as desiring symptomatic relief only rather than over-all help, and as having not only a poor understanding of the psychotherapeutic process but also a lack of desire for psychotherapy. The true nature of his problem in terms of such aspects as degree of manifest anxiety or amount of obvious secondary gain yielded by the *illness*, does not appear to be related to social class.

This has important implications, for it suggests that such measures as reducing the cost of therapy or increasing the availability of treatment will not necessarily result in a greater number of lower class patients being ready to take advantage of therapeutic opportunity or being accepted for or benefiting from such treatment. On the other hand, it has been demonstrated that lower class clients who are properly prepared and whose expectations are more congruent with those of the therapist, do stay in therapy as long and benefit from therapy as much as upper class clients.

Miller and Mishler (1964) also stress the importance of initial patient characteristics in the type of treatment sought and received. They point out that, in arguments that the lower class is being short-changed in *not* receiving the better or more intensive forms of treatment, there "seems to be an assumption that it is the psychiatrist who relatively completely controls the type of treatment given. It may be that patients search out psychiatrists (or other professionals) who will give them their preferred type of treatment and reject non-preferred treatments . . . The selective process and pressures emanating from the patient cannot be ignored in a full account of the biased pattern of psychiatric treatment."

There is little doubt that preferred type of treatment does differ as a function of social class (or its determinants). Hollingshead and Redlich (1958) in their classic book, *Social Class and Mental Illness,* report that the most frequent source of difficulty for Class V patients lies in their looking for (and wanting) an authoritarian attitude on the part of the psychiatrist. This tendency, coupled with an insistence that their troubles are a physical illness and with a lack of confidence in a "talking" treatment, creates a formidable barrier indeed against traditional therapeutic procedure and gain. These attitudes toward therapy are consistent with and undoubtedly stem from the larger pattern of values and child-rearing practices of the lower class. Bronfenbrenner (1958), in summarizing studies in this area, concludes that lower class parents are more apt to concentrate on overt acts and consequences, to employ greater physical punishment, and generally to emphasize the maintenance of order and obedience, resulting in a more authoritarian parent-child relationship. In contrast, middle class parents give greater attention to internal dynamics and show more concern over their child's *motives and feelings,* leading to a more acceptant and equalitarian relationship.

Here two points can be made: (1) Members of the lower classes are more likely to adopt an attitude of apathy toward their problems and exhibit a pattern of "learned helplessness" in the face of difficulty. A meager income and lack of education undoubtedly place them in a position where they actually have much less control over their external environment and much less opportunity to learn how to achieve control than their upper-class counterparts. In addition, their position within their own families has fostered an attitude of submission and obedience rather than equal participation and learned mastery, whereas their own motives, feelings, and actions have resulted in positive gains for themselves as individuals. (2) When they do seek outside help, they seem to be looking for an authoritarian relationship wherein the therapist will assume responsibility for solving their difficulties by giving them direct advice, medication, or some other immediate "cure."

Regardless of their origin, it is small wonder that the foregoing factors complicate the patient-therapist relationship, and unless corrected, frequently result in disappointment, premature termination, or prolonged frustration. Orne and Wender (1968) succinctly describe the plight of such a patient (as well as that of his therapist):

> Perhaps he has been referred by a medical or surgical clinic, a social agency, or the courts. He does not know anyone who has ever been in psychotherapy and has had little exposure to psychological novels or causal "psychologizing." He has no concrete idea of what to expect and may well think that psychiatrists are dangerous and powerful people who deal with crazy folks. In the ensuing inaction there will be a clear lack of mutually complementary role expectations between himself and the psychiatrist. The result is easy to caricature, but it has a familiar ring.
>
> The patient, relying on the only model in his experience which is appropriate, acts as if the psychiatrist were another medical doctor. Having briefly stated his presenting complaint, he expects to be asked further questions. The psychiatrist, on the other hand, wanting to get at the patient's feelings, makes little or no response and listens attentively. The patient waits expectantly to be asked questions while the therapist waits for the patient to say more. Both parties in the interaction become increasingly uncomfortable. When the level of anxiety becomes sufficiently high the psychiatrist may ask some questions to elicit factual information or the patient may repeat the recital of his difficulties and his pleas for help in different ways. At the end of the first hour, both parties are thoroughly dissatisfied.
>
> The patient, who has come for help, advice, and treatment, wonders what the doctor really wants. He is confused and feels that somehow he has failed. His doubts about the availability of help from psychiatrists are reinforced, and his belief that his problem is really medical may be stronger. He usually feels worse than when he came and takes this to mean that treatment is not only ineffectual but actually harmful. He will return only because he feels he must, or perhaps

because he has already been through several other medical clinics and this is the end of the line.

The psychiatrist, who is usually a resident, is equally dissatisfied. He may have some choice thoughts about why he has been assigned another untreatable patient with no capacity for insight or insufficient intelligence for treatment. He thinks: "Perhaps things will improve in further sessions, but I doubt it." But he has little choice except to go on seeing the patient.

In this manner, both patient and psychiatrist may continue unhappily for some time: the patient needing and wanting help, the psychiatrist willing to provide it, but both frustrated by a lack of communication. Eventually, the predictions which have been made privately by both parties come true, and the patient fails to keep his appointments. After perfunctory attempts to induce him to come, he is assigned to drug therapy or discontinued with a sigh of relief and an appropriate note on his chart indicating why he is unable to benefit from the treatment (pp. 1205-1206).

It is clear that psychotherapy, quite unlike any medical treatment, presupposes attitudes, motivations, and expectations which have a profound bearing on the inception, continuation, progress, and outcome of the therapeutic enterprise. Until fairly recently it was the practice either to select patients to fit a particular method of psychotherapy or to ignore the problem of the patient's suitability. The latter course typically resulted in exceedingly high dropout rates which have been a common phenomenon at mental health clinics. In recent years various efforts have been made to tailor therapeutic services to fit the needs, expectations, and capabilities of the client. Crisis call centers, store-front agencies, indigenous or paraprofessional helpers, and many others are examples of this trend. A somewhat different approach (the one to which this chapter is devoted) is represented by attempts *to produce changes in the attitudes and expectations of prospective clients,* thereby rendering them increasingly amenable to more or less "traditional" therapeutic procedures which over the years have demonstrated their utility—in this case, group psychotherapy.

ROLE INDUCTION: CONCEPT AND TECHNIQUES

How can one produce a better alignment between the patient's feelings, attitudes, and expectations about psychotherapy on the one hand and the experiences he actually faces as a patient on the other? A common sense approach to the problem would be simply to inform him as to what psychotherapy is about and what it is like to be a patient. The object here is to induct the person into the patient role or to provide him with "anticipatory socialization for psychotherapy."* To accomplish this goal one might expose the patient to a role induction interview (RII) prior to psychotherapy, in which the patient is told what he needs to know. Such an interview might be conducted either by the therapist himself (Orne and Wender, 1968) or by another trained individual (Hoehn-Saric, Frank, Imber, Nash, Stone and Battle, 1964). Another approach consists of vicarious therapy pretraining, in

*Credit for the pioneer effort in this area belongs to Dr. Martin T. Orne.

which prospective patients listen to a tape recording illustrating "good" patient behavior in group therapy prior to the beginning of actual group therapy (Truax, 1966). More recently, Truax has employed videotapes for the same purpose.

Does a role induction interview have a favorable effect on the course and outcome of psychotherapy with clinic patients? To investigate this problem Hoehn-Saric *et al.* (1964), working at the Henry Phipps Psychiatric Clinic at Johns Hopkins Hospital, compared two groups of neurotic outpatients (each group comprised of twenty patients) on a variety of in-therapy and outcome measures. Their results unequivocally favored the experimental group which had received the RII. The experimental group exhibited better in-therapy behavior; it had a better attendance rate; and therapists rated the experimental group more favorably with respect to establishing and maintaining a therapeutic relationship. Of even greater importance are the better outcome measures for the experimental group. The latter included: therapist's rating of improvement; patient's rating of mean target symptom improvement; and social effectiveness ratings. The authors concluded that the RII could become a valuable tool in psychotherapy. A five-year follow-up of clients participating in the role induction study, to be published soon, will examine long-term effects of therapy outcome (Liberman, Frank, Hoehn-Saric, Stone, Imber, and Pande, in press).

In addition to producing better outcomes, the RII gave evidence of increasing the interpersonal attraction between patient and therapist which, as past research (Goldstein, 1962; Wallach and Strupp, 1960) has shown, is an important prerequisite for successful therapy. Lower-class patients, in particular, often fail to appeal to therapists (Hollingshead and Redlich, 1958); consequently, as the patient's motivation for therapy is increased, he may become more attractive to the therapist, hence eliciting greater commitment, interest, and effort on the therapist's part (Strupp, 1960). Only in recent years has the importance of this point begun to be fully appreciated.

The vicarious training procedure (VTP) developed by Truax, likewise produced encouraging results. Truax (1966) found that the use of VTP had major therapeutic benefits for outpatients, modest therapeutic benefit for hospitalized mental patients, and no therapeutic benefit on institutionalized juvenile delinquents. So far no results pertaining to the videotaped version have been reported. (For additional reports of the work with VTP by Truax and his colleagues, see: Truax, Shapiro and Wargo, 1968; Truax, Wargo and Volksdorf, 1970; Truax, Wargo, Carkhuff, Kodman, and Moles, 1966).

Present Research Goals

The role induction procedures investigated to date clearly emerged as promising techniques meriting further research. In particular, it seemed desirable to explore whether it might be possible to develop a role induction instrument which would combine the advantages of an individual interview with mass administration. Considerable savings in time and manpower might thus be effected. With these objectives in mind, the research project reported in these pages was designed and carried out. The ensuing presentation includes two parts: (1) development of a new role induction instrument; and (2) systematic evaluation of the new role induction technique under field conditions.

DEVELOPMENT OF ROLE INDUCTION FILM

"Turning Point": A Role Induction Film

The anticipatory socialization interview (Orne and Wender, 1968) was designed to serve three major purposes: (1) to provide some rational basis for the patient to accept psychotherapy as a means of helping him deal with his problem, recognizing that talking is not seen by most patients as a treatment modality; (2) to clarify the role of patient and therapist in the course of treatment; and (3) to provide a general outline of the course of therapy and its vicissitudes, with particular emphasis on the clarification of the patient's negative and hostile feelings. In addition to these broad objectives, we considered it desirable to convey numerous points of information designed to create more positive and realistic attitudes concerning the psychotherapeutic enterprise. Thus the role induction should prepare the patient:*

1. To express personal feelings to a mental health professional.
2. To recognize that talking about troublesome feelings can be useful.
3. To understand that change requires work that he must do himself.
4. To accept the knowledge that some of his difficulties are self-inflicted, through inadequate thinking and defensive attitudes.
5. To understand that some physical ailments can be, in part at least, caused by psychological stresses.
6. To realize that there are adaptive and maladaptive ways of expressing anger, hostility, resentment, and agression.
7. To accept peers as potential allies and friends instead of enemies.
8. To expect no miracles and understand that personality change takes time.
9. To accept the knowledge that medication provides no solution to problems in living.
10. To learn that difficulties in living are common, and that they can be dealt with more effectively by talking about them than by hiding them.
11. To expect that there are no "cures" for life's difficulties, only more or less adequate ways of dealing with them.

After preliminary explorations to determine optimal approaches to a new role induction instrument, we arrived at the conclusion that a documentary

---

*Some of the points are noted by Riessman, Cohen, and Pearl (1964).

film might be the most effective vehicle for creating positive attitudes toward mental health services in prospective patients. Following the collection and study of interview data from patients seen at a local outpatient clinic, the project staff developed a general plan for the contents and format of the projected film and a script was written by a member of the project staff. The film was titled *Turning Point.**

Synopsis

The film is a dramatic story dealing with the life of a truck driver. Tom Sevier is a man in his early thirties whose major problem, as depicted in the film, is a volatile temper which leads to open conflict with authority figures, notably his boss, as well as with co-workers and his wife. Following a violent verbal interchange with the boss, he gets fired from his job. Prospects for help from a mental health clinic, where Tom is seen in a preliminary interview by a social worker, impress Tom as dim. His pattern of uncontrolled aggressiveness leads to dismissal from several other jobs, and Tom's wife and children leave him after one of his provocations. Tom reaches a state of despondency, turns to alcohol, and eventually contemplates suicide. Recalling a friendly interaction with a patient whom he had encountered at the clinic, he returns and joins a therapy group. A series of scenes showing the therapy group in action demonstrates how in the context of this experience Tom gains some understanding of his own contribution to the difficulties in his life. The film ends as Tom succeeds in applying these insights: he regains his original job and works out a more satisfactory relationship with his wife. (Black and white, 16 mm, running time 32 minutes).

The film appeared to have several potential advantages as a role induction instrument, including: direct human appeal to a wide audience, particularly to members of the lower income group who are seen as the prime target audience; dramatic impact; and a realistic presentation of the nature and extent of benefits a prospective client of the target population may expect from mental health services, especially from group psychotherapy.

The following section describes our efforts at evaluating the utility and effectiveness of this film.

EVALUATION OF ROLE INDUCTION FILM

Research Design and Procedures

The purpose of this phase was to evaluate the role induction film whose development has been described in the preceding section. To this end, it seemed highly desirable to assess its advantages or drawbacks under conditions which approximated as closely and realistically as possible the field conditions under which such an instrument would ordinarily be used. There-

---

*Herschel N. Pollard (Vanderbilt University) served as writer and production coordinator. H. Thomas Bell (Design Center, Inc., Washington, D.C.) was film director for the project.

fore, it was decided to set up a series of therapy groups composed of typical members of the target population, and to systematically compare the effects of varying induction procedures upon the course and outcome of group therapy.

General Design

It is stipulated that each of four experienced psychotherapists would treat three groups of clients for twelve weekly sessions, each group initially being composed of approximately ten individuals. Each group was introduced to group psychotherapy by one of the following procedures:

1. The role induction film developed as part of this project.

2. A role induction interview patterned after the Anticipatory Socialization Interview developed by Orne as adapted by the investigators at the Henry Phipps Psychiatric Clinic, Johns Hopkins Hospital (see preceding section). This procedure was followed in order to carry out a direct comparison between the relative effects of the film and the interview.

3. A neutral film, intended as a control, was included to equalize the interest and attention devoted to prospective patients receiving the foregoing procedures. It occupied a comparable amount of time but contained no information relevant to the induction process.

Assessments were made at specified times. The general plan of the experimental design is summarized in these pages. It is important to emphasize that each therapist treated three groups, one under each of the induction procedures. Therapists and clients were unaware of the design and the purpose of the study.

Hypothesis and Aims

The general hypothesis of the research may be stated as follows: In group pschyotherapy programs aimed at rehabilitating lower-class clients, a preliminary role induction procedure (a psychiatric interview or a film especially designed for the purpose) will favorably affect the clients' attitudes, motivations, expectancies, attendance, in-therapy behavior, and therapeutic outcome.

The research reported here was clearly exploratory. We examined in detail the extent of the foregoing effects as well as the relative efficacy of the two role induction procedures, while pursuing our primary aim of evaluating the usefulness and effectiveness of the Role Induction Film developed as part of the project.

Clients

In order to recruit the requisite number of clients, we worked closely with the Tennessee Vocational Rehabilitation Service and numerous community service agencies in the Nashville area. Emphasis was placed on lower income clients who were in need of psychological counseling to reach their rehabilita-

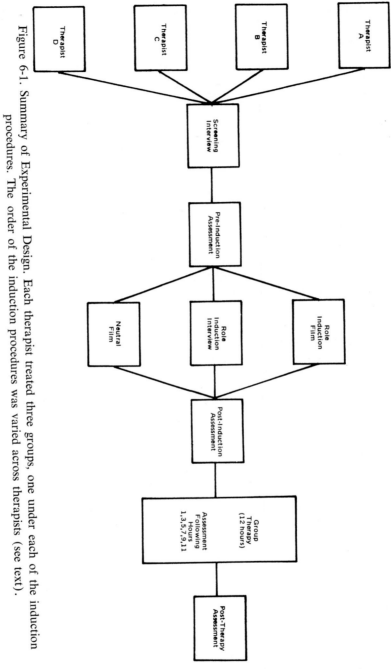

Figure 6-1. Summary of Experimental Design. Each therapist treated three groups, one under each of the induction procedures. The order of the induction procedures was varied across therapists (see text).

tion objectives and yet had minimal motivation to seek and accept mental health services.

A total of 122 clients were selected from twelve community agencies to participate in the role induction evaluation. The sample population proved to be well balanced by sex and by race, containing similar proportions of males and females and of Blacks and Whites. The average age was twenty-nine. Although clients ranged from 17 to 65 years of age, the majority were young adults in their twenties or thirties. The educational level ranged from fourth grade through college, with the average years of education completed falling at 10.8. Again, the heaviest clustering was around the mean.

Therapists

In searching for persons who would assume the leadership in the therapy groups, we stipulated that candidates should be individuals with considerable experience in group psychotherapy, particularly with clients similar to those constituting the target population.

Four persons meeting these criteria were selected: three were male clinical psychologists holding the Ph.D. degree; one was a psychiatric nurse with comparable training and experience. All were actively working as therapists and highly competent. The therapists were paid a regular professional fee for their participation in the program.

Induction Techniques

Role Induction Film

The Role Induction film, *Turning Point,* the development of which has been described in the preceding section, was shown to groups of prospective clients in accordance with the stipulations of the experimental design. Clients were simply informed that they were to see a motion picture; no further instructions were given.

Role Induction Interview

All interviews were conducted by an experienced psychiatrist who met with designated groups of prospective patients at their first scheduled meeting.* He was thoroughly familiar with the points to be covered in such an interview (as enumerated earlier) but freely adapted them to his own style and to the needs of the clients as he perceived them. Clients were encouraged to ask questions about group psychotherapy or other relevant concerns. The interviews were conducted in a professional manner, yet in keeping with the clients' level of understanding and sophistication.

Neutral (Control) Film

As already indicated, the neutral film was intended to have some relevance to prospective clients but at the same time was not to constitute an induction procedure in its own right. After screening a number of available mental health films, we selected a motion picture dealing with teen-age marriage as

---

*Dr. Charles E. Wells, Associate Professor of Psychiatry and Neurology, Vanderbilt University. A transcript of a sample interview, and the question and answer session that followed, can be found in Strupp and Bloxom, 1971.

an appropriate neutral film. The instructions accompanying the presentation were minimal and paralleled those of the role induction film.

Procedures

In order to evaluate the effectiveness of the role induction procedures in as natural and typical a setting as possible, the study included two parallel phases, called the therapy phase and the research phase. Separate personnel were employed in each phase. By separating the therapy and research aspects of our work, rather than administering the various instruments within the therapy setting, we hoped to obtain more open and honest responses and to avoid interference with the therapeutic process.

The Therapy Phase

The first step in instituting the therapy phase was the recruitment of patients from various agencies in the community who were working with members of the target population. We offered to provide a free twelve-week group therapy program to any clients who were in need of such services but for reasons of inadequate resources or lack of interest had not received therapeutic aid. The therapy program was incorporated into the agency's framework, with the clients maintaining their primary contact with the agency. The agency, project staff, and therapist worked together to arrange such details as type of group, therapist, and optimal meeting place for each client.

After receiving agency referrals, a member of the project staff contacted each client to explain the program in more detail and to invite him to a screening interview with his proposed therapist. Following this interview, appropriate clients were given an appointment for their first group meeting, which was the role induction meeting described above. At the conclusion of the role induction session, each client was given a written schedule for his therapy group meetings.

The therapy group meetings were scheduled once a week for twelve consecutive weeks. Each meeting lasted one to one and one-half hours, depending on the preference of the individual therapist. Therapists were encouraged to conduct group meetings in accordance with their preferred style. No restrictions were imposed on the therapists' activities, with the exception of the request that all sessions be recorded on audio tape. The therapeutic techniques employed by the group leaders may be characterized as broadly electric.

The Research Phase—Client Participation

At the time of initial contact, the research aspects of the therapy program were described and the client's participation solicited. From the client's point of view, the research phase was comprised of ten data collection sessions, spaced throughout the therapy program. Each data collection session lasted approximately one half hour, during which the client was asked to fill out an appropriate set of ratings presented to him in booklet form. Clients were paid one dollar for each completed booklet. The decision to pay clients cooperating in the research was intended to compensate them for their time and effort as well as to provide an incentive for completing the forms.

The Research Phase—Therapist Participation

The therapists' role in the research phase consisted of filling out information and evaluation forms at designated intervals in the therapy program. These measures required approximately ten to fifteen minutes of therapist time for each client. Each set of rating forms was distributed to the therapist at the appropriate time and collected immediately upon completion.

Research Instruments

A battery of tests and rating instruments was developed for the purpose of carrying out the appropriate assessments. Many of the measures employed to assess in-therapy behavior and therapeutic outcome were selected on the basis of their demonstrated utility in earlier research at the Phipps Psychiatric Clinic of Johns Hopkins University. When necessary, these instruments were modified for group psychotherapy, and the wording was simplified for lower-class patients. In addition, an intensive review of the literature was conducted for the purpose of selecting instruments relevant to the present study. Published scales were used whenever possible. Several additional measures were constructed by the project staff to extend or explore in greater depth the findings of earlier research in this area (see Hoehn-Saric *et al.*, 1964; Sloane, Cristol, Pepernik and Staples, 1970; Yalom, Houts, Newell and Rand, 1967). The complete text of all research instruments, their source of origin, and the schedule of administration can be found in Strupp and Bloxom, 1971.

Results*

Statistical Procedures

A least-squares analysis of variance was employed to isolate main effects for the three role induction conditions, the four therapists, and repeated measures over time, as well as to examine for interactions of these variables. Results discussed in this chapter are primarily those derived from examination of the role induction condition main effects and condition by repeated measures interactions. Correlations were calculated by the Pearson Product-Moment method. The 5 percent level of confidence was the criterion of significance.

Pre-Induction Comparability of Clients

Table 6-I presents the initial comparability of clients in the three role induction conditions on demographic variables, verbal ability, social desir-

---

*A complete report of the results from the evaluation study can be found in Strupp and Bloxom, 1971, just referred to; only brief highlights will be reported here. Please note that all differences reported in this section were significant beyond the .05 level, unless otherwise stated.

ability, severity of disturbance, prognosis in therapy, suitability as a candi-

TABLE 6-I*

PRE-INDUCTION COMPARABILITY OF CLIENTS

		Induction Condition		
	Total Sample	Film	Interview	Neutral
Client Attributes:				
Sex: Male	45%	50%	45%	40%
Female	55%	50%	55%	60%
Race: White	56%	59%	40%	70%
Black	44%	41%	60%	30%
Age (mean)	29.1	31.9	25.3	30.2
Education (mean)	10.8	10.6	10.9	10.8
Verbal ability	22.7	20.1	21.8	26.3*
Social desirability scale	18.1		No difference	
Severity of Disturbance:				
Therapist's rating of severity of disturbance	2.9		No difference	
Client's report of symptom discomfort	14.6		No difference	
Target symptom severity	3.4		No difference	
Prognosis:				
Client's prognosis in the therapy program	3.0		No difference	
Suitability for Therapy:				
Client's attractiveness for psychotherapy	3.1		No difference	
Self disclosure	19.1		No difference	
Client anticipates active role in conversation	3.4		No difference	
Motivation to Begin Therapy:				
Client wants to begin therapy	2.0		No difference	
Estimated length of stay in therapy	1.7		No difference	
Outcome of Screening Interview:				
Client's satisfaction with screening interview	3.1		No difference	
Quality of screening interview interaction	2.9		No difference	
Client's comfort in screening interview	2.4		No difference	

*Statistically significant condition difference (p ≤.05).

date for therapy, motivation to begin therapy sessions, and outcome of the screening interview. There were no group differences among clients in the three role induction conditions on any of the therapy-related measures. There were a few group differences with respect to client attributes. Clients in the neutral group obtained higher scores on the test of verbal ability and there was a higher proportion of White clients in this group. The interview group contained a higher proportion of Black clients and had a lower mean age. Overall, we considered the three groups as initially well matched. It is important to note that the clients in the induction film group did not differ from the client population as a whole on any of the pre-induction measures.

Immediate Effects of Induction Procedures

Clients' Attitudes Toward Induction

Clients who received either of the role induction procedures enjoyed their initial role induction meeting more than those in the neutral condition, and they considered the session as more helpful in preparing them to benefit from the group sessions to follow. The induction experience, clearly a crucial first contact, enabled the client to enter his group therapy sessions with a more favorable and hopeful attitude toward the treatment program. The film induction was evidently as effective as the personal interview in instilling these attitudes.

It is equally clear that these attitudes and expectancies were based on more than the possible *entertainment value* of the induction procedure. Significant positive correlations were found between items assessing the degree to which the client enjoyed and expected to benefit from the role induction process and other measures of positive expectations, such as willingness to begin the treatment program, anticipated satisfaction with the first therapy session, estimated global improvement, and realistic expectations of improvement. Moreover, these attitudes and expectancies were found to be significantly associated with subsequent measures of in-therapy behavior and satisfaction, such as client's satisfaction with progress in therapy, and therapist ratings of the client's appropriate in-therapy behavior. Post-therapy measures of outcome still reflected the strong influence of these early attitudes and expectancies in the significant correlations found for such items as client's gain in self-understanding, global improvement, and the therapist's satisfaction with the client's progress in therapy.

It is also important to note that clients who were in greatest need of help, as evidenced by therapists' ratings of the severity of their disturbances, tended to experience the most positive reaction to the role induction procedures.

Motivation to Begin Group Sessions

In order to assess the immediate effects of the role induction procedures on the client's motivation to enter group psychotherapy, ratings were obtained from the therapists both before and after the induction session. Major results, presented in Figure 6-2, may be summarized as follows:

1. Therapists' ratings of the client's willingness to begin treatment showed changes in the direction of increased willingness for clients who had either viewed the role induction film or participated in the role induction interview; clients in the neutral condition were rated as less willing to begin therapy. The difference between the positive and negative changes were statistically significant beyond the .05 level.

2. Three additional therapist ratings related to the client's motivation to enter therapy provided further evidence favoring one or both of the induction procedures over the neutral film. However, on one of the items (the therapists' rating of the degree to which the client considered group psychotherapy the proper treatment for him), the film group showed an increment in motivation whereas the interview group showed a marked decrease. This finding suggests that the film may be superior in some ways to the interview as an induction procedure for group psychotherapy. However, as subsequent results will indicate, this seemingly adverse effect of the interview procedure was apparently transient.

It is evident that either the film or the interview induction procedure was consistently associated with increased motivation to enter group therapy,

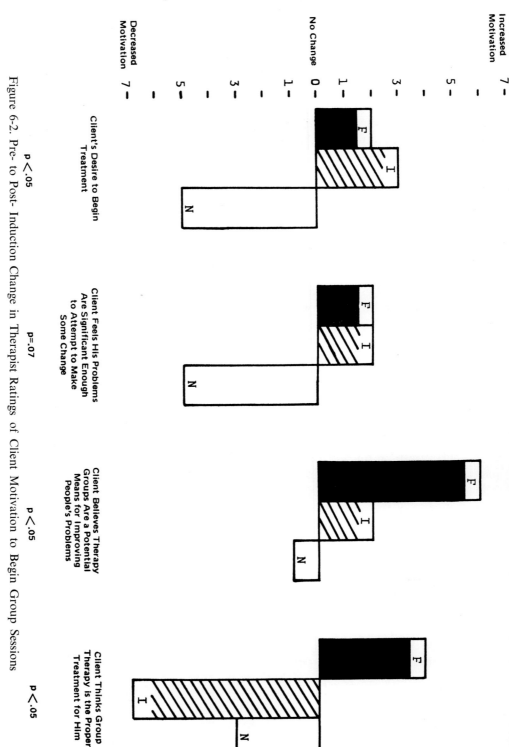

Figure 6-2. Pre- to Post- Induction Change in Therapist Ratings of Client Motivation to Begin Group Sessions

whereas decrements in motivation were observed for clients who had viewed the neutral film. On every measure the induction film equaled or surpassed the interview in bringing about these motivational changes in the clients. In addition, it should be emphasized that the changes must have been exhibited in the clients' overt behavior, which provided the basis for the therapists' ratings. The therapists, it will be recalled, remained unaware of the content or the purpose of the role induction meeting; thus, the foregoing results are based on "blind" ratings made at the time of the screening interview and following the first therapy session.

Knowledge of Therapy and Client-Therapist Roles

Measures were administered both before and after the induction procedures to assess the client's understanding of group therapy as a treatment modality and, more specifically, his perception of the respective roles of the client and the therapist in the treatment process. The major findings are summarized below:

1. Both role induction procedures effected a favorable change in the client's understanding of the therapy process and his role in it, while clients in the neutral condition showed either negligible or unfavorable changes in this area.

2. A specific component of the favorable change (for clients receiving either of the role induction procedures) was the increased expectancy of playing an active role in the therapy process (initiating and continuing discussion). At the same time, the therapist tended to be seen as functioning in a guiding role rather than offering direct suggestions and solutions to the client's problems. Those in the neutral condition showed no change in expectancies concerning their participation; rather, there were marked increments in their expectancy that the therapist would offer direct suggestions and answers to their problems.

3. In addition to the more restrained role expected of the therapist, clients participating in either of the role induction procedures showed a significant increase in their expectancy that they would find their therapist reassuring. Clients in the neutral condition showed no change in this expectancy.

Estimated Post-Therapy Improvement

Estimates of the client's prognosis in the treatment program (rated by therapist) and his expected global improvement (rated by client) were obtained before and after the induction session. In ratings made after the induction, both therapists and clients expected a significantly greater improvement for clients who had participated in one of the role induction procedures. Clients who had viewed the induction film expected greater improvement than those who had participated in the interview. Comparable prognostic ratings by therapists favored the two induction groups over the neutral group. The pre-induction ratings showed no differences between groups.

Thus the two role induction procedures clearly resulted in greater expectations of improvement. The film was most effective in raising the clients' expectations, although the two role induction procedures appeared to have similar effects in terms of therapists' ratings. Clients in the neutral condition showed a lower expectancy of improvement, both in terms of therapists' and self ratings.

Symptom Discomfort

A twenty-five item Discomfort Scale was completed by the clients prior to their induction session and a week later (before their first therapy session). This scale yielded a total discomfort score as well as subscale scores for somatic, anxiety, and depression symptoms. All clients showed a significant drop in discomfort following the induction. This decrease was apparent in each of the subscale scores as well as in the total score, and it was equal for the neutral, film and interview groups. In keeping with the findings of other research (Frank, Nash, Stone and Imber, 1963), the act of entering the treatment program proved comforting to the clients, regardless of the specific content of the induction meeting.

The foregoing increase in comfort was evidently manifested in the clients' subsequent behavior, since ratings made by the therapists closely paralleled those of the clients. Therapists rated the clients' severity of disturbance before the induction meeting and again after the first therapy session. The later ratings indicated a significantly lower level of disturbance across all clients. Again, the magnitude of this decrease was equal across all induction groups.

It was evident that entering a therapeutic program produced a significant decrease in the discomfort reported by clients and in the level of disturbance rated by therapists; however, the specific content of the induction procedures was not sufficiently powerful to produce any differential changes between groups.

Therapist Ratings of Client Attractiveness

At the time of the screening interview, therapists rated each client on his attractiveness for psychotherapy. There were no differences on this rating among clients assigned to the various role induction procedures. After the first therapy session, the therapists again rated each client's attractiveness. At this time, clients in the film and interview groups were rated as more attractive than those in the neutral group. The level of attractiveness had risen for clients in the two induction groups, while remaining substantially the same for clients in the neutral group. We may conclude that participating in either of the role induction procedures made the client more attractive to his therapist. The film was equally or slightly more effective than the interview in this respect.

In-Therapy Effects of Induction Procedures

Client's Satisfaction with Therapy Sessions

Clients rated their satisfaction with the group therapy sessions at several points throughout the program (Post-Sessions 1, 3, 5, 7, 9, and 11). Their Post-Session 1 responses are presented in Figure 6-3. Clients in the two role induction groups reported a significantly greater satisfaction with their first therapy session than did those in the neutral induction condition. Similar group differences appeared in the ratings made following each of the subsequent sessions. In addition, there was a slight tendency for all clients to report a higher level of satisfaction by the end of the therapy program as seen

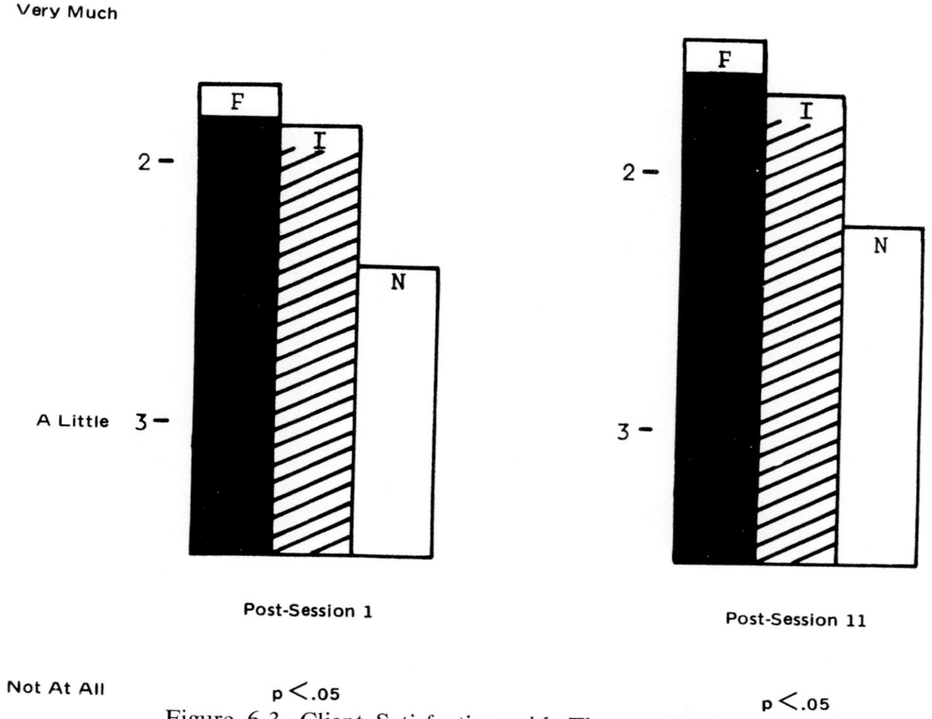

Figure 6-3. Client Satisfaction with Therapy Sessions

in the Post-Session 11 ratings in Figure 6-3. These ratings indicate that the effects of the role induction procedures were reflected not only in the immediate post-induction assessments but later in therapy as well.

Client's Progress in Therapy and Perceived Improvement

Clients' satisfaction with their progress in therapy was assessed following Sessions 1, 3, 5, 7, 9, and 11. Ratings were made on a 5-point scale, ranging from "Displeased" to "Very Much Pleased." Although all clients expressed some satisfaction with their progress, the degree of satisfaction reported was significantly different among clients experiencing the various role induction procedures. Figure 6-4 shows the effect of the induction condition over all therapy sessions. We note that the film induction group reported the greatest satisfaction, the interview group an intermediate level, and the neutral group reported the lowest level of satisfaction. This effect of the induction condition, favoring the film and interview induction groups, was found at each of the separate data collection sessions. The group differences were significant following Session 1 ($p = .04$), became even more pronounced following Sessions 3, 5, 7, and 9 ($p = .02$), and were still quite evident following Session 11 ($p = .01$).

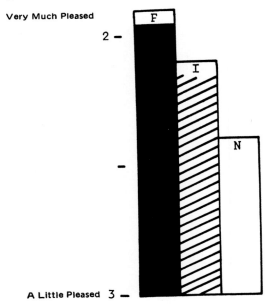

Effect of the Induction Condition Over All Therapy Sessions

$p < .05$

Figure 6-4. Client Satisfaction with Progress in Therapy

When we examined *changes* in the client's level of satisfaction over time, we found that the ratings of clients in the neutral group tended to fluctuate around their initial level, while clients in the film and interview induction groups became more satisfied with their progress as the therapy program continued. This increase in satisfaction was most pronounced during the first half of the therapy program for clients who had viewed the induction film, while it did not appear until the latter half of the therapy program for clients who had participated in the induction interview.

Clients assessed how they "get along with others" at several points throughout the therapy program. Although the induction conditions appeared to have no demonstrable effect on the *level* of satisfaction reported by clients, there was a significant difference among groups in their *change* scores on this item. When we examined the change in satisfaction between ratings made at Session 1 and ratings made at Session 11, we found that clients who participated in the film or interview induction procedures showed a significant increase in their satisfaction with their interpersonal relations, while clients in the neutral condition remained relatively unchanged. Again, this increase in satisfaction appeared early in the therapy program for clients in the film induction group, and later in the program for clients in the interview group.

On alternate sessions, clients were asked, "How much do you feel you are in control of and can change the way you are now?" All clients reported feelings of greater control as the therapy program progressed. The greatest changes occurred following Session 3, with ratings remaining fairly constant thereafter. There were no significant differences in the initial ratings or change scores on this item among clients from the three role induction groups.

Taken together, these findings indicate that:

1. Clients who participated in the film or interview induction procedures reported greater satisfaction with their progress in therapy than those in the neutral condition. The highest level of satisfaction was reported by clients in the film induction group, and they reported satisfaction earlier in the therapy program.

2. Clients in the neutral condition did not report appreciable improvements in their interpersonal relations, in contrast to clients in both the film and interview induction groups who reported increased ability to get along with others over the course of the therapy program. The induction film was as facilitative as the interview in increasing the clients' interpersonal effectiveness, and its benefits were apparent earlier in the therapy program.

3. The group therapy sessions evidently produced a greater sense of mastery and self-control for all clients. Moreover, the specific training provided by the induction film and interview apparently better enabled the clients to translate this potential into positive changes. This was evidenced by the higher ratings of general progress and ability in getting along with others reported by clients in the two induction groups. The induction film was superior to the interview in facilitating these changes at an earlier stage in the therapy program; the neutral induction procedure was least effective.

Therapist Ratings of Clients' In-Therapy Behavior

Therapists were asked to rate each client's in-therapy behavior following Session 1 and again at the end of the therapy program. The 5-point scale ranged from "Very Appropriate" to "Very Inappropriate." Figure 6-5 shows the comparative ratings of appropriate in-therapy behavior during Session 1 and during all therapy sessions for clients in each of the three role induction groups. During Session 1, clients who had viewed the induction film exhibited the most "appropriate" behavior. Clients who had participated in the induction interview received an intermediate rating, while the behavior of clients in the neutral procedure was considered least appropriate. These group differences were statistically significant. Post-therapy ratings of the

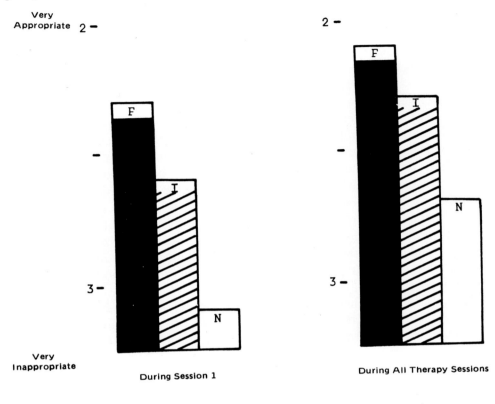

Figure 6-5. Appropriateness of Client's Behavior

clients' behavior throughout all therapy sessions revealed two points of interest:

1. The *level* of appropriateness was greater than at Session 1 for all clients, indicating that they were learning more appropriate in-therapy behavior as the sessions progressed. There was a slight tendency for clients with the lowest initial ratings to show the greatest increases. Thus clients were becoming more similar in this respect as they participated in a greater number of therapy sessions.

2. The rank ordering of clients in the three role induction groups, which appeared in the Session 1 ratings, remained unchanged, and the difference among groups was still statistically significant.

Thus, throughout the therapy program clients in the two role induction conditions exhibited more *appropriate* therapy behavior than those in the neutral condition, and the induction film was most effective in facilitating this behavior.

Some more specific aspects of clients' in-therapy behavior were measured by the Therapy Behavior Scale (descriptions of sixteen desirable and fifteen undesirable behaviors which a client might exhibit during his therapy sessions). Therapists rated the prevalence of each behavior on a 3-point scale, following Sessions 1, 3, 5, 7, 9, and 11. The scale range was 0-62, with *lower* scores indicating more desirable behaviors. Figure 6-6 shows that at all points in the therapy program there were significant group differences, attributable to the different induction procedures. Clients who had participated in the film or interview induction procedures exhibited much more desirable be-

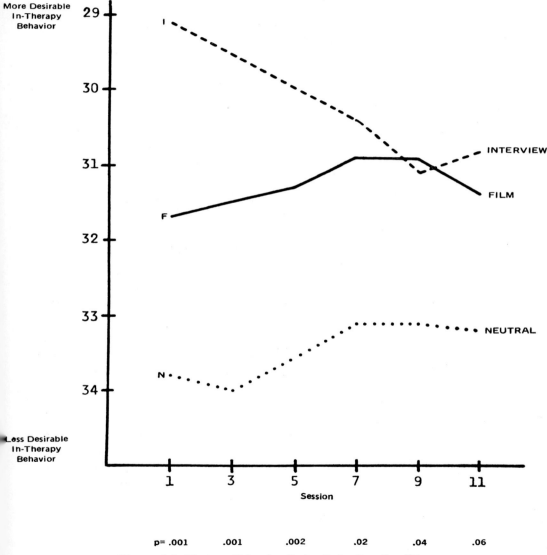

Figure 6-6. Therapy Behavior Scale: Induction Condition
Main Effects Across Time

havior than those in the neutral induction condition. The effects of the induction conditions were greatest at Session 1 ($p = .001$), and gradually diminished as the therapy program progressed to Session 11 ($p = .06$).

In summary, clients who had viewed the role induction film or had participated in the induction interview demonstrated more desirable in-therapy behavior throughout the therapy program than clients in the neutral condition. The greatest differences were noted at the first therapy session, with clients in all groups growing more similar in behavior as therapy progressed.

Attendance

There were no statistically significant differences among clients from the three role induction groups on any of the attendance indices. This may be partly a function of the nature of client recruitment and of the overall structure of the therapy program. It will be remembered that clients in the program were already participating in, and maintaining their primary contact with, another rehabilitation agency or program. Therefore, termination from the parent program usually necessitated termination from our therapy program as well, since continued attendance at the group sessions was no longer feasible. Major reasons for leaving an agency were obtaining a job or parole, a change of residence, or hospitalization for physical complaints. Only 6 percent of the client population reported as a reason for termination that they did not wish to continue therapy, while 35 percent terminated because they had left their parent agency. Though the resulting attrition rate is quite marked, it is fairly typical for therapy programs with similar client populations (see Bahn and Norman, 1959; Baum, Felzer, D'Zmura, and Shumaker, 1966; Brandt, 1965; and Kotkov and Meadow, 1952).

Because of the numerous artifacts affecting attendance, direct comparisons between the induction groups seemed to be of questionable validity. Clearly, there were many reasons for termination beyond those of motivation and satisfaction with the progress of therapy. These factors become especially apparent in group therapy where the therapy hour cannot always be rescheduled to correspond to a specific individual's changing circumstances and needs.

Outcome Effects of Induction Procedures

To assess the effects of the induction procedures on therapeutic outcome, several measures were obtained immediately following the last therapy session (Session 12). These included the client's retrospective impression of his induction procedure; therapist ratings of client's attractiveness for psychotherapy; client and therapist ratings of therapy outcome; and client's satisfaction with the treatment program.

Estimated Helpfulness of the Induction Procedure

Clients were asked to rate, in retrospect, how helpful the induction procedure had been in the group meetings that followed. Figure 6-7 shows that clients who had participated in the role induction film or interview considered the induction significantly more helpful than did clients in the neutral procedure. Figure 6-7 also compares these post-therapy ratings with similar ratings made prior to the beginning of therapy. Although significant beyond the .001 level at both points in time, the differences among induction groups were marked in the post-therapy ratings. This greater difference seems to be due to the significantly lower post-therapy ratings of clients in the neutral condition. The post-therapy ratings of the interview group were somewhat lower, while those of the induction film group remained about the same. Thus clients who had received some role induction training rated these procedures as more helpful than clients in the neutral procedure. Furthermore, the induction film was considered the most helpful procedure in terms of the retrospective post-therapy ratings.

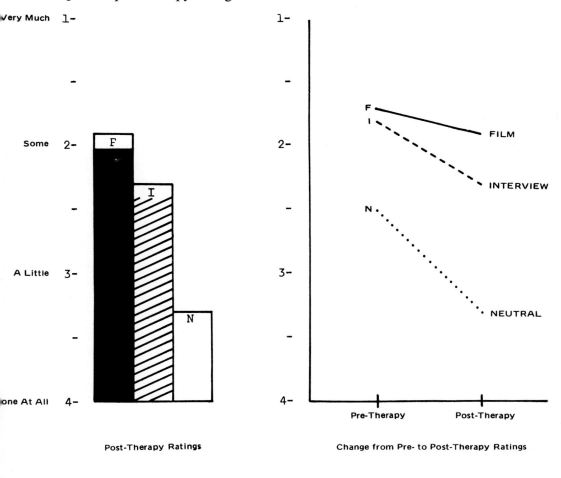

Figure 6-7. Helpfulness of Induction Procedure

Therapist Ratings of Client Attractiveness

Therapists judged each client's attractiveness for psychotherapy by rating on a 5-point scale how closely the client compared to what the therapist believed was an *ideal* client. Clients in the two role induction conditions were considered significantly more attractive than those in the neutral condition in these post-therapy ratings. It will be remembered that similar ratings were made by the therapists prior to the role induction and again following Session 1. We examined changes in the therapists' ratings of attractiveness over time and found: the pre-induction ratings revealed no differences among clients; the post-induction ratings showed a significant difference among groups, resulting from an increase in attractiveness for clients in the film and interview groups and no change for clients in the neutral group; post-therapy ratings revealed a decrease in attractiveness for all clients, regardless of induction condition, but there were still significant group differences in level of attractiveness which favored the clients in the two role induction groups.

It appears that the role induction training enhanced the client's attractiveness to the therapist. This effect was most marked early in therapy, but was still present (relative to the neutral group) in the post-therapy ratings. The induction film and interview procedures seemed equally effective in this respect.

Client Ratings of Post-Therapy Improvement

Immediately following Session 12, clients were asked to make several ratings of their improvement during therapy. Figure 6-8 presents data for three of these measures: global improvement, improvement in specific target symptoms, and self-understanding achieved through therapy.

Global improvement was rated on a 5-point scale ranging from "Greatly Improved" to "Worse Than Before." (cf. Figure 6-9). While most clients indicated moderate improvement as a result of therapy, the ratings of clients in the role induction film and interview conditions were significantly higher than those of clients in the neutral condition. The film was equal, or slightly superior, to the interview in initiating a therapy program which culminated in ratings of greater global improvement.

Specific target symptoms were obtained by asking clients, prior to their induction meeting and again before and after their first therapy session, to list the three things they would most like to change during the course of therapy. Following Session 12, each client rated the degree of change accomplished in these areas. Ratings were made on a 5-point scale ranging from "Great Change for the Better" to "Worse than Before." Although all clients reported some positive change in these target areas, clients who had viewed the role induction film reported significantly greater improvement than clients in the interview and neutral conditions. (It may be noted that the level of improvement in specific target symptoms was somewhat lower than the level of global improvement.)

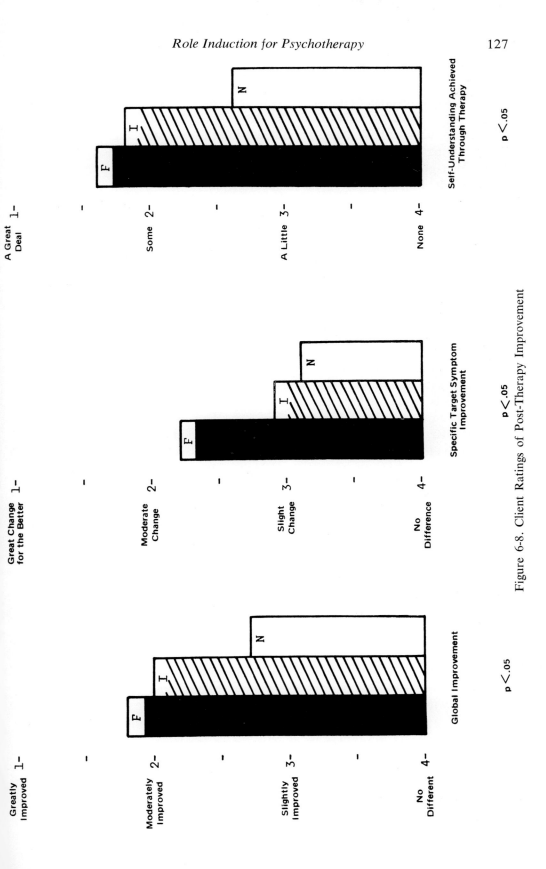

Figure 6-8. Client Ratings of Post-Therapy Improvement

To assess **self-understanding** achieved through therapy, clients were asked to rate how much they had learned about themselves since coming to the group therapy sessions. These post-therapy ratings were made on a 5-point scale ranging from "A Great Deal" to "Know Less than Before." As seen in Figure 6-8, all clients reported an increase in self-understanding. Clients who had participated in either of the two role induction procedures felt they had achieved a greater self-understanding than clients in the neutral condition, and the induction film was equal, or superior, to the interview in this respect.

In summary, all clients reported **substantial improvement** in all areas measured. Significant induction group differences were reflected in the ratings of global improvement, improvement in specific target symptoms, and self-understanding achieved through therapy. All group differences favored the two role induction conditions over the neutral condition, with the role induction film appearing somewhat more effective than the interview procedure.

Therapist Ratings of Post-Therapy Improvement

Following Session 12, therapists completed several measures of the clients' post-therapy improvement. These included: Global improvement, specific improvement in discomfort, self-awareness, interpersonal behavior, and symptoms; and satisfaction with the clients' progress in therapy.

Therapists tended to rate clients as improved both in terms of global ratings and more specific assessments; however, there were no statistically significant differences among the three treatment conditions. When the therapists' evaluations were compared with the clients' self-ratings, it was seen that the self-ratings generally reflected higher levels of improvement.

Figure 6-9 presents the percentage figures of clients rated as "Improved," "No Change," or "Worse" by themselves and their therapists, for each of the three role induction conditions. As in the mean levels of improvement, there were significant induction group differences in the client ratings but not in the therapist ratings, and greater improvement was reported by clients than by therapists. However, this generalization does not hold for clients in the neutral condition: here client and therapist ratings of "Improved" were comparable, but 30 percent of the clients rated themselves as "Worse" compared to only 7 percent who were so regarded by their therapists.

A possible explanation for these discrepancies is that clients and therapists were using different base lines for improvement. Perhaps clients compared their post-therapy state with their entire recent history before entering therapy. Therapists were only in a position to compare the clients' post-therapy performance with their performance in the early therapy sessions. (With the exception of a brief screening interview, this was the first time the therapists had an opportunity to observe the clients.) This becomes very relevant when we remember that clients showed a great deal of change immediately following their induction session, and these changes were more marked and broader in scope for clients in the induction film and interview conditions. On some

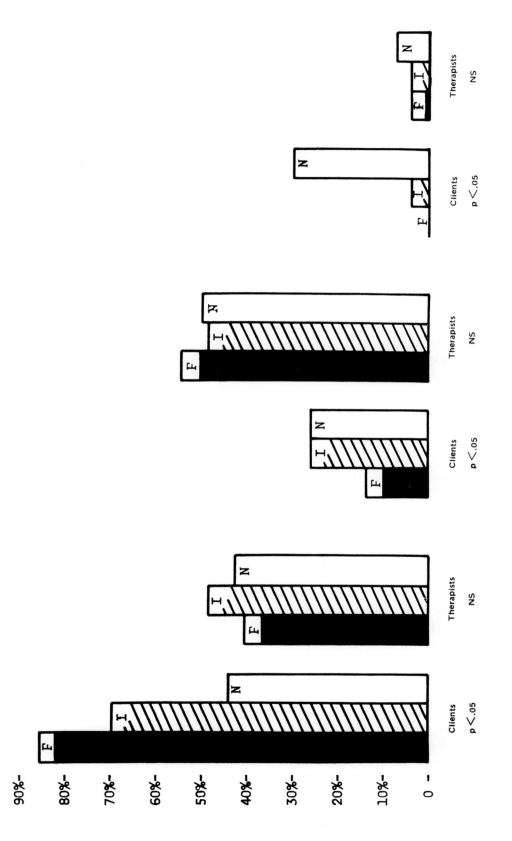

IMPROVED NO CHANGE WORSE

Figure 6-9. Post-Therapy Global Improvement: Comparison of Client and Therapist Ratings

measures, such as appropriate in-therapy behavior, clients in the two role induction conditions were able to begin their first therapy session at a very high level, which gradually decreased throughout therapy, while clients in the neutral condition began the first session at a lower level, which gradually increased to the level exhibited by all clients at the end of the therapy program. On other measures, such as symptom discomfort, all clients showed a significant positive change immediately after their induction session, and maintained this level throughout therapy.

If the therapists used client behavior in the first therapy session as part of the base line from which they judged subsequent improvement (as they surely must have in the absence of any other extensive data), it becomes obvious that much of the gain experienced by the clients would be lost in the therapists' improvement scores, and this loss would be greater for clients in the induction film and interview groups. This could explain the client-therapist discrepancies in both degree of improvement and differences between conditions. Other possibilities are that therapists were more cautious in their assessments (using a broader spectrum of patients as a standard), and that clients' ratings were inflated by placebo effects and the desire to please the researchers.

Further evidence of the therapists' relative lack of enthusiasm about the therapeutic outcome is found in their ratings of satisfaction with the clients' progress. They reported only modest levels of satisfaction, with no significant differences among the three induction groups.

In summary, therapists tended to rate clients as mildly improved, regardless of the induction procedure. The therapists' ratings of improvement were generally lower than those of the clients across all areas measured, and revealed none of the significant induction group differences observed in the clients' ratings. It was suggested that these client-therapist discrepancies could have resulted from the use of different base lines for assessing improvements.

Clients' Satisfaction with the Treatment Program

It will be recalled that clients in the induction film and interview groups were more satisfied with their therapy sessions than clients in the neutral group. These differences were apparent at Session 1 (Figure 6-3) and remained statistically significant throughout the therapy program. As a follow-up clients were asked after the last therapy session whether they would recommend the group meetings to a friend. Of the clients in the induction film group, 85 percent said they would recommend the group therapy sessions, compared to 77 percent of the interview group and only 63 percent of the neutral group. These differences were significant beyond the .05 level. We may conclude that clients who had participated in one of the role induction procedures were more satisfied with their therapy program than clients in the neutral condition.

DISCUSSION AND CONCLUSIONS

Evaluation of Results

Measures Reflecting Role Induction Benefits

In overview, we have presented consistent evidence that a role induction procedure facilitates a favorable therapy experience for lower-class clients. The effects of two comparable techniques (a structures interview and a sound film) were evident immediately following the induction session. They were reflected in the clients' attitudes toward the induction process, knowledge of group therapy including the respective roles of client and therapist, motivation to begin group therapy, expected improvement from therapy, and clients' attractiveness to their therapists. The changes were maintained throughout therapy as measured by numerous indices of satisfaction, progress, and in-therapy behavior. Perhaps most important, the clients' self-ratings of therapy outcome, improvement in specific target symptoms, and self-understanding achieved through therapy, as well as satisfaction with the treatment program, were enhanced by the role induction sessions. Similarly, therapists' post-therapy ratings of the clients' attractiveness favored those clients who had been exposed to the role induction training.

Not a single measure favored clients in the neutral group. It is important to emphasize that clients in the neutral condition had been initially comparable to those in the two role induction conditions, except that the former group had higher verbal ability and a greater proportion of Whites— attributes typically associated with *better* therapy performance and outcome.

Relative Effectiveness of Two Role Induction Techniques

In general, participation in either of the two role induction procedures was clearly more beneficial than the neutral procedure. However, there were some differential effects of the two role induction techniques. The interview seemed to be superior in conveying a detailed knowledge of the process of group therapy. This was reflected in the clients' immediate post-induction ratings of their knowledge about the type of groups being offered and in the therapists' ratings of specific behaviors during the early therapy sessions.

By contrast, the film was superior over a wider range of measures. These included the clients' confidence in group therapy as a potential means of dealing with emotional problems in general as well as the belief that group therapy was the proper treatment for them. (The interview seemed to have an inhibiting effect on the latter measure: while it may have imparted a more detailed account of the client's role in therapy, it also seemed to arouse considerable anxiety or ambivalence about his actual participation in the therapy process.) Clients who viewed the film reported higher expectations of improvement and they were rated by their therapists as having more realistic expectations about therapeutic change. During therapy, they reported greater satisfaction with their progress and their therapists rated them as exhibiting more appropriate behavior in therapy. At the end of therapy, clients in the film condition reported greater improvement in target symptoms, and they expressed greater satisfaction with the therapy program as well as with the helpfulness of the induction procedure.

Thus the role induction film seems to be a superior technique for introducing clients to group therapy as a treatment modality from which they might reasonably expect to benefit. To this must be added the efficiency of the film technique, the obvious advantage of a standardized procedure readily available for mass administration, and wide audience appeal to both men and women from the lower socio-economic groups. Moreover, viewing a film in familiar surroundings is undoubtedly a highly acceptable first step for a reluctant or defensive client which might pave the way for a more relaxed face-to-face encounter with mental health professionals.

Measures Not Reflecting Role Induction Benefits

While the vast majority of measures completed by both clients and therapists showed the foregoing differential effects, certain areas of measurement yielded inconclusive results. These were (1) attendance, (2) therapist ratings of therapy outcome, and (3) client ratings of symptom discomfort.

ATTENDANCE: Earlier research produced conflicting evidence on the effects of role induction on attendance of therapy sessions. Hoehn-Saric *et al.* (1964) reported significantly better attendance for clients who had participated in a role induction interview and remained at least until Session 4. These clients had been selected from applicants to an outpatient clinic and were seen in individual therapy. Sloane *et al.* (1970), studying patients from a similar outpatient clinic and assigned to individual therapy, found no differences in number of sessions attended or in percent of appointments kept. Likewise, Yalom *et al.* (1967), working with middle-class clients at a university outpatient clinic, reported no differences in attendance of group therapy sessions.

In the present study, the clients' continuing relationship with their parent agencies was probably a determining factor in therapy attendance. Two-thirds of the clients terminating from the therapy program did so because they were discharged by the parent agency and therefore attendance at the therapy sessions was no longer feasible; only about one-tenth of those terminating left therapy because they were not satisfied with the groups. In addition, attendance in the present study was found to be unrelated to satisfaction or improvement in therapy.

Some general observations concerning the problem of attrition may be in order. First, the seemingly high dropout rate (54 percent of the original sample were not in attendance at Session 12) is well within the range (30 to 65 percent) reported in previous studies (Baum *et al.,* 1966; Bahn and

Norman, 1959; Brandt, 1965; Frank, Gliedman, Imber, Nash, and Stone, 1957; Kotkov and Meadow, 1952; Nash, Frank, Gliedman, Imber, and Stone, 1957; Overall and Aronson, 1963) with lower-class clients reported as having a dropout rate of 57 percent after an initial interview and before the first meeting with the therapist. The criterion employed in this study, any client who attended the induction session but was not in attendance at Session 12, yielded the *maximum* possible dropout rate. Secondly, it must be remembered that clients in the present study were of lower socio-economic status with minimal motivation for psychotherapy; many were highly resistant to discussions about "mental health" and had rejected repeated attempts to guide them toward therapy. This fact, coupled with the findings of Frank *et al.* (1957) that lower-class clients exhibit a dropout rate double that of middle-class clients and that the dropout rate for group therapy is three times that for individual therapy, strongly suggests that attendance in this study was relatively encouraging.

THERAPISTS' RATINGS OF OUTCOME: While clients' self-ratings of therapy outcome showed clear-cut differences favoring the role induction procedures, therapists' ratings failed to do so. In this connection, it may be recalled that clients in general were more enthusiastic in their reports of positive changes than the therapists, whose evaluations were perhaps more realistic and objective. The only previous investigation of a role induction technique in which comparable ratings by therapists were employed (Hoehn-Saric *et al.,* 1964) showed statistically significant differences in the predicted direction. Since there were numerous differences between the two studies, the divergent findings are difficult to interpret. However, possible factors include: (1) therapists' level of experience (ratings in the Hoehn-Saric study were made by psychiatric residents whereas in the present one, more experienced therapists were used); and (2) time of final evaluation (Hoehn-Saric assessed improvement for all clients at the time of termination irrespective of when it occurred, whereas in the present study only clients in attendance at the end of the program were assessed).

SYMPTOM DISCOMFORT: This was a third area which showed no differential changes attributable to the induction variable. Regardless of the induction procedure, all clients showed immediate symptom improvement which persisted throughout the course of therapy. The improvement related to the number of symptoms reported as well as to their severity. These findings are consistent with earlier research (Frank *et al.*, 1963; Hoehn-Saric *et al.*, 1964; Stone, Frank, Nash, and Imber, 1961) in which the Discomfort Scale typically registered prompt improvement following psychiatric intervention, but failed to discriminate between different treatment conditions. As noted by Stone *et al.* (1961), symptoms of anxiety and depression appear to be characteristically relieved by an expectation of help.

Relation of Results to Previous Research

Three major studies employing a role induction interview as a preparation for psychotherapy have been reported in the literature (Hoehn-Saric *et al.,* 1964; Sloane *et al.,* 1970; and Yalom *et al.,* 1967). Direct comparisons are difficult because each study varied considerably in terms of the specific content of the induction interview; furthermore, there were differences relating to clients and therapists (e.g., experience level), as well as major variables and measuring instruments. Despite the numerous divergences, all studies found a role induction technique to have significant beneficial effects on one or more of the major variables investigated.

It is interesting to note that when the four relevant studies (including the present one) are ranked with respect to (1) magnitude of effects attributable to the role induction procedure and (2) clients' level of sophistication about psychotherapy, there emerges a direct inverse relationship. In other words, the least sophisticated clients showed the greatest response to role induction. To stress the importance of the client variable in the outcome of these studies does not, of course, rule out the influence of other factors such as content of the induction interviews, therapists' level of experience, and assessment techniques. Bergin (1971) documents the relevance of the latter two factors and concludes that nearly three times as many studies involving experienced therapists yield positive results as those employing unexperienced therapists, and that separate outcome factors often emerge as a function of the rater and of the assessment instrument.

Comparing the present study to predecessors, which led to its inception, the following contributions may be noted:

1. A wider range of variables was studied and more systematic attention was paid to effects immediately following the induction procedure as well as to changes occurring early in therapy.

2. A less motivated, lower-class population was employed. Most of the clients studied were in need of rehabilitation as preparation for employment and independent living.

3. A new role induction procedure (the role induction film), suitable for mass administration, was shown to be an efficient and economical technique. On the basis of a variety of assessments, it proved to be at least as effective as a personal interview preceding psychotherapy, and in many respects it was superior. The findings were quite consistent and clear-cut. With few exceptions, the desirability of systematically preparing clients for psychotherapy again receiving strong empirical support.

Implications

A clear perception of the field of mental health is still obscured for many by a haze of mystery and a lack of information. Even among highly educated individuals, there is not always a clear understanding of the process and goals of psychotherapy, the roles the client and therapist are expected to play, and the kinds of expectations one might reasonably entertain. Nunnally (1961), in surveying popular conceptions of mental health, uncovered several areas (especially those of therapy process and the role of the therapist) in which the views of the general public were inconsistent with current therapeutic practice. In addition, studies of outpatients and prospective clients have revealed similar misconceptions (Garfield and Wolpin, 1963; Overall and Aronson, 1963). Levitt (1966) concluded that one of the most pervasive misconceptions of psychotherapy is the expectancy that the therapist will take an active, directive role in isolating the problem and prescribing a cure, with the client assuming a passive role once he has stated his complaints. The findings of the present study support this conclusion.

The client's dearth of accurate information concerning psychotherapy becomes critical when we consider its consequences for successful participation in any therapeutic encounter. A host of recent studies have shown that initial client variables are of overriding importance for the successful outcome of therapy. Cartwright (1963), among others, stated: "How far the patient can go in using the opportunity of psychotherapy for making positive personality changes is largely predetermined by the kind of structure he brings to the experience."

To bring about a better alignment between the client's expectations and the realities of psychotherapy, several efforts have been made in recent years (Bach, 1954; Bettis, Malamud, and Malamud, 1949; Berzon and Solomon, 1966; Berzon, Reisel, and Davis, 1969; Hoehn-Saric *et al.,* 1964; Leitenberg, Agras, Barlow, and Oliveau, 1969; Malamud and Machover, 1965; Martin and Shewmaker, 1962; Nash, Hoehn-Saric, Battle, Stone, and Imber, 1965; Oliveau, Agras, Leitenberg, Moore, and Wright, 1969; Orne and Wender, 1968; Sloane *et al.,* 1970; Spinks, 1969; Truax, 1966; Truax *et al.,* 1968; Truax *et al.,* 1966; Truax *et al.,* 1970; Yalom *et al.,* 1967). Similarly, the goal of the procedures studied here was to equip the client with the structure, information, and expectations that would enable him to achieve maximum benefit from the group therapy program he was about to enter.

The results provided a convincing demonstration that the role induction procedures employed were successful in removing misconceptions and in instilling accurate information concerning psychotherapy, the psychotherapist, and the client's role in the therapeutic endeavor. Moreover, they made the client's role in therapy more meaningful and satisfying and led to a more favorable outcome. The role induction film developed as part of this study proved to be a highly effective technique, and in certain respects appeared to be superior to a comparable interview with a psychiatrist. These results are particularly encouraging since we purposely focused on prospective clients who have traditionally been regarded as a high-risk group.

Why does a role induction procedure work and how does it achieve beneficial results? Studies to isolate the components have met with little success to date (Imber, Pande, Frank, Hoehn-Saric, Stone, and Wargo, 1970; Sloane *et al.*, 1970). To approach the problem of *why* the role induction seems to work, it may be more profitable to think in terms of a learning experience. The content of the role induction interview or film covers a wide range of relevant information. Consequently, a client who accepts this information is equipped with more realistic expectations concerning the process of therapy, his role vis-a-vis the therapist and other clients, the meaning of improvement, and the steps he must take to benefit from the experience. These changed expectations produce complementary changes in attitudes, motivations, and behavior which make him more attractive to the therapist and in other respects enhance his likelihood of success. Coupled with the symptomatic relief a client typically experiences upon entering therapy, the foregoing factors may potentiate a favorable therapy outcome.

In conclusion, the primary contribution of a role induction procedure is (1) to provide accurate information concerning the process of therapy; (2) to dispel misconceptions and prejudice which are abundant in all strata of the population, but particularly among unsophisticated persons; (3) to enhance the prospective client's motivation for psychotherapeutic change; and, perhaps more important, (4) to pave the way for a more realistic view concerning emotional problems in living and their resolution. The latter entails an acceptance of the position that the individual must take a more *active* role in mastering his problems, assume greater responsibility for himself and his place in the world, and oppose the tendency for dependency and passivity. These lessons obviously cannot be learned in a single session or by viewing a film. Nevertheless, the motion picture developed for this purpose appears to be an excellent vehicle for initiating the process.

Relevance of Findings for Social Agencies Today

The general concept of role induction is neither unique nor new. Most of what we call socialization is at least in part a form of "role induction" for living as an individual in society. We see it in operation as children play house, school teacher, nurse, or fireman. We try to model appropriate behavior for those around us; we prepare children for their first visit to the dentist; we give job descriptions to new applicants; in numerous ways we are constantly attempting to prepare ourselves and others for the various roles we are required to play in everyday life.

Forms of role induction have been successfully employed by social agencies in recent years as they prepare clients for new careers, engage in role playing before job interviews, and encourage participation in related activities. Role induction would seem appropriate, and often necessary, anytime a client is being referred out from an agency to another facility or program. It would be equally useful in agency intake procedures to help new clients understand their role and responsibilities as a rehabilitation client. For the rehabilitation counselor to have goals and motivation for achieving these goals is not sufficient (or certainly not efficient) when these goals involve change and effort on the part of the client. The motivation and goals must be *the client's own* for real progress to ensue. The greater the community of goals and agreement on techniques necessary to achieve these goals, the more readily and efficiently these goals will be achieved. The client is not the pawn in rehabilitation work, but the player. He must know the rules of the game and have the will or desire to play.

Though the concept and procedures of role induction have been in our repertory for some time, they are not being utilized as widely or as well as they might be in many areas; one of these is the preparation of clients for participation in psychotherapy. The importance of adequately preparing clients for the experience of psychotherapy is frequently an issue of relevance to counselors working in social agencies, since they are often confronted with the task of creating an awareness in their clients of the need for psychotherapeutic help. Thus, it is frequently the counselor who provides the client with his initial exposure to the area. And it is frequently the counselor who feels some responsibility to bring the client into contact with a trained therapist. This responsibility should not be construed solely as a need to persuade, coerce, or otherwise deliver the client to the door of the therapist. The expectancy that the "expert" will then take over and perform his "cure" as simply and directly as administering a shot of penicillin or an inoculation against measles is not a realistic one. A therapist simply cannot operate this way. The problems with which he deals are more varied, more complex, and less well understood. They have been building up over the course of a lifetime and their remediation, likewise, requires a considerable amount of time and effort. Misinformation or false expectations may substantially hamper this progress. The "try it, you'll like it" approach to initiating therapy not only fails to prepare the client, it is often misleading. Clearly, a more informative approach is needed.

The project described in this chapter had attempted to document the importance of this information and the crucial nature of early contacts between social agencies and prospective candidates for psychotherapy. We have attempted to provide agency workers with an efficient and effective tool for introducing prospective clients to the process and goals of psychotherapy. Our results demonstrated the utility of the role induction film, *Turning Point,* for this purpose.

In addition to its primary function of preparing the prospective client for psychotherapy, the film may prove useful for other purposes. Although the need for more adequate information is most acute among those currently in need of psychotherapy (especially if they are poorly educated or from the lower socio-economic classes), many other individuals can benefit from it. Accordingly, the film may serve a useful function in (1) educating the families of prospective clients, (2) training agency workers who will be dealing with these clients and their families, and (3) providing general information to the community.

In addition to clarifying the process of psychotherapy, the film serves to dispel misconceptions and prejudices which are abundant in all strata of the population but are particularly prevalent among relatively unsophisticated and uneducated persons. It clarifies the meaning of emotional problems in living as well as the procedures used for dealing with them, and it strongly emphasizes the need for *active* participation on the client's part in learning to cope with difficulties of which he had traditionally seen himself as the victim. Thus, the film paves the way for a conception of mental health in terms of mastery, competence, and self-direction.

REFERENCES

Bach, G. R.: *Intensive Group Psychotherapy*. New York, Ronald Press, 1954.

Bahn, A. K. and Norman, V. B.: First national report on patients in mental health clinics. *Public Health Report, 79*:943, 1959.

Baum, O. E., Felzer, S. B., D'Zmura, T. L. and Shumaker, E.: Psychotherapy, dropouts and lower socioeconomic patients. *American Journal of Orthopsychiatry, 36*:629-635, 1966.

Bergin, A. E.: The evaluation of therapeutic outcomes. In Bergin, A. E. and Garfield, S. L. (Eds.), *Handbook of Psychotherapy and Behavior Change*: *An Empirical Analysis*. New York, Wiley, pp. 217-270, 1971.

Berzon, B., Reisel, J. and Davis, D. P.: Peer: An audio tape program for self-directed small groups. *Journal of Humanistic Psychology, 9*:71-86, 1969.

Berzon, B. and Solomon, L. N.: The self-directed therapeutic group: Three studies. *Journal of Counseling Psychology, 13*:491-497, 1966.

Bettis, M. D., Malamud, D. I. and Malamud, R. F.: Deepening a group's insight into human relations. *Journal of Clinical Psychology, 5*:114-122, 1949.

Brandt, L. W.: Studies of "dropout" patients in psychotherapy: A review of findings. *Psychotherapy, 2*:6-12, 1965.

Brill, N. Q. and Storrow, H. A.: Social class and psychiatric treatment. *Archives of General Psychiatry, 3*:340-344, 1960.

Bronfenbrenner, U.: Socialization and social class through time and space. In Maccoby, E. E., Newcomb, T. M. and Hartley, E. L. (Eds.), *Readings in Social Psychology*. New York, Henry Holt and Co., 1958.

Cartwright, R. D.: Two conceptual schemes applied to four psychotherapy cases. Paper presented at the meeting of the American Psychological Association, 1963.

Frank, J. D., Gliedman, L. H., Imber, S. D., Nash, E. H. and Stone, A. R.: Why patients leave psychotherapy. *AMA Archives of Neurology and Psychiatry, 77*:283-299, 1957.

Frank, J. D., Nash, E. H., Stone, A. R. and Imber, S. D.: Immediate and long-term symptomatic course of psychiatric outpatients. *The American Journal of Psychiatry, 120*:429-439, 1963.

Garfield, S. L. and Wolpin, M.: Expectations regarding psychotherapy. *Journal of Nervous and Mental Disease, 137*:353-362, 1963.

Goldstein, A. P.: *Therapist-Patient Expectancies in Psychotherapy*. New York, Pergamon Press, 1962.

Hoehn-Saric, R., Frank, J. D., Imber, S. D., Nash, E. H., Stone, A. R. and Battle,

C. C.: Systematic preparation of patients for psychotherapy: I. Effects of therapy behavior and outcome. *Journal of Psychiatric Research, 2*:267-281, 1964.

Hollingshead, A. B. and Redlich, F. C.: *Social Class and Mental Illness: A Community Study.* New York, Wiley, 1958.

Imber, S. D., Pande, S. K., Frank, J. D., Hoehn-Saric, R., Stone, A. R. and Wargo, D. G.: Time-focused role induction. *Journal of Nervous and Mental Disease, 150*:27-30, 1970.

Joint Commission on Mental Illness and Health. *Action for Mental Health.* New York, Basic Books, 1961.

Kotkov, B. and Meadow, A.: Rorschach criteria for continuing group therapy. *The International Journal of Group Psychotherapy, 2*:324-333, 1952.

Leitenberg, H., Agras, W. S., Barlow, D. H. and Oliveau, D. C.: Contribution of selective positive reinforcement and therapeutic instructions to systematic desensitization therapy. *Journal of Abnormal Psychology, 74*:113-118, 1969.

Levitt, E. E.: Psychotherapy research and the expectation-reality discrepancy. *Psychotherapy, 3*:163-166, 1966.

Libermann, B. L., Frank, J. D., Hoehn-Saric, R., Stone, A. R., Imber, S. D. and Pande S. K.: Patterns of change in treated psychoneurotic patients: A five-year follow-up investigation of the systematic preparation of patients for psychotherapy. In press.

Malamud, D. I. and Machover, S.: *Toward Self Understanding: Group Techniques in Self Confrontation.* Springfield, Thomas, 1965.

Martin, H. and Shewmaker, K.: Written instructions in group psychotherapy. *Group Psychotherapy, 15*:24-29, 1962.

Miller, S. M. and Mishler, E. G.: Social class, mental illness, and American psychiatry: An expository review. In Riessman, F., Cohen, J. and Pearl, A. (Eds.), *Mental Health of the Poor: New Treatment Approaches for Low Income People.* New York, The Free Press, 1964.

Nash, E. H., Frank, J. D., Gliedman, L. H., Imber, S. D. and Stone, A. R.: Some factors related to patients remaining in group psychotherapy. *The International Journal of Group Psychotherapy, 7*:264-274, 1957.

Nash, E. H., Hoehn-Saric, R., Battle, C. C., Stone, A. R. and Imber, S. D.: Systematic preparation of patients for short-term psychotherapy: II. Relation to characteristics of patient, therapist and psychotherapeutic process. *Journal of Nervous and Mental Disease, 140*:374-383, 1965.

Nunnally, J. C.: *Popular Conceptions of Mental Health.* New York, Holt, Rinehart & Winston, 1961.

Oliveau, D. C., Agras, W. S., Leitenberg, H., Moore, R. C. and Wright, D. E.: Systematic desensitization, therapeutically oriented instructions and selective positive reinforcement. *Behavior Research and Therapy, 7*:27-33, 1969.

Orne, M. T. and Wender, P. H.: Anticipatory socialization for psychotherapy: Method and rationale. *The American Journal of Psychiatry, 124*:1202-1212, 1968.

Overall, B. and Aronson, H.: Expectations of psychotherapy in patients of lower socioeconomic class. *American Journal of Orthopsychiatry, 33*:421-430, 1963.

Riessman, F., Cohen, J. and Pearl, A.: *Mental Health of the Poor: New Treatment Approaches for Low Income People.* New York, The Free Press, 1964.

Rosenthal, D. and Frank, J. D.: The fate of psychiatric clinic outpatients assigned to psychotherapy. *Journal of Nervous and Mental Disease, 127*:330-343, 1958.

Sloane, R. B., Cristol, A. H., Pepernik, M. C. and Staples, F. R.: Role preparation and expectation of improvement in psychotherapy. *Journal of Nervous and Mental Disease, 150*:18-26, 1970.

Spinks, N. J.: The effects of male and female models in vicarious therapy pretraining on the self-concept of institutionalized juvenile delinquents in group counseling. Unpublished doctoral dissertation, Florida State University, 1969.

Stone, A. R., Frank, J. D., Nash, E. H. and Imber, S. D.: An intensive five-year follow-up study of treated psychiatric outpatients. *Journal of Nervous and Mental Disease, 133*:410-422, 1961.

Strupp, H. H.: *Psychotherapists in Action.* New York, Grune & Stratton, 1960.

Strupp, H. H. and Bloxom, A. L.: Preparing the Lower-Class Patient for Psychotherapy: Development and Evaluation of a Role Induction Procedure. Final report for Research and Demonstration Grant No. 15-P-55164 to the Social and Rehabilitation Service of the Department of Health, Education and Welfare, September 1971.

Szasz, T. S.: *The Myth of Mental Illness.* New York, Hoeber-Harper, 1961.

Truax, C. B.: *Counseling and Psychotherapy: Process and Outcome.* (Final Report: V.R.A. Research and Demonstration Grant No. 906-P) University of Arkansas, Arkansas Rehabilitation Research and Training Center, June 1966.

Truax, C. B., Shapiro, J. G. and Wargo, D. G.: The effects of alternate sessions and vicarious therapy pretraining on group psychotherapy. *The International Journal of Group Psychotherapy, 18*:186-198, 1968.

Truax, C. B., Wargo, D. G., Carkhuff, R. R., Kodman, F. and Moles, E. A.: Changes in self-concepts during group psychotherapy as a function of alternate sessions and vicarious therapy pretraining in institutionalized juvenile delinquents. *Journal of Consulting Psychology, 30*:309-314, 1966.

Truax, C. B., Wargo, D. G. and Volksdorf, N. R.: Antecedents to outcome in group counseling with institutionalized juvenile delinquents: Effects of therapeutic conditions, patient self-exploration, alternate sessions, and vicarious therapy pretraining. *Journal of Abnormal Psychology, 76*:235-242, 1970.

Wallach, M. S. and Strupp, H. H.: Psychotherapists' clinical judgments and attitudes toward patients. *Journal of Consulting Psychology, 24*:316-323, 1960.

Yalom, I. D., Houts, P. S., Newell, G. and Rand, K. H.: Preparations of patients for group therapy. *Archives of General Psychiatry, 17*:416-427, 1967.

Chapter 7

MOTIVATING THE CULTURALLY DEPRIVED

John Goss Skelton, Jr.

E LIMINATION of poverty was virtually set as a national goal with the implementation of the Economic Opportunity Act of 1964. Since then, an ever-increasing emphasis has been placed upon work with the disadvantaged. In many respects, this emphasis has evolved into what comes close to being a moral commitment. While concepts such as "the disadvantaged," "culturally deprived," "socio-economically depressed," and the "culturally different" have crept into the vernacular, these terms are most often restricted to meaningful usage only within the context of those in the various rehabilitation and habilitation agencies, programs, and other organizations designated as a part of the *helping* professions.

In spite of the national urgency relative to helping the disadvantaged, the concomitant encouragement of research, and subsequent publication thereof in scientific journals—all this to substantiate the efficacy of *helping methods* —pitifully few books, articles, reports, papers, pamphlets, or workshops have actually come to grips with the problem. In fact, not even the essential ingredients that spell any degree of effectiveness or success with regard to counseling techniques, therapeutic methods, or modalities needed to bring about positive change in the disabled disadvantaged, have been identified. Consequently, relatively little is known about ways and means of motivating those who until now have had little cause to be motivated.

Where, then, can the rehabilitation counselor turn for help when he is confronted with the task of motivating the culturally deprived? The sources are few. This chapter will attempt to define the nature of the problem, outline the search for counseling techniques utilized to help solve it, and describe some characteristics of the type of counselor who could be effective in working with this segment of the population.

The Nature of the Problem

Working with the culturally disadvantaged client presents probably the most challenging and difficult problem the rehabilitation counselor faces. Primarily, this counselor is dealing with massive feelings of alienation. By middle class standards, the culturally disadvantaged may be thought of as mentally ill. Fromm (1964) states that the terms *normal* and *healthy* seem

141

to be useful in two ways. First, from the standpoint of a functioning society, he believes that one can call a person normal or healthy if he is able to fulfill the social role he is to take in that given society. More concretely, Fromm says that this means that the healthy individual is able to work in the fashion which is required in that particular society, and furthermore is able to participate in the reproduction of society, i.e., that he can raise a family. Secondly, from the standpoint of the individual, he says that health or normalcy are looked upon as the optimum of growth and happiness of the individual.

Further, if the structure of a given society were such that it offered the optimum possibility for individual happiness, both viewpoints would coincide. However, this is not the case in most societies, including our own. Not only do these differ in the degree to which they promote the aims of individual growth; Fromm feels that there is discrepancy between the aims of the smooth functioning of society and of full development of the individual. This fact, Fromm observes, makes it imperative to differentiate sharply between the two concepts of health: the one being governed by social necessities, the other by values and norms concerning the aim of individual existence.

Relative to blacks, in a recent conversation with Mannie (1972), there was found to be support for the theory of mental illness for most disadvantaged blacks:

> When you live through all of the kinds of problems that they have to live through, you just can't come out with a healthy mind . . . I think very often we (blacks) are accused of being paranoid, and by middle class standards, we are paranoid. But, I suppose by our standards, we are not. (*From an interview*)

Mannie sees alienation as the prime etiological factor in psychosis:

> The number one factor to driving any man insane is to cut him off from his group, from other people who are like him. Any time you convince a person that he doesn't belong, you have inflicted a lethal blow to his personality structure.

In this case, she is talking about the total community, and not just the black subculture.

Some sociologists and anthropologists feel that much of the deviant behavior of the black poor is actually normative and transmitted in the socialization process, but Parker and Kleiner (1970) appear to conclude that the transmission of this deviancy attitude serves to maintain the mental health of those living in a severely disadvantaged social situation. This seems to support the theory that, by middle class standards, the culturally disadvantaged perhaps are mentally ill in terms of the socialization process.

A client from a Mexican-American background, on the other hand, may precipitate the counselor into unique factors embedded in the values and beliefs of that culture. It is not altogether atypical in the Southwest, especially among those Mexican-Americans who are poorly educated, to harbor some belief in witchcraft, or some degree of belief therein.

Although most Mexican-Americans will only speak of knowing someone

who believes in witchcraft, the counselor may come face to
reality, as did the counselor in the case reviewed below. A M.
can social case worker from a small Texas town had an automo.
after which punitive and financial damages were being sought by
During the course of the evaluation, to demonstrate damage from
dent, it developed that this social case worker was known in he.
as a *bruja* (witch). She apparently held many of the townspeople, i.
some of the Anglo-Americans, in the grips of fear relative to her *powers*.
For the most part, she seemed to use these *powers* only to extort large financial contributions for community projects and her church, for which the priest
of her parish was eternally and ecstatically grateful. However, it seemed the
bruja held one high ambition. She had always aspired to become a member
of the church's altar society (almost the equivalent of an exclusive club in
that town), which up to that time had been almost exclusively controlled by
the Anglo women of the community and few monied *senoras*. Presumably,
the *bruja* had delivered verbal threats through an intermediary (seemingly a
necessity in a successful hexing operation) that various kinds of evils would
befall the group, particularly its president, were she excluded from membership. The priest frankly wanted the *bruja* excluded because of her trouble-
making reputation; but he, like Pontius Pilate, washed his hands of the whole
affair and quickly, and maybe wisely, turned his attention exclusively toward
the spiritual affairs of the church.

The point to be made is that the *bruja's* influence even found its way into
a large medical complex in a metropolitan city of 800,000 people some 200
miles away from her home. Seeing a frail woman of some 40 years, it was
difficult to believe that this rather neatly groomed, almost elegantly-behaved
individual could terrify so many people, including a few hospital staff members, who demonstrated, even in jest some hesitancy in ultimately labeling
her difficulties as largely hysterical and malingering in nature. Yet, this
story is true.

The unfortunate part of the story is that no one dared to be creative or
to help either this woman, or her community. With concentrated effort the
woman could probably have been integrated into the community as an
effective and positive contributing societal force.

An inexperienced counselor confronted with the task of understanding
and motivating the black or the Mexican-American client, then, must look
into the cultural background, the values and beliefs of that subculture, before
he can work effectively toward the rehabilitation of the client. Unless he is
aware of and utilizes the unique nuances of that culture in his plan of
motivation, he may reap only frustration and failure for his efforts. If he
accepts the challenge, and studies the culture and his client, he may find
this area the most fascinating and rewarding one in the field of rehabilitation.

The Search for Meaningful Techniques
of Counseling the Culturally Disadvantaged

Ayers (1970), in his earlier observations, states that there is a dearth of literature dealing with the ingredients of, and techniques available for creating a counseling relationship with the disadvantaged client. Relative to an early work concerning cultural difference and medical care, Saunders (1954) sees two major biases which can hamper effectiveness in working with the culturally disadvantaged: rationalism and ethnocentrism. In this instance, he is referring to the Spanish-speaking Americans of the Southwest, but the biases of rationalism and ethnocentrism probably hold true for other disadvantaged groups.

The rationalistic bias, according to Saunders, can, in this instance, lead medical men and women working in cross-cultural situations, to see their own behavior as being highly determined by rational considerations. By the same process they view the actions of persons from another culture as exhibiting behavior resulting from irrationality, ignorance or stupidity, merely because it happens to differ from their own.

Ethnocentrism, on the other hand, may result in the universal tendency of human beings to think that their ways of thinking, acting, and believing are the only right, proper, and natural ones and to regard the beliefs and practices of other people as strange, bizarre, or unenlightened. Among several examples cited, Saunders talks about the Texan seated before his thick, red steak and the Hindu who looks upon the eating of beef as a sacrilege, as likely each to view the other as some sort of barbarian. Or, the monogamous wives pondering the sad state of the polygamous wife who must share her husband with five other women, while Mrs. Polygamy pities the plight of Mrs. Monogamy who has to tolerate her husband all by herself.

Senter (1947) has pointed out that folk practitioners in the Southwest, treating patients who have been *embrujado* (placed under the influence of witchcraft), utilize an approach and procedures very similar to those familiar to psychotherapists, or psychotherapeutically-oriented professionals, in their counseling methods. The illness is actually seen by both as a function of the maladjustment of the individual to some aspect of his environment. Bychowski (1970) states the theoretical differences and positions rather clearly. Being middle class leads to inner flight, or neuroses. Being lower class leads to acting out, unusual behavior or outer flight. Thus, the counselor focuses upon the individual and his neuroses, while the *albolaria* focuses upon dealing with the *bruja*. In many cases, the latter method of treatment may prove more effective with certain individuals. Utilizing this approach in counseling, a beautiful young woman was able to wrest free from the lesbian hold another had upon her by working through the cultural ethos rather than by attacking the neurosis.

A young man, accused of assault with intent to murder six persons in a small town dance hall "because something came over me" following peer *brujo* threats, is now functioning effectively in society: he no longer believes his fate is tied into destiny. He no longer considers himself a victim of those about him.

A counterpoint to witchcraft in the black community is the case of a black child who was *psychotic* because his god, James Brown, told him to engage in weird behavior. The counselor *talked* with James Brown, and told the child that James Brown had told him that the child had simply misunderstood James Brown. In this last case, the counselor used a variation of a true story a rabbi had told years earlier about a Gentile woman who came to him, seeking conversion to Judaism. "God told me to come and see you," she explained. In reply, the rabbi answered her, "Well, if God told you to come, how come He didn't tell me you were coming?"

The traditional methods often will not work with the culturally disadvantaged. Truax and Carkhuff (1967) claim that essential ingredients of successful therapy or counseling, are emphatic understanding of the counseled, non-possessive warmth for the counseled, and therapist authenticity or genuineness.

Empathy has long been a central tool in most dynamic psychotherapies. Empathy is not some diagnostic and external understanding, but a truly emphatic understanding of the subject, as described by Fleiss (1942) in this excerpt:

> it depends essentially on his (the counselor or therapist's) ability to put himself in the latter's place, to step into his shoes and to obtain in this way inside knowledge that is almost first-hand. The common name for such a procedure is empathy.

From a client-centered therapy point of view, Schlien (1961) suggests:

> That technique is "reflection", particularly reflection of feeling rather than content. At most points in communication where others would interpret, probe, advise, escape, we reflect . . . Reflection can be, in the hand of an imitating movie, a dull, wooden mockery. On paper it often looks particularly so. Yet it can also be profound, intimate, empathically understanding response, requiring great skill and sensitivity and intense involvement.

Warmth is considered necessary in any trusting relationship and even more crucial for the counseling and therapeutic relationship, which focuses upon the client's guilt-ridden feelings, inadequacies and other facets. Rogers, *et al.* (1951, 1957, 1967), has emphasized this nonpossessive warmth for the client as being without "if's and's or but's".

Wolpe (1958) further elaborates:

> All that the patient says is accepted without question or criticism. He is given to feelings that the therapist is unreservedly at his side. This happens not because the therapist is expressly trying to appear sympathetic, but as a natural outcome of a completely non-moralizing objective approach to the behavior of human organisms.

Genuineness, according to the Truax and Carkhuff position, implies most basically a direct personal encounter, a meeting on a person-to-person basis without defensiveness, or a retreat into facades or roles, and so in this sense an openness to experience. They further feel that there is no substitute for genuineness in the psychotherapeutic relationship. The therapist may think he can fool the patient. Humans can tell the difference between insincere warmth and true warmth. They feel that genuineness is not easy to define: it implies the very difficult task of being quite intimately acquainted with ourselves, and of being able to recognize and accept as well as respect ourselves as a whole containing both good and bad. In essence, the *phony* or artificial person is soon discovered.

Warmth, empathy, and genuineness, these three aspects permeate virtually all theories of psychotherapy and counseling, and also relate to everyday experiences. Shoben (1953) points out: "If warmth, permissiveness, safety and understanding seem to be prerequisites of any desirable human relationship rather than being peculiar properties of the psychotherapeutic interaction, this is precisely the case."

Truax and Carkhuff found that all types of *help-seekers* respond favorably when these elements of empathy, nonpossessing warmth and therapist genuineness are strongly present and analogously respond unfavorably when they are absent. The distinction to be made, of course, is that most of the disadvantaged cannot be classified as help-seekers. It is the *helpers*, under the presumed national mandate of 1964 to eliminate poverty, who are seeking. This places an entirely different emphasis upon just what type of help is to be extended or expected.

Thus, the demand for creativity and innovativeness upon the part of the counselor is at a premium. No longer can the counselor be tied to his office. No longer can the feasibility of early closure and implied quotas, and diagnostic categories (Silver, 1967; Skelton, 1967) be used exclusively as criteria for acceptance practices, particularly within the rehabilitation process.

In discussing internal versus external locus of control, McDonald (1970) concludes that research literature points to membership in socially disadvantaged and minority groups as conductive to the development of external control orientations. Suggesting how this can be used competitively as a motivating factor with students, for example, Rogers (1971) generally concurs: "The competitive attitude underlying achievement appears to be absent in the Mexican-American culture, and, at the lower levels of acculturation, striving to excell over classmates may result in disapproval by the group." She suggests that it is possible to use the group identity to arouse competition with other groups, such as other classes in the same school or between schools. The individual student's desire to achieve, she says, can be stimulated by the press to contribute to his own group's goals.

Relative to locus of control, it seems to be mostly external in the disadvantaged. Where traditional counseling and therapeutic approaches have failed, simple, honest, direct methods with "activity" counseling as a focal point, are most effective. As trite as it may appear, a chat over a cup of coffee outside the office surroundings can surmount hours of heretofore marked resistance. Even the exchange of a token mint candy clearly means more to the disadvantaged than "therapeutic acceptance" to "convey" an attitude of friendliness.

Activity can take many forms: a visit to the neighborhood, the school, on the job, etc. Activity can include the conjoint involvement of myriad community resources, government, private or United Fund agencies. The church, for example, is the center of much of black life, and counselors might do well to spend some time meeting the individuals who minister to the spiritual needs of the people they are trying to help. One counselor in a Texas city can work miracles in a particular school district because she has taken the time to attend church services and community events in the district. Another counselor in that same district, far better qualified in both theory and academic training, is unable to marshal any type of leadership because something is basically missing in her relationship with people. This "something" goes beyond emphatic understanding, nonpossessive warmth and genuineness. Call it caring, honesty, simplicity, innovativeness, or whatever. Maybe it can be termed cooperative guidance, but it works!

So many counselors, in all types of work situations, even excluding those working with the disadvantaged, feel that they must "go it alone." Somehow, ego demands prove so great that the sense of "I did it" distorts the reality and possibilities of success. It really is unimportant who takes the credit. Several years back, a vocational rehabilitation counselor and a psychologist embarked on an experimental group venture with male federal drug offenders. The program was carried to their families, to the neighborhood, to the office, anywhere. Where Mexican-Americans were exclusive members of the group, the members were allowed to speak whatever language they felt comfortable in using. They voted for types of programs and materials they would like to discuss. Every innovation was used to motivate these men. It appeared to prove successful; at least the Minnesota Multiphasic Personality Text pre-and-post "therapy" profiles suggested that benefits were obtained with at least one small group of men who because of minimally sufficient education and language ability were able to complete the MMPI form. The ingredients which created positive movement and change are not known. But it is known that the counselor and the psychologist *wanted* the project to be successful.

With group therapy and counseling programs at a local "halfway" house for women, a school teacher was brought in to talk about feminine hygiene (specifically birth control methods), play stereo albums of popular music, and ask for interpretations, utilize psychodrama (an activity psychotherapy), arrange social outings, hair styling and make-up sessions, as well as traditional "therapeutic" involvement. This technique proved to be successful. There are endless ways to innovate and create if one is willing to break out of the mold of traditional counseling techniques and therapeutic methods.

Some Characteristics of the Counselor
Effective With the Culturally Disadvantaged

After reviewing the nature of the multifold problem of counseling the culturally disadvantaged, and examining the search for meaningful techniques of working with them, one is struck with the idea of unique counselor traits essential to effective counseling with these individuals. Mannie (1972) observed, relative to disadvantaged blacks, that the most effective counselors she knows are those people who have never seen the inside of a school room:

> I have come a long way with counseling and guidance from many people and most of these people have been formally uneducated. People who have said things to me that were more helpful were not professors in college. I am not sure that the trained ones are at all effective in counseling the disadvantaged. I am really not suggesting that we don't get training, but I am suggesting that we can change our models. It might be profitable as counselors for us to observe some of these para-professionals as they relate quite effectively with others.
> *(From an Interview).*

Rioch (1965), in her almost classical although heretical study at the National Institute of Mental Health at Bethesda, Maryland, proved quite dramatically that non-formally trained college-educated housewives can function quite effectively in the role of psychotherapists, and in many instances have proved more effective than the professionals, i.e., psychiatrist, psychologist, and psychiatric social workers. Her thesis was not to shift all psychotherapeutic endeavors to the non-professional, but under the supervision of professionals, to strongly encourage the use of para-professionals where indicated.

In its recommendation for a national mental health program, the Joint Commission on Mental Illness and Health (1960) came to similar conclusions that nonmedical, nondoctorally-trained counselors with aptitude, sound training, practical experience and demonstrable competence should even be permitted to do general, short-term psychotherapy under the auspices of recognized health agencies. Many mental health centers about the country are following through with the recommendations of the Commission, often with startling success.

The use of para-professionals and sub-professionals seems clearly indicated in counseling of the disadvantaged. It takes an especially skilled, academically trained counselor, versed in multi-cultures and perhaps even possessing bi- tri- or multi-lingual talents to understand some of the nuances of the culture if the gap is to be bridged. Often colleges, even with massive field trips and poverty internship placements, simply are not able to train, at this point in time, the kind, and certainly not the number of individuals who could function successfully in culturally disadvantaged areas. Perhaps it is not desirable to do so. In fact, too many academic programs, as they are now constituted, "screen out" some of the very ingredients that (from the research reviewed) tend to make effective counselors for the culturally disadvantaged.

The Rioch approach would appear to be the most effective direction for the moment, at least in terms of meeting immediate manpower needs. It would be highly desirable, it would seem, if counselors of all colors could be completely weaned from ethnocentric and rationalistic positions.

This recommendation is not advocating the abandonment of academic training and theory. A theoretical basis and a framework from which to operate are essential. In working with the neurotic and psychotic through the years, theories have been developed and models and techniques conducive to positive change advanced. This same procedure must be relived with the culturally disadvantaged as the focal point. This will take highly trained, creative and dedicated individuals.

In the meantime, the counselor characteristics of warmth, empathy, and genuineness must be kept firmly in mind. The biases of rationalism and ethnocentrism must be avoided. But most of all counselors who are creative, dare to be innovative, and who carry the battle of motivation to the client and his family in activities and as a model must be encouraged. Counseling the culturally disadvantaged is not an eight-hour-a-day job. Training and learning do not terminate with the award of the sheepskin or a year of experience. It is an endless, ever dynamic, and challenging quest.

REFERENCES

Ayers, George E.: The disadvantaged, an analysis of factors affecting the counseling relationship. *Rehabilitation Literature, 31*:194-199, 1970.

Bychowski, Gustav: Psycho-analytic reflections on the psychiatry of the poor. *International Journal of Psycho-Analysis, 51*:4, 1970.

Fleiss, R.: The metapsychology of the analyst. *Psychol Quart, 11*:42, 1942.

Fromm, Erich: *Escape from Freedom.* New York, Holt, Rinehart and Winston, p. 138, 1964.

Joint Commission on Mental Illness and Health: *Action for Mental Health.* New York, Basic Books, 1961.

Mannie, Virginia D., (Consultant, Guidance and Counseling, The Education Service Center, Region 20), Interview. San Antonio, Texas, February 11, 1972.

McDonald, A. P.: Internal-external locus of control: A promising rehabilitation variable. *Journal of Counseling Psychology, 18*:2, 1970.

Parker, Seymour and Kleiner, Robert J.: The culture of poverty: An adjustive dimension. *American Anthropologist, 72*:3, 1970.

Rioch, Margaret J.: Changing concepts in the training of therapists. *Journal of Consulting Psychology, 30*(4): 290-292, 1966.

Rogers, C. R.: *Client-Centered Therapy.* Boston, Houghton Mifflin Co., 1951.

Rogers, C. R.: The necessary and sufficient conditions of therapeutic personality change. *Journal of Consulting Psychology, 21*:95-103, 1957.

Rogers, C. R. and Truax, C. B.: The therapeutic conditions antecedent to change: A theoretical view. In Rogers, C. R., Gendlin, E. T., Kiesler, D. and Truax, C. B. (Eds.), *The Therapeutic Relationship and Its Impact: A Study of Psychotherapy With Schizophrenics.* Madison, University of Wisconsin Press, 1967.

Rogers, Dorothy: Personality traits and academic achievement among Mexican-American students. Unpublished doctoral dissertation, University of Texas, 1971.

Saunders, Lyle: *Cultural Differences and Medical Care.* New York, Russell Sage Foundation, 1954.

Schlien, J. M.: *Psychotherapy of the psychoses.* New York, Basic Books, p. 302, 1961.

Senter, Donovan: Witches and psychiatrist. *Psychiatry, Journal of the Biology and Pathology of Interpersonal Relations,* pp. 10, 49-56, 1947.

Shoben, E. J.: *Psychotherapy: Theory and Research.* New York, Ronald Press, p. 126, 1953.

Skelton, John G.: Acceptance practices in a medically-oriented vocational rehabilitation project. Unpublished doctoral dissertation, Texas Tech University, 1967.

Truax, Charles B. and Carkhuff, Robert R.: *Toward Effective Counseling and Psychotherapy: Training and Practice.* Chicago, Aldine Publishing Co., 1967.

Wolpe, J.: *Psychotherapy by Reciprocal Inhibition.* Palo Alto, Calif., Stanford University Press, p. 106, 1958.

(PART THREE)

THE ADDICTED

ALCOHOL ADDICTION:

REHABILITATION OF THE ALCOHOLIC
ALCOHOLISM

CHEMICAL ADDICTION:

THE DRUG ABUSE PROGRAM OF THE
  TEXAS REHABILITATION COMMISSION

THE EFFECTS OF MOOD ALTERING DRUGS:
  PLEASURES AND PITFALLS

CLINICAL AND COUNSELING PROBLEMS
  IN DRUG DEPENDENCE

Chapter 8

REHABILITATION OF THE ALCOHOLIC

GEORGE V. CLARK

THE VOCATIONAL REHABILITATION Act Amendments of 1965 provide a way whereby the services available to disabled individuals in Texas through the Texas Rehabilitation Commission, could be extended to persons suffering from alcoholism. The flexibility that the 1965 amendments brought into the Vocational Rehabilitation Act affords an opportunity for alterations in State and local Vocational Rehabilitation programs to meet the needs of clients with vocational handicaps resulting from physical or mental disability. Prior to the above mentioned amendments of the Vocational Rehabilitation Act, the potential existing in Vocational Rehabilitation programs could not be utilized to provide financial support for services to persons handicapped by alcoholism.

The Texas Rehabilitation Commission extended services to the alcoholic client shortly after the 1965 amendments. Major emphasis was placed on referrals from inpatient treatment programs. Since the majority of the treatment programs were located in State Hospitals, the Texas Rehabilitation Commission's first major thrust was programming in the State Hospital setting. During the initial stages of serving persons handicapped by alcoholism, it was felt that those persons (alcoholics) who had been through an inpatient treatment program were "better" candidates for the adjunct services of Vocational Rehabilitation. Having overcome much of the "growing pains" resulting from extending services to alcoholics, and discovering the feasibility of serving alcoholics, services to alcoholics are becoming more and more community based. The emphasis currently being placed on community Vocational Rehabilitation programs for alcoholics is positively effected by the development of Mental Health and Mental Retardation Centers and other local support programs. It is not difficult to see a de-emphasizing of long-term inpatient care in favor of short-term inpatient care for detoxification and longer term support services after the treatment of the acute illness. Thus, the Texas Rehabilitation Commission is placing more counselors in local community settings, with a primary responsibility for serving those persons disabled by the abuse of alcohol. This is in no way suggesting a *cut back in hospital* programs, but rather is to be viewed as an *expansion* of the

153

overall program, thereby making Vocational Rehabilitation services available and accessible to a greater number of persons victimized by alcoholism.

Eligibility for Rehabilitation

Alcoholism is recognized as an extremely complex problem with cultural, psychological, physiological and spiritual overtones. Alcoholics Anonymous showed us that recovery is possible for the person handicapped by alcoholism. It is apparent now that services provided by Vocational Rehabilitation can help the alcoholic resume a normal place in society, becoming again self-supporting, self-respecting, good citizens, good husbands and good parents. However, in considering the alcoholic for Vocational Rehabilitation services, eligibility and feasibility are of great importance (Texas Rehabilitation Commission Manual, 1972).

> A diagnosis of alcoholism establishes the presence of a disability. This diagnosis may be accepted from any licensed physician who certifies that a person has a recent history of alcoholism. If the addiction to alcohol is well established and there appears to be no underlying disorder, a psychiatric and/or psychologic examination is not required unless recommended by the examining physician or medical consultant. A psychiatric evaluation must be obtained if it appears that the person has severe emotional problems. An individual with alcoholism may be eligible for six months' extended evaluation.
>
> All applicants with a diagnosis of alcoholism who are accepted for Vocational Rehabilitation must be engaged in a therapeutic program during the Vocational Rehabilitation process. The concept of therapy includes that provided by such a program as Alcoholics Anonymous. The provision of Vocational Rehabilitation services to the alcoholic individual is based on his demonstration and indicated ability to maintain abstinence from alcohol and accept ongoing treatment and programming (p. 1).

Alcoholics, as in the case of any other applicant for Vocational Rehabilitation services, must meet the eligibility requirements. The applicant must have a physical or mental disability; there must be a substantial handicap to employment; and there must be a reasonable expectation that rehabilitation services may render the individual fit to engage in gainful employment.

> The third criterion is concerned primarily with *vocational* prognosis. Rehabilitation services are provided "to assist personally and economically dependent individuals with impairments (physical, mental, emotional, educational, cultural, etc.) in the achievement of the highest level of personal and economic independence possible." This does not mean that it must be determined that every applicant will eventually be able to work on a full-time job; neither does it mean that Vocational Rehabilitation is a one-time service. It does mean that improvement in ability to function is a goal of the state rehabilitation agency and that services are offered in order to assist impaired individuals in their efforts to attain the highest possible level of independence.
>
> A few reasonable questions to ask in regard to the prospective alcoholic client would be:
>
> 1. Is rehabilitation for this person feasible?
> 2. Will he be able to profit from services rendered?
> 3. Can he participate in a rehabilitation program that places emphasis on his vocational potential; and, if he does, is there at least a fair chance that the end result will be a productive person who receives personal and economic benefit from his own productivity?

A man may be too disabled to be eligible for rehabilitation services, or he may not be disabled enough to be eligible. The rehabilitation counselor must determine the eligibility of each applicant; and once he determines that a substantial handicap for employment exists, his next task is to decide whether or not the barrier that lies between the applicant and employment can be removed or markedly reduced. This latter task is often referred to as "determination of feasibility" (pp. 1-2).

The counselor may have little, if any, problem *making* an alcoholic eligible for Vocational Rehabilitation services, but the matter of *feasibility* is of great significance when considering an application on a potential client handicapped by alcoholism. Vocational Rehabilitation counselors often find themselves closing clients in statuses other than "26" (rehabilitated) because the client was not feasible when the counselor accepted the client for services. Age, physical condition and retirement status are samples of concerns that enter the picture when determining feasibility. Unfortunately, many times alcoholics' age is a barrier to employment. This is not a barrier in all instances, but in enough instances for the counselor to be concerned as thinking is given to placement of a client in gainful employment.

There are also instances when the client's health, even after he has obtained sobriety will not permit him to function in the competitive labor market. Many alcoholics suffer from emphysema badly enough for special consideration to be given them in employment.

Retired persons may not be feasible for Vocational Rehabilitation services. This is not to establish a blanket policy for retirees; however, the counselor needs some assurance that he may obtain a justifiable rehabilitant once services are rendered. Many retirees suffering from alcoholism are even more difficult to rehabilitate because of a consistent, if not substantial, income. Placing retired persons may prove to be difficult because the retired may have no desire for job placement.

It must be pointed out that many alcoholics are not physically disabled and that many of them have some kind of job skill. This means that they may not require much assistance oftentimes in terms of case service money. However, they require a great deal in terms of personal relationships, counselor time and emotional energy.

In the light of the immediately above statement, emphasis is placed on counseling the alcoholic in the remainder of this chapter.

Carl Jung (Clinebell, 1968) is quoted as having said,

Learn your theories as well as you can, then put them aside when you touch the miracle of the living soul. Not theories, but your own creative individuality alone must decide! (p. 214)

Learn your theories, yes; but what is this "other" that has led a great doctor to suggest that when you are dealing with "the miracle of a living soul," theories are to be put aside—this "other" that takes precedence over theories and techniques.

The effective utilization of one's own "creative individuality" in counseling situations is determined, in Clinebell's words, by "a relationship characterized by warmth, genuineness, acceptance, caring and trust." This is especially true in counseling alcoholics.

An In-Depth Relationship

First and foremost in counseling involvement is the establishment of a relationship rather than a direct approach to the solution of the problem. The building of a "relationship bridge," as Clinebell (p . 214) puts it, over which the alcoholic brings feelings and gains knowledge of himself in a meaningful and hopefully helpful way seems to be imperative in every way. The building of this bridge opens up communication between the alcoholic and his counselor. The building of this bridge begins when the alcoholic feels that the counselor is interested in him and in his problems and is listening in depth and relating with his being. When the counselor gives himself totally to the experience, experiencing and recognizing the intrinsic human dignity of the alcoholic, the warmth and regard that the alcoholic feels and reacts to will cause his confidence and outgoingness to flourish and further tend to develop within the counselor an interest in what the alcoholic is concerned about. And this is the beginning of a therapeutic involvement.

At some time very early in the counseling of the alcoholic, the counselor must face his own attitudes toward the alcoholic and toward alcoholism. It is hardly possible to escape emotional involvement as he begins to direct any serious thought toward working with the alcoholic. There are searching questions the counselor will often direct to himself. "Am I convinced that the alcoholic is a sick person and is suffering from the disease of alcoholism? Is my feeling toward the alcoholic one of love? Or is my feeling that of indifference or rejection?" Facing this reality within ourselves is one of the most basic requirements for anyone who counsels people who have serious drinking problems. Alcoholics are such experts at being phonies that they are also experts at spotting phonies. If the counselor is wearing a mask, it will soon be discovered by the alcoholic and this usually ends in an unhealthful and unhelpful involvement; no "relationship bridge" is likely to be built.

Further, insecurity and feelings of ambivalence about the use of, and the user of, beverage alcohol, tends to allow the counselor to slip into the alcoholic's own confusion.

The alcoholic is in need of, and in many instances in quest of, a situation wherein such basic needs as status, acceptance, "structure" and healthy dependency can be fulfilled; and this is the ideal sought in building a relationship. All too often, and very easily, we find ourselves unable to bend, not flexible, and rigid in thinking, principles and dogma. The principles that prove to be applicable and helpful in one situation may be completely irrelevant in another experience. Resorting to rigidities, most especially as regards the counselor's own patterns of behavior or his principles, may tend to lead into attempting a sale to the alcoholic in some manipulative fashion of what has proven helpful for someone else. There is a need for the counselor to be open enough so as not to push down his current interpretation or some original plan that may prove to be inappropriate and totally inadequate. The alcoholic needs someone who understands how he feels and cares about him and his feelings. The alcoholic needs someone who can help him become aware of what the possibilities and nature of alcoholism are; but he, the alcoholic, receives little if any help from rigid counselors with preconceived ideas of who, or rather what, the alcoholic is and of what the alcoholic needs individually for attaining and maintaining sobriety.

One of the greatest needs of the alcoholic is the need for someone who is free to let the alcoholic be free, someone who can let the alcoholic make decisions that appear to be, from the counselor's point of view, not in the alcoholic's best interests, John Keller, in his book *Ministering to Alcoholics* (1966), put it this way:

> (The alcoholic) needs someone who is free to let him go—who can love him enough to completely let him go to the bottom, like unto the love of the father in the story of the prodigal son. He does need someone who is free to let the problem prove itself to him. He does need someone who is free to let him experience the inner pain and natural results of his drinking without imposing other pain upon him. He does need someone who can let the problem be his problem and at the same time seek to motivate him to responsible action (p. 69).

We who counsel alcoholics need to be able to give, for we cannot maintain human relationships without giving. The word "giving" is used in the sense of giving up something for the benefit of another. This kind of giving involves giving up energy, time, or things, in order to fulfill the other person's needs and desires. This kind of giving implies an awareness of the alcoholic as being a human person like one's self, rather than merely an object. Real giving represents to some extent an identification with the interests of the alcoholic. This makes giving, to a great extent, an act of love, and because it is reminiscent of living, it kindles responsiveness. This giving on the part of the counselor of alcoholics is not some sort of interchange of material things and favors, but rather in addition to time and energy, the giving of praise, understanding, affection, approval, encouragement, and an acceptance of the alcoholic's weakness along with respect for his strengths.

Chaplain George Dominick of the Georgian Clinic in Atlanta, Georgia, states, "As we move into a depth relationship with the alcoholic, it becomes increasingly clear that he is acting out in his own way those same inner conflicts which others of us act out in other ways . . . a pervasive sense of inner dividedness" that all humans share in common.

This pull of the two selves as seen in the alcoholic, the counselor must also recognize and accept in himself; otherwise he will be more limited in his ability to counsel alcoholics effectively. This kind of self-awareness on the part of the counselor enables him to allow the alcoholic to have, if not the same worth, at least more worth in the eyes of the counselor; and it points up the fact that the alcoholic is a person, and a person of great worth, maybe differing in talents, abilities, etc., but of equal worth as a human being and child of God.

Channeling Feelings

It was mentioned earlier that the counselor, to be of greatest effect, must relate with his full being. An area that needs to be mentioned is that of our feelings and emotions as counselor with regard to the feelings of the alcoholic. Our feelings are essentially motivators. They are forces prodding us to action. Things happen around us or within our bodies, and in response to these things we feel emotion: anger, fear, joy, guilt, shame, and envy. Emotions are experienced as tension; tension is generally unpleasant; thereby we are moved to act in a way to remove the tension. Recognition, acceptance, and willingness to share or express feelings all play a great part in counseling alcoholics. Many things verbalized may not be the same as what is conveyed on a feeling level, and more often than not, feelings, which can be picked up by persons as sensitive as alcoholics, betray and give more information about the counselor than he sometimes wants to convey. Whether the counselor and the alcoholic accept or deny their feelings, they both are in on the fact that feelings are present and unless the feelings are accepted and dealt with in some appropriate fashion, they will create a wall between the counselor and the alcoholic.

There are some very crucial times when the counselor's feelings about the alcoholic may get in the way. "Success needs" sometimes may, consciously or unconsciously, cause the counselor to "hang on" to the alcoholic who is exhibiting some independent action, decision-making, or the like, especially if the alcoholic has become some kind of special person for the counselor. The alcoholic may be filling the counselor's ego need; and the counselor is not able to let the alcoholic go, thus fostering an unhealthy dependency.

Another time when feelings may cause trouble is when verbalization of feelings on the part of the counselor may threaten, possibly to the point of breaking, what is felt to be a good relationship. Honest feelings about an alcoholic are not reflected for fear the alcoholic may lose confidence and not seek a sharing relationship again. Several things may be going on at this time. It may be that the counselor cannot tolerate the idea of failure and thus cannot allow the alcoholic the freedom to fail and miss the opportunity for both the counselor and the alcoholic to grow from the experience. It is likely to help the alcoholic's growth toward his full potential for personhood, constructive relationships, and productive living when the alcoholic experiences, in his relationship with the counselor, a freedom that allows for some independent action and decision-making on the part of the alcoholic. The relationship can begin to move in a helpful direction when the counselor can reflect negative as well as positive observations to the alcoholic about the alcoholic and tell him how things are seen and felt by the counselor at that particular time. If the counselor can run the risk of sharing some of his own feelings about himself, when necessary and hopefully helpful, the alcoholic is likely to feel relieved when he discovers that his counselor is a human being in the full sense of being human.

The need in counseling is to get something done and to see some results. This falls into the category of "success needs." This need to point to an accomplishment may cause, oftentimes, a push for results; and the counselor, in giving in to this need, may—consciously on unconsciously—push the sale of a patented product, a ready-made plan that may not have any relevancy for this specific case. This kind of action may cause the alcoholic to be less open and limit the possibility of his self-discovery and growth. The discoveries the alcoholic makes about himself are the most helpful and most lasting. The counselor should avoid attempting to give or have all the answers, but rather should function as a partner who aids in setting up a situation where possibly some guidelines may be found as he and the alcoholic venture deeper and more meaningfully into their involvement with each other, both giving and taking.

The counselor of alcoholics is doing himself and the alcoholic a great service if he forms a habit of constantly searching his own feelings, admitting them to himself and accepting them; in so doing the counselor is more likely to be immediately aware of himself in the counseling situation. If the counselor avoids or denies his emotions, he may find himself acting on them without knowing that they are motivating his actions; and he might do or say things damaging to the counselor setting—things he may regret later.

When dealing with the emotions of the alcoholic, the counselor may do one or more of three things. First, when the counselor encounters emotion in the alcoholic, he may encourage its expression. In a heightened state of tension the alcoholic is hardly ready, willing, or able to deal honestly with anything other than the feelings causing this tension, and this is also true of the counselor. It does not matter what the feeling or emotion is; when the counselor encounters the emotion, he should not avoid it but should get the alcoholic to talk about it, if possible, at that time; if the alcoholic refuses or is unable to talk then and there, it may help to make him aware of the fact that the counselor is aware of the alcoholic's feelings.

Second, the counselor may make the alcoholic aware of the alcoholic's feelings. Sometimes an alcoholic may not deal with his feelings because he lacks conscious awareness of what he is feeling at the moment. This, combined with an unconscious desire to conceal the emotion both from himself and from others, works against his expressing himself. When this is happening it may prove valuable for the counselor to make the alcoholic aware of what he is feeling. The counselor may or may not tell the alcoholic directly, depending upon where they are in the relationship and upon whether or not the relationship is strong enough to survive this kind of confrontation. If the counselor is not ready to risk the relationship with direct confrontation, the counselor can suggest that the alcoholic's behavior seems to indicate that he has this feeling and that his feeling is quite understandable. This could create a situation wherein the alcoholic becomes aware of his feelings.

Third, the counselor can accept the alcoholic's feelings without criticizing them. "It is all right to feel the way you feel; it is natural to have these feelings, and you do not have to be losing control as long as you are aware of and accept these emotions." Once the alcoholic feels that he is not going to be criticized for his feelings, he may be better able to get them out, diminishing tension and thus enabling him to appraise the problem more realistically.

Emotions may not be controllable, but to be aware of and to accept the feelings, may prove to be appropriate ways of dealing with them. Feelings are extremely helpful in a counseling situation when the counselor comes to be aware of and can trust his own emotions. Generally, bringing one's feelings as counselor, as well as the alcoholic's feelings, out into the open as much as possible, proves to be very valuable in counseling with alcoholics. Clinebell (1968) puts it this way:

> What is crucial is that one's (the counselor's) responses be an expression of a genuine fellow feeling and growing understanding on the counselor's part (p. 217).

REFERENCES

Arrell, V. M.: State rehabilitation and the alcoholic. *Texas Journal on Alcoholism,* pp. 7-8, 1970.

Clinebell, H. J.: *Understanding the Alcoholic.* New York, Abingdon Press, 1968.

Dominick, George P.: The Clergyman and the Alcoholic. Paper presented at the Texas Summer Studies on Alcoholism, Austin, Texas, 1968.

Keller, John E.: *Ministering to Alcoholics.* Minneapolis, Augsburg Publishing House, 1966.

Texas Rehabilitation Commission: *Rehabilitation Services Manual.* No. 02-4, February 1972.

Chapter 9

ALCOHOLISM

HARRY G. DAVIS AND PRESTON E. HARRISON

HISTORY AND PHILOSOPHY

THE DEBILITATING EFFECTS of alcohol have been recognized for quite some time. However, not until recent years has an integrated and organized attempt been developed to aid in the recovery of those persons crippled by the excessive use of alcohol. It was not until 1934 that a self-help nonprofessional group of recovered alcoholics called Alcoholics Anonymous (AA) began actively working in this field of rehabilitation. The historical facts and the names to be introduced below are quite well known to anyone who has been acquainted with AA. Knowledge of this movement and its philosophies is essential in understanding the alcoholic through any methodology.

The events leading up to this "foundation group" began in 1934 when Dr. Silkworth pronounced Bill W. a chronic and hopeless alcoholic. Ebby T., a member of the Oxford Group,* is credited with aiding Bill W. in his recovery from alcoholism. He presented to Bill W. an example of his own sobriety and William James' book, *Varieties of Religious Experience.* Following what he called a *miraculous religious experience,* Bill W. was then able to remain sober. Bill W.'s attempts to aid other alcoholics using the principles of the Oxford Group met with total failure. Bill W. and Dr. Bob found a common bond in the inability to tolerate alcohol. These two along with eighteen other men formed the first AA group in June of 1935. The four absolutes and the desire of the Oxford Group to reach all individuals gave way to the first six of the now twelve steps of AA and to the specific purpose of helping alcoholics to remain sober. Recognizing the alcoholic's problem, sharing of group experiences, relying on God as he is individually perceived, and aiding others in recovery, were the working principles of that first group. The basic philosophies have not changed but simply been extended.

In 1937, following the break with the Oxford Group, AA began to expand. In 1939 the first edition of *Alcoholics Anonymous* was printed, and a one-room New York office was opened and operated through volunteers.

---

*Oxford Group, a universal brotherhood for moral improvement with four absolute principles as its foundation: (1) absolute love, (2) absolute purity, (3) absolute unselfishness, and (4) absolute honesty (Alcoholics-Anonymous Comes of Age, 1957, p. 161).

AA's public acceptance created many public relations problems. AA was presented as a way of life. It was not to be confused with a new religious cult, nor was it to infringe on medical boundaries. A working relationship with the fields of religion and medicine was established and has become increasingly effective through the present time. It was also necessary to determine how best to cooperate with radio, television, press, and motion pictures. Employee-employer relationships and related fields, such as alcohol education, research and rehabilitation were other areas needing policy or at least guidelines. The basic practices and attitudes of AA emerged through a trial and error process, and the public relation policies at that time have evolved into the twelve AA traditions. Those traditions are (W. 1957, p. 78):

1. Our common welfare would come first; personal recovery depends upon AA unity.
2. For our group purpose there is but one ultimate authority—a loving God as He may express Himself in our group conscience. Our leaders are but trusted servants; they do not govern.
3. The only requirement for AA membership is a sincere desire to stop drinking.
4. Each group should be autonomous, except in matters affecting other groups or AA as a whole.
5. Each group has but one primary purpose: to carry its message to the alcoholic who still suffers.
6. An AA group ought never endorse, finance or lend the AA name to any related facility or outside enterprise, lest problems of money, property, and prestige divert us from our primary purpose.
7. Every AA group ought to be fully self-supporting, declining outside contributions.
8. Alcoholics Anonymous should remain forever nonprofessional, but our service centers may employ special workers.
9. AA, as such, ought never be organized; but we may create service boards or committees directly responsible to those they serve.
10. Alcoholics Anonymous has no opinion on outside issues; hence, the AA name ought never to be drawn into public controversy.
11. Our public relations policy is based on attraction rather than promotion; we need always maintain personal anonymity at the level of press, radio, films, and TV (p. 78).
12. Anonymity is the spiritual foundation of our traditions, ever reminding us to place principles before personalities.

In 1955, twenty years following the offical founding of AA, a conference was held in St. Louis, Missouri, commemorating its birth. The General Service Council of AA was to be named as the permanent successor to the co-founders of AA (W., 1957, p. 1). This conference was highlighted by the advancements and acceptance of AA in the areas of industry, prison systems, and state hospitals (W., 1957, p. 5).

Tiebout (1955) points out that research and treatment in the field of alcoholism has repeatedly met with failure. He attributes this failure to a lack of understanding concerning the basic philosophies of AA. Investigators have approached the problem from an orientation specific to their own profession without considering a specialized AA approach. This outlook usually results in fruitless efforts to explain causality and does not deal with the disease entity as it is manifested in the individual. He adds that investigators usually quit after one attempt in this specialized field of study.

The most successful treatment of the alcoholic has, in the past, been given by recovered alcoholics. Most authorities agree that any individual who works with an alcoholic patient or client must have a thorough knowledge of the workings of AA, as well as a dynamic approach to problem drinking.

At the present time, alcoholism is listed as the nation's third leading health problem, second only to mental illness and cardiovascular disease (Block, 1962, p. 19). In 1955 the estimated number of alcoholics in the United States was approximately five million. In 1965, a statistical survey published by the National Council on Alcoholism (NCA) approximated this figure at six million. In 1971 the National Institute on Alcohol Abuse and Alcoholism estimated the number of alcoholics in the United States at nine million.

The primary source of help for those who seek it, is AA. Local chapters exist in almost every city with a fairly large population. There is no accurate method of determining the size of membership, but it is estimated that there are over three hundred thousand members in AA today (Block, 1962, p. 152). There is a markedly higher number of individuals estimated to have a severe drinking problem than there are individuals who seek help for such difficulties.

Definitions and Drinking Patterns in Alcoholism

Block (1962) reviews some of the more accepted definitions of this disease. They are as follows:

E. M. Jellinek, former consultant to the World Council of Alcohol: Alcoholism is a progressive disease characterized by uncontrollable drinking.
Howard J. Clinebell: An alcoholic is anyone whose drinking interferes frequently or continuously with any other important life adjustment or interpersonal relationship.
Harold W. Lovell, former President of the NCA: Alcoholism is a condition characterized by uncontrollable compulsive drinking.
Marty Mann, Founder and Executive Director of NCA: The disease which manifests itself chiefly by the uncontrollable drinking of the victim, who is known as the alcoholic.
World Health Organization's Expert Committee: Any form of drinking which in its extent goes beyond the tradition and customary "dietary" use or the ordinary compliance with the social customs of the whole community concerned, irrespective of the etiological factors leading to such behavior, and irrespective also to the extent of which such etiological factors are dependent upon heredity, constitution, or acquired physiopathological and metabolic influences (pp. 20-21).

Block (1962) continues that alcoholism is a deviate pattern of social behavior. He adds to the above mentioned definitions, the phrase "continuing adverse effects upon the individual or his family or the community." The major impact of the importance of the social implications is further stressed by Bacon (1962). It is his opinion that cultural and subcultural mores determine the recognition of the problem, the stigma attached, and the avenue taken for treatment or non-treatment. Bacon feels that one cannot speak of alcoholism in general, but rather of specific groups of alcoholics. He adds that symptoms are constantly changing as an individual reaches a different stage and that the symptoms become more pronounced as the disease progresses.

Murphy (1961) reviewed some of Jellinek's major works. He states that Jellinek is considered the foremost authority on alcoholism. Jellinek distinguishes the five major types of alcoholics as: (1) Alpha: Alcohol is primarily used to relieve psychological threat or pain. This pattern is not totally uncontrollable, abstaining is not unattainable, and the pattern is not progressive. (2) Beta: In this group numerous physical symptoms occur with the dependence on alcohol. (3) Gamma: There is increased tissue tolerance to alcohol and adaptive cell metabolism. Withdrawal symptoms and craving occur. A loss of control is present, and the disease progresses from psychological to physical. Marked behavior changes occur. This is the most common type of alcoholism found in the United States. (4) Delta: This group is differentiated only from the Gamma type in that the loss of control is replaced by the inability to abstain. (5) Epsilon: This category describes the periodic alcoholic. An individual in this category formerly was more commonly classified as dipsomaniac. Less information is available on this group than the other four.

Fox (1957) approaches the typology on a more behavioral, or causal basis. The following trichotomy separates (a) those individuals who began drinking following some traumatic or crisis incident, (b) those persons who drink to relieve neurotic symptoms acquired somewhat later in life, and (c) those essential alcoholics who began drinking early due to pathological reasons or for no apparent reason.

Bolman (1965) dichotomizes the alcoholic population with terms of essential and reactive alcoholism. Essential alcoholism exists where no apparent cause can be found, and the drinking pattern starts very early in life. The reactive alcoholic, conversely, has at one time been able to function adequately in an adult situation for at least some short time, but following some unpleasant event or events, has turned to drinking for escape.

Review of the Literature

The recent literature on alcoholism shows a wide variety of approaches to examining the problem. Many studies have been concerned with identifying special physical, personality, motivational, intellectual, and familial characteristics of alcoholics. Other investigators have attempted to differentiate the alcoholic population from a normal group. This approach has been carried further by attempting to show distinct groups within the total population of alcoholics. There have also been several attempts to associate particular characteristics with participation, success and failure in therapy programs. Finally, numerous hypothetical constructions based on various personality theories have been tested.

Even though the problem of alcoholism has been approached from various areas, little agreement is shared on alcoholic personality types. It is widely agreed that therapeutic treatment programs are valuable; however, it is not evident what changes occur in this treatment. Also, no particular criteria associated with successful alcoholic rehabilitation are apparent from the current studies.

Variables Associated with Alcoholism

The past several years have seen an increased interest in associating certain variables with the cause of alcoholism and the continued use of alcohol. Many of the variables assumed to be correlated with alcoholism are not frequently replicated in other studies. It will be shown later, however, that the factor of dependence is quite common in studies on alcoholism. There seems to be a positive correlation between a high dependency need and successful alcoholic rehabilitation.

Viaille (1963), in a search of the literature through 1960, states that there is a poverty of information in this area. He attempted to relate a number of variables to successful or non-successful alcoholic rehabilitation, but he found no particular situation variable associated with the ability to remain sober.

Moore and Ramseur (1960) gathered biographical data on one hundred hospitalized alcoholics and their families. They found that no particular variable could be isolated as a direct result of alcoholism. They did, however, find several interesting common characteristics in their sample of alcoholics, such as a high average intellectual level and an extremely unstable work history. Seventy-three percent were considered alcoholic before the age of thirty, and the home situation was very unstable and divorce more common than not. Finally, most of the subjects began drinking in the adolescent years.

Fitzhugh (1965) found that although alcoholic subjects did not differ from controls on a general intelligence factor, they did do more poorly on tasks involving abstraction and adaptive abilities. He also found that older alcoholics did significantly poorer work than younger alcoholics on these same tasks.

Mechanic (1962) in a study of attitudes among hospitalized alcoholics, found that those individuals who expressed intentions to drink again had fathers who did not drink. Further, they viewed the community as not disapproving of drinking, and this group fell at the lower end of the dependency variable.

Hershenson (1965) using self-report instruments with twenty male alcoholic subjects found that the need for self-identity was associated with a need for excessive drinking during stress situations. With the intake of alcohol, the identity need seemed to become less threatening. The subjects expressed that they did not desire to drink in the face of stress, but the crisis did lead to drinking more readily and that this first drink led to drunkenness.

Alcoholic Groups and the Normal Population

The most widely psychometric device employed in research with the alcoholic has been the Minnesota Multiphasic Personality Inventory (MMPI). Manson (1949) administered this test to 123 alcoholics and compared them to a similar group of normal subjects. Within the group of alcoholics there were active drinkers and AA members. He could find no significant differences between these two groups; but when these groups were combined and compared with a normal population, he found a significantly higher *Pd* scale in the alcoholic population. This study suggested that although this test could differentiate the alcoholic from the normal, subgroups of alcoholics did not differ significantly. Rosen (1960), using the same test with varied groups of alcoholics, such as private clinics, hospitals, skid row bums, and adolescent problem drinkers, did find significant difference between these groups. He concluded that grouping all alcoholics as a single unit for experimental purposes constituted a definite sampling error.

Heartzen and Hill (1959) administered the MMPI to two hundred alcoholics, two hundred drug addicts, and two hundred criminals in an attempt to identify specific characteristics with specific groups. A factor analysis of all six hundred profiles showed a first order factor which they called undifferentiated psychopathology. All three groups loaded on the *Pd* scale. Further, they found a second order, bipolar factor. The alcoholics loaded heavily on the *D, Pd* negative end, while the criminals loaded heavily on the *Pd, Ma* positive end, and the drug addicts fell between these two groups. The authors concluded from these results that alcoholics as a group were more neurotic, while criminals showed a more clearly psychopathic pattern. Such findings could explain why alcoholics as an unselected group would significantly differ from a normal population, especially on the *Pd* scale of the MMPI. This study also suggests the necessity of accounting for criminal records in any given sample of alcoholics.

MacAndrews and Geertsma (1963), after reviewing the literature, stated that the MMPI has been more effective than all other measures, including projective techniques, in assessing personality characteristics of the alcoholic. From these studies they believe that the *Pd* scale has yielded more results than the other MMPI scales. They administered the MMPI to two hundred male hospitalized alcoholics and two hundred male non-alcoholics from a private clinic. All of the subjects were volunteers. A factor analysis of the *Pd* scale showed five distinct factors: (1) desurgency, (2) acceptance by others, (3) discontent with family situations, (4) social deviance, and (5) remorseful intrapunitiveness. The alcoholic group scored significantly higher on factors (4) and (5). When the three most discriminating items were removed from these factors, the mean significance disappeared. Those items were: (1) used alcohol excessively, (2) have been in trouble with the law, and (3) have not lived the right kind of life.

MacAndrews (1965), using the identical groups as those mentioned widely used alcoholic scales derived from the MMPI by Hampton, Holmes, Hoyett, and Sedlacek. They found that out of 191 items shared by all three scales, only seven items were common to all three. These scales had been shown to differentiate alcoholics from a normal population. MacAndrews and Geertsma applied each of the three scales to a group of three hundred male psychiatric patients. It was found that none of the three scales could significantly differentiate the two groups. It was concluded that these scales were not actually measuring alcoholism but were general measures of mal-adjustment.

MacAndrews (1965), using the identical groups as those mentioned above, attempted to differentiate alcoholics from a general psychiatric population. An item analysis from the MMPI was computed. Fifty-one items were found significant in isolating the alcoholic group. Two of the items dealt directly with drinking and were therefore deleted. The forty-nine item scale was able to differentiate the two groups at the .001 level of confidence. It was concluded that this scale would be of clinical value since it could discriminate between patient groups rather than simply differentiating a normal population from a maladjusted population.

From the studies using the MMPI mentioned previously, it is difficult to assign any particular set of personality characteristics or symptoms to the alcoholic. The ability to differentiate the alcoholic from the normal population has not proven to add much information to the area. If this is the case, it might then be profitable to review some of the studies that attempt to demonstrate drinkers as a separate group.

Seiden (1960) administered the Bender Gestalt to a matched group of fifty AA members and fifty alcoholics who were not AA members. Using the Pascal and Suttle scoring method, he found significant differences between the two groups. This study would support the sampling error postulate mentioned previously by Rosen (1960). Seiden concluded that the AA members show a greater degree of ego strength, and further postulated that the degree of ego strength might be related to the length of sobriety.

Williams (1965) investigated the self-concept variable in an attempt to explain causality in alcoholics. The subjects were college students consisting of those individuals who had a drinking problem and those persons who had no difficulty with alcohol. The problem drinkers were highly self-critical with lowered self-acceptance and a wide discrepancy in self-ideal self. This finding would, in part, support Seiden's conclusions. Wine and Edwards (1964) attempted to isolate personality factors in temperate and intemperate groups. Seventy-eight male hospitalized patients were administered the Comrey Dependence Scale. While this factor did not differentiate the groups, two variables included in the factor did show significance. The intemperate group was significantly higher on shyness and anxiety.

Another attempt to dichotomize AA members was done by Machover, Puzzo, and Plumeau (1962). They administered the Alport Vernon Lindsey study of values to twenty-three AA members of long sobriety, twenty-three AA members of periodic sobriety, and a matched control group. No differences in value structure could be found; however, the alcoholics as a group showed significantly more scatter, suggesting to the authors a more neurotic profile than the control group. Ramsey, Jansen, and Sommer (1963) administered the same test to forty-seven hospitalized alcoholics before and after therapy. Individual psychotherapy with the use of LSD 25 was the treatment variable. The only significant difference found was post-therapy increase in religious values. These profiles were compared with Machover's (1962) hospital population. Both groups showed low esthetic values, and the hospital group showed higher peaks on religious and social values.

Testing Specific Postulates

Aside from experimental studies attempting to differentiate alcoholics from normal subjects and to isolate particular sub-groups of alcoholics, there are several studies investigating specific hypothetical constructs. Gibbins and Walters (1961), following the psychoanalytic assumptions that alcoholism is a function of latent homosexuality, tested male groups of sixteen homosexuals, thirteen alcoholics, and twenty controls. The subjects were shown a series of sex symbols and responded either masculine or feminine. The homosexuals differed significantly from the normals, but the alcoholics did not differ significantly from either group. The authors felt that the psychoanalytic theory of homosexual tendencies in alcoholics could not be confirmed. They did, however, point out that the results did warrant more investigation. Meer and Ammons (1963), from another psychoanalytic point of view, studied identification processes in alcoholics. They administered the Photo Preference Test to three groups of male subjects consisting of 145 alcoholics jailed for being drunk, 67 hospitalized alcoholics, and 77 controls. Factor analysis did not differentiate the alcoholics from the control subjects on one of the factors which was the family-parental attitude factor. They showed negative attitude toward older men, interpreted as rejection of the father, and positive attitude of older women, interpreted as searching for the symbolic mother. These results suggested dependency and fear of competition. The authors postulated that many of the alcoholics failed to learn how to achieve gratification in an environment that demands successful striving for realistic goals. They believe that this finding may be due basically to the alcoholic's inability to make an adequate masculine identity.

Vogel (1961) states that the failure of research to show particular personality traits leads one to think that alcoholism is simply a symptom and not a disease. He examined the relationship between drinking patterns and introversion-extraversion by administering the Maudsley Personality Inventory to fifty-eight hospitalized alcoholics. Introverts tended to show steady and solitary drinking patterns. Extraverts were associated with periodic solitary drinking with frequently more blackouts than the introverts.

Griener (1961) attempted to clarify one reason for the alcoholic's abnormalities. He tested twenty AA members and twenty nonalcoholics of college level on recall of pleasant and unpleasant words associated with nonsense syllables. He found that the AA members showed a significantly higher recall rate of unpleasant words than did the control group. This inhibited recall may be a lowered ability for selective forgetting of anxiety provoking words, therefore a psychologically damaging process. It might be assumed, however, that this AA group is a representative sample of successful rehabilitation and that such a psychological set is actually a good prognostic sign in the treatment of alcoholism.

Another method of assessing personality traits, other than objective or projective tests, was demonstrated by Bailey (1965) using perceptual approaches. He administered the Witkin Rod and Frame Test to AA members, a group of patients diagnosed as chronic brain syndrome (CBS) with psychosis, and a group of normal subjects. The AA members and CBS both differed significantly from the normal group in what the author called field dependency. He believes, however, that the suggestion that dependent individuals are predisposed to alcoholism is yet premature. Voth (1963) believes that perceptual performance does suggest basic personality structure. He tested 473 hospitalized alcoholics and 432 normal subjects with the autokinetic stimulus. The alcoholics perceived five times as much movement as did the normal subjects. The author states that these results support those mentioned by Bailey (1965) and further agrees that alcoholics are field dependent, indicating that suggestibility reflects dependency, and that alcoholics react more frequently on this trait than normal subjects.

Voth (1965), with a similar, but slightly increased sample, found that those alcoholics who show a lower suggestibility tend to escape from the hospital and are more frequently readmitted than those alcoholics who show more movement perception on the autokinetic task. This finding leads the author to believe that suggestible and dependent alcoholics show better prognostic indications than do the more independent group. Coopersmith (1963) studied the perceptual defense structure of hospitalized alcoholics and normal subjects. Emotionally loaded and neutral words were presented to subjects at both the prethreshold and threshold level with GSR recordings and verbal responses following each word. The alcoholics showed more threat at the prerecognition level and also became more verbally defensive at the recognition level. The author postulates that this over-responding pattern is, in part, due to the alcoholic's limited defense system. The alcoholic shows more sensitivity to threat without the capacity to discriminate selectively threatening from nonthreatening stimuli. A higher degree of dependence on external stimuli is suggested as one reason that an individual turns to alcohol. Alcohol seems to lessen the intensity of such stimuli.

Alcoholic Treatment Programs and Their Results

Although experimentation concerning personality structure of the alcoholic is not conclusive, many of the inferences drawn from these studies can be applied to treatment programs and many new hypotheses tested. Slicer (1965), Bolman (1965), and many others suggest that the overcrowded conditions, especially in the state mental hospitals, make it increasingly necessary to identify those patients who have optimal chances for at least partial recovery. Each year brings a large increase in the number of alcoholics admitted to state hospital treatment programs. Matkom (1965) reviews several studies showing representative increases. In the New York state hospital system, the rate increased fourfold from 1957 through 1960. In Wisconsin, alcoholics presently comprise 25 percent of first-admission patients. Spern, Morrow, and Peterson (1965) report in all first admission patients. Alcoholic males account for as high as 40 percent and females 15 percent of this population. The male alcoholics are the leading first-admission diagnoses while the females rank third. These percentages have increased since 1945, 22 and 5 percent respectively. Alcoholic admissions are usually short term as compared to those patients with other diagnoses. Spern *et al.,* (1965) point out that 90 percent of the alcoholic patients are back in society within three months, and 96 percent are returned within six months.

Male-Female Ratios

The admission trends through the present time have shown the rate of male alcoholics far exceeding that of female alcoholics. Research in the field of alcoholism has reflected such tendencies by either selecting all male populations or combining both males and females in one sample.

Although the overall number of males yet exceeds that of females, the female percentage of increase over the past several years is slightly higher than the male. Voth (1963) estimated the ratio at about eight to one, male over female. In a later estimate, Locke and Duvall (1965) reported a four or five to one ratio. Bailey (1965), in a community survey of problem drinkers, found a 3.6 to one ratio. Spern *et al.,* (1965) estimate that the male to female ratio is steadily closing and at present is approximately three to one.

In 1962, the Texas State Hospital System admitted 2,294 patients to the alcoholic treatment program. Of this number 1,932 were male while 362 were female. This figure indicates a ratio of almost six to one. Block (1962) suggests that there is little doubt that females will become more a part of the treatment program. He states that little differences have been found in the personality patterns of male and female alcoholics in the Sixteen Personality Factor Questionnaire (16PF). Distler, May, and Tuma (1964) found that in order to differentiate response to hospital treatment, male and female schizophrenics had to be examined as separate groups. Little attention has been paid to this area in the field of alcoholism.

Belfer, Shader, Carroll, and Harmatz (1971) state that the number of female alcoholics is steadily increasing and further add that the differences in male and female alcoholics might suggest treatment specific to that group. As an example of this specialty need, these authors postulate that the drinking pattern in some females is directly related to the premenstrual cycle and did report good results in a limited number of patients using anti-anxiety agents, chlordiazepoxide and diazepam, when the premenstrual cycle occurs. These authors further suggested that female alcoholics show a higher level of anxiety as well as more pronounced depressive features, as opposed to male alcoholics. Their review of the literature through 1970 did indicate that more experimental data is needed.

Type of Program

Matkom (1965) pointed out that alcoholics are proud of their symptoms of heavy drinking and need the fellowship of others with similar problems. Most of the programs reported in the literature provide group and individual psychotherapy (Bolman, 1965; Mindlin, 1964; Strayer, 1961; and Pattison, 1966), some few use hypnotherapy (Ramsey, Jensen, and Sommer, 1963; and Reinhart, 1965), while some use conditioned reflex therapy (Kapner, 1965; and Clancy, 1964). Also many programs have employed the use of LSD 25 (Smart and Storm, 1954, and Jensen, 1962); others have tried the use of such drugs as disulfiram (Chambers and Schultz, 1964; and Wedel, 1965). It is generally seen, however, that the AA approach is the core of the alcoholic treatment programs. Bolman (1965) found that if the patient had the choice, only about 6 percent would volunteer for the other therapies.

Voth (1963) summarizes a state hospital setting. He states the program is educational in nature with a rather direct approach. A didactic approach with analogies and suggestions seems to yield the best results. Specificities, rather than abstractions, are more meaningful to the alcoholic. A reality orientation is stressed. Resentment, hostility, and self-castigation are suggested to be the difficult areas for the alcoholic. It is postulated by Voth that if the central structure of the alcoholic personality were known, the method of treatment could become more controlled and scientific.

Many of the state hospital treatment programs for alcoholics are based on the philosophies of AA. Most of the counselors are active AA members and are not necessarily professionally trained. Alcoholic patients can enter the state hospital program by either court or voluntary admission. Those patients who have a history of excessive drinking are accepted in the special program if other treatment plans are not indicated. Although many individuals show resistance to the alcoholic treatment program, final acceptance is on a personal basis as can be found in the preamble of Alcoholics Anonymous (Block, 1962, p. 145).

> Alcoholics Anonymous is a fellowship of men and women who share their experience, strength, and hope with each other that they may solve their common problem and help others to recover from alcoholism.
> The only requirement for membership is a desire to stop drinking. There are no

dues or fees for A. A. membership. It is self-supporting through contributions. A. A. is not allied with any sect, denomination, political group, organization, or institution; does not wish to engage in any controversy; neither endorses nor opposes any causes. Its primary cause is to stay sober and help other alcoholics to achieve sobriety.

The goals and methods of the program are laid down by the famous twelve steps of AA (Anonymous, 1954, pp. 71-72).

1. We admitted we were powerless over alcohol, that our lives had become unmanageable.
2. Came to believe that a Power greater than ourselves could restore us to sanity.
3. Made a decision to turn our will and our lives over to the care of God as we understood Him.
4. Made a searching and fearless moral inventory of ourselves.
5. Admitted to God, to ourselves, and to another human being the exact nature of our wrongs.
6. Were entirely ready to have God remove all these defects of character.
7. Humbly asked Him to remove our shortcomings.
8. Made a list of all persons we had harmed, and became willing to make amends to them all.
9. Made direct amends to such people wherever possible, except when to do so would injure them or others.
10. Continued to take personal inventory and when we were wrong promptly admitted it.
11. Sought through prayer and meditation to improve our conscious contact with God as we understood Him praying only for knowledge of His will for us and the power to carry that out.
12. Having had a spiritual awakening as the result of those steps we tried to carry this message to alcoholics, and to practice these principles in all our affairs (p. 145).

Although formal religion is not practiced in AA, belief in a Higher Power is ever present. The Serenity Prayer is considered the creed of the alcoholic (Anonymous, 1957, p. 196).

God grant us the serenity to accept things we cannot change, courage to change the things we can, and wisdom to know the difference (p. 196).

Fox (1968) emphasizes the strong role that is played by the AA philosophy, along with group techniques, but states that a multidisciplinary approach is essential to any adequate treatment program. She summarizes the effectiveness of each of the modalities comprising a comprehensive approach to the treatment of alcoholism.

Fox believes that group psychotherapy, along with AA, is the most effective and elicits the most far-reaching positive results. She includes in the modality, the various related techniques, such as psychodrama, role reversal, etc. She feels that hypnotherapy is only useful in an adjunctive manner for relaxation and temporary anxiety reduction. She believes that disulfiram programs are relatively unproductive when they are a major emphasis of treatment. She does point out, however, that this drug does aid in reducing the number of traumatic decisions that an alcoholic must make each day. If the alcoholic decides to take disulfiram in the morning, the necessity of further decisions concerning whether or not he will drink during that day are eliminated. LSD studies offer some promise, but Fox believes a moratorium on this drug is necessary until the question of chromosomal damage is clarified.

PROGNOSIS

In an attempt to discover which psychological areas were more related to improvement, several studies were completed. Armstrong and Hoyt (1963) attempted to measure changes in personality in hospitalized alcoholics. They administered the IES before and after therapy to twenty-five male alcoholics. The time between testing was three weeks. They found that the self-concept remained constant. Alcoholics were guilt-ridden on admission; then later, a slight suppression of the super ego was manifested. Ego strength increased to some degree, but not significantly. They could find no difference between those who attended group therapy and those who attended only the AA meetings. The authors suggest that many alcoholics are psychopathic, and for this reason, show no basic personality changes over a short period of time.

Another point of view that would directly affect the structure of a treatment program is presented by Clancy (1961). He believes that alcoholism is a symptom rather than a disease. It is stressed that the alcoholic consciously employs denial and rationalization in order not to quit drinking. Therefore, it is necessary to deal directly with these defenses before therapy can be effective. Strayer (1961) supported this position by stating that confrontation is a necessity in a group therapy program for alcoholics.

A means of examining the above mentioned position was employed by Moore and Murphy (1960). These authors administered a five-point rating scale of denial to one hundred institutionalized male alcoholics. The ratings were completed by staff members with a score of four (meaning complete denial) and zero (meaning complete acceptance). The sixty-five patients who were considered generally unimproved showed a 3.2 score on admission and also a 3.2 at discharge. The thirty-five patients who were rated as generally improved on a similar four-point scale, scored 2.7 at admission and 2.1 at discharge. Those patients who showed the most improvement after a follow-up (105 on the scale) received a score of 2.7 at admission and 1.3 upon discharge.

An important variable pointed out earlier was success as it was related to the length of stay in therapy. Davis and Dittman (1963) demonstrated that court referred alcoholics voluntarily attended therapy as well as non-alcoholic, psychiatric self-referred patients. Demone (1963), working with a sample of two hundred alcoholics from a correctional institution, supported this position. He speculated that with the proper encouragement from a team approach, alcoholics from this particular population could be successfully treated.

It is pointed out by Blane and Meyers (1963) that the alcoholic who is overtly dependent will stay longer in therapy and relate better to the therapist. They implied that perhaps a different approach should be taken with the patient who does not show this particular dependency. If one follows the position of the writers mentioned above, a guarded prognosis would have to be given to those patients showing denial of the problem or a low degree of dependency.

Karp, Witkin, and Goodenough (1965) examined the postulate that dependency correlated with the degree of alcoholism. They administered the Rod and Frame and the Imbedded Figures Test to groups of active and recovered alcoholics. The two groups could not be significantly differentiated. They concluded that dependency does not decrease with sobriety, but is a precondition for alcoholism. Although this finding may be a route to the causality problem, it does not lend support to establishing prognostic values.

Zax, Marsey, and Biggs (1961) stated that those patients who are self-referred and who show more stability in the marriage relationship, remain longer in treatment. Corotto's (1963) findings reflect a different viewpoint concerning this stability factor among alcoholics. He administered the California Psychological Inventory to a group of hospitalized, male alcoholics. A group of sixty-one subjects who volunteered for further treatment was compared with a group of 114 who requested discharge after the thirty day commitment. Nine of the eighteen scales significantly differentiated the groups. The non-volunteers scored significantly higher on: (1) well being, (2) socialization, (3) self-tolerance, (4) tolerance, (5) good impression achievement via conformance, and (6) psychological mindness scale. This author postulates that volunteers seem to be less socially and psychologically well-adjusted. This finding should be an important consideration in the planning of a treatment program.

Dittman (1968) states that there are no specific rules for prognosis, but through his experience he postulates several generalities. The homeless, divorced, physically ill, unemployed, poor, uneducated, non-achievers and minority groups have the poorest prognosis. The alcoholic past fifty has a better prognosis than the younger, probably because he cannot stand the physical abuse of drinking.

In most cases, the primary concern of an individual who has been drinking excessively for a long period of time is physical restoration. The patient must be relatively free of the extreme physical symptoms produced by prolonged drinking before any type of counseling can begin. Previously, in many cases, it was advisable for the family of the alcoholic to have the patient hospitalized if he or she would not willingly consent to treatment. An increasing problem in the treatment and care of the alcoholic was the revolving door policy of many facilities that admitted alcoholic patients for a short time period. Such treatment policies were simply the physical restoration of the patient without considering the many social-psychological components of the alcoholic patient. Instead of hospitalization, many alcoholics were being jailed in their acute stages of intoxication with inadequate, or in many instances, no treatment facilities available to them. Following the case of Easter *vs* the District of Columbia (1966), it was ruled that alcoholics were to be treated as sick persons and not criminals, and that when an individual was confined for intoxication, treatment facilities must be available.

Following this court decision, a detoxification unit, that was later to be used as a model for many such centers, was established in Washington, D.C. The purpose of the seventy-five bed center is essentially to arrest and improve the physical deterioration of the acutely ill alcoholic, and in addition, to motivate the patient to seek further help for the problem. The maximum length of stay in this center is seventy-two hours, during which time the patient receives vitamins, tranquilizers, and anti-convulsants, if a need is indicated. The patients are introduced to, and do attend, the AA meetings, as well as group psychotherapy conducted at this center by a social worker and an R.N. Since most alcoholics who have been on a prolonged drinking episode have poor nutritional habits, the center employs a nutritionist who assists the patients in planning a proper diet. Before the patient is discharged, he or she meets with the staff for discharge planning and usually is urged to seek further help from a mental health center or AA.

This detoxification center won the American Psychiatric Association Silver Award for its pioneering efforts in this area. It was shown that alcoholics in the acute phases of their illness could be successfully treated without hospitalization or incarceration (Hammersley, 1971).

Not all of those individuals seeking help for an alcoholic problem enter the state hospital or even spend several days in a detoxification unit. AA does provide a crisis intervention program handled by its members. Those individuals receiving help through these means many times do not seek further professional assistance, especially if the AA program is successful. Some local community mental health centers also receive and treat alcoholics on an out-patient basis. Such treatment centers are only successful when they offer a gamit of services including group and/or individual therapy, social services, and vocational rehabilitation services. The patient also can be referred for physical care if and when it becomes necessary.

Vogel (1961) suggests that alcoholics are better treated in a mixed group with patients who have problems other than alcoholism. He includes both neurotic and psychotic categories in this treatment philosophy. This mixed group prevents the repetitive discussion of drinking habits and escapades as a defense against dealing with some of the underlying causes. Most treatment programs, both in-patient and out-patient, however, consider alcoholic patients as a homogeneous group, and comprise therapy groups accordingly. Any definite direction or informative research in this therapeutic area is not available at present. When the alcoholic comes for therapy, it is vital to accept him as soon as possible. With these individuals, delay is rejection and the alcoholic will probably return to his previous drinking habits. Whether or not the alcoholic is to begin therapy while still drinking is determined by the individual therapist. If the drinking pattern is not too destructive then therapy can begin; but if the drinking habit is too pronounced, he is usually told to come back when he is sober.

Sobriety is not the only goal of therapy as it can only be maintained if the maladaptive behavior is improved. Most workers in the field of alcoholism follow the assumption that the goal of therapy is the arrest of the disease and not cure. For some time following disuse of alcohol, fantasies and dreams of deprivation are quite common and should not be viewed in a negative light by either the patient or therapist.

In 1939, Tiebout (1955), who is considered the first professional to affiliate with AA, postulated one essential to sobriety. To this author, the surrender-compliance hypothesis is all important. Compliance is the verbal and superficial acceptance of the problem that one is an alcoholic. Surrender is necessary for sobriety, and in order to remain sober, an alcoholic must fully, emotionally, and totally accept that he or she is an alcoholic and cannot take even one drink. To Tiebout, true acceptance comes from the admission to oneself and others that he or she is an alcoholic, and such surrender comprises the basic essential of sobriety.

Bell (1965) suggests that the first two years of sobriety are the most difficult and those individuals who have passed this point in treatment can be considered as very good candidates for rehabilitation services.

Presently, in most of the alcoholic treatment and rehabilitation programs, at least two factions have the possibility of clashing with each other. These broad disciplines are those individuals supporting the more traditional AA views and attitudes, and those professional disciplines advocating psychotherapeutic approaches in their multiple forms. One of these treatment procedures certainly does not contra-indicate the other; in fact, many experts agree that the simultaneous application of these treatments is preferable. It is important, however, that workers in the field of alcoholism understand the historical difficulties in bringing these elements together and the probability that the potential for alienation of these groups could be quite detrimental to treatment outcome.

REFERENCES

Alumbaugh, R. V., Davis, H. G., and Sweney, A.B.: A comparison of methods of constructing predictive instruments. *Educational and Psychological Measurement, 29*:369-651, 1969.

Anonymous: *Alcoholics Anonymous.* New York, Alcoholics Anonymous, 1954.

Anonymous: *Alcoholics Anonymous Comes of Age,* 1957.

Armstrong, R. G., and Hoyt, D. D.: Personality structure of male alcoholics as reflected in the IES test. *Quart J Stud Alcohol, 24*:239-249, 1963.

Atwell, C. R., and Wells, P. L.: *Wide Range Vocabulary Test.* New York, Psychological Corp., 1937.

Bacon, S. D.: Socia! setting conducive to the alcoholic. *A Manual on Alcoholism.* American Medical Association, pp. 61-74, 1962.

Bailey, M. B., Haberman, P. W., and Alkane, H.: The epidemiology of alcoholism in an urban residential area. *Quart J Stud Alcohol, 22*:187-393, 1965.

Belfer, M. L., Shader, R. I., Carroll, M., and Harmatz, J. S., Alcoholism in women. *Archives of General Psychiatry, 25*(No. 6):540, 1971.

Bell, R. G.: Defensive thinking in alcoholic addicts. *Canad Med Assoc J, 92*:228-236, 1965.

Bernstein, A. S., Klein, E. R., Barger, L. and Cohen, J.: Relationship between institution, other demographic variables, and the structure of intelligence in chronic schizophrenics. *J Consult Psychol, 29*:320-324, 1965.

Blane, H. T., and Meyers, W. R.: Behavioral dependence and length of stay in psychotherapy among alcoholics. *Quart J Stud Alcohol, 24*:503-511, 1963.

Block, M. A.: *Alcoholism: Its Facets and Phases.* New York, John Day, 1962.

Bolman, W. M.: Abstinence versus permissiveness in the psychotherapy of alcoholism. *Arch Gen Psychiatry,* Vol. 12, 1965.

C., Bill: The growth and effectiveness of Alcoholics Anonymous in a southwestern city. *Quart J Stud Alcohol, 26*:279-285, 1965.

Cattell, R. B.: *Handbook for the Sixteen Personality Factor Questionnaire.* Champaign, Ill., Institute for Personality and Ability Testing, 1957.

Chambers, J. F., and Schultz, J. D.: Double-blind study of three drugs in the treatment of acute alcoholic states. *Quart J Stud Alcohol, 25*:10-18, 1964.

Clancy, J.: Motivation conflicts of the alcohol addict. *Quart J Stud Alcohol, 25*: 511-519, 1964.

Coopersmith, S.: Adaptive reactions of alcoholics and nonalcoholics. *Quart J Stud Alcohol, 24*:495-503, 1963.

Corotto, L. V.: An exploratory study of the personality characteristic of alcoholic patients who volunteer for continued treatment. *Quart J Stud Alcohol, 24*: 432-443, 1963.

Davis, F. M., and Dittman, K. S.: The effect of court referral and disulfiram on motivation of alcoholics: A preliminary. *Quart J Stud Alcohol, 24*:495-503, 1963.

Davis, Harry G., Rich, Charles, C.: Concurrent validity of MMPI alcoholism scales. *Journal of Clinical Psychology, 25*(No. 4):425-426.

Demone, H. W., Jr.: Experiments in referrals to alcoholism clinic. *Quart J Stud Alcohol, 24*:295-503, 1963.

Distler, L. S., May, P. R. A., and Tuma, A. H.: Anxiety and ego strength as predictors of response to treatment in schizophrenic patients. *J Consult Psychol, 28*:170-177, 1964.

Dittman, K.: Do we have a specific treatment for alcoholism? *International Journal of Psychiatry, 5*(No. 1):48-53, 1968.

Edwards, A. A.: *Statistical Methods for the Behavioral Sciences.* New York, Newhart and Co., 1954.

Fitzhugh, L. C., Fitzhugh, K. B., and Reitan, R. M.: Adaptive abilities and intellectual functioning of hospitalized alcoholics: Further considerations. *Quart J Stud Alcohol, 26*:393-401, 1965.

Fox, Ruth: A multidisciplinary approach to the treatment of alcoholism. *International Journal of Psychiatry, 5*(No. 1):34-44, 1968a.

Fox, Ruth: Reply to the critics. *International Journal of Psychiatry, 5*(No. 1): 65-71, 1968b.

Fox, Ruth: Treatment of alcoholism. In Himwick, E. E., (Ed.), *Alcoholism.* Washington, American Association for the Advancement of Sciences, Publication No. 47, 1957.

Fuller, G. B.: Research in alcoholism with the 16 P. F. Test. *IPAT Bull,* Vol. 12, 1965.

Gibbins, R., and Walters, J.: Latent homosexuality in alcoholics. *Quart J Stud Alcohol, 22*:501-560, 1961.

Goldstein, I. B.: A comparison between Taylor's and Freeman's Manifest Anxiety. *J Consult Psychol, 27*:466, 1963.

Griener, D. S.: Selective forgetting in alcoholics. *Quart J Stud Alcohol, 22*:580-587, 1961.

Griffith, R. M.: Rorschach water percepts: A study in conflicting results. *J American Psychol Assoc, 15*:307-311, 1961.

Hammersley, Donald W.: Silver award: Emergency care for alcoholics—The Alcohol Detoxification Center, Washington, D.C. *Hospital and Community Psychiatry, 22*(No. 10):302-305, 1971.

Heartzen, E. A., and Hill, H. F.: Effects of morphine and phenobarbital on differential MMPI profiles. *J Clin Psychol, 15*:434-437, 1959.

Hershenson, D. S.: Stress-induced use of alcohol by problem drinkers as a function of their sense of identity. *Quart J Stud Alcohol, 25*:213-222, 1965.

Jellinek, E. M.: *The Diseases Concept of Alcoholism.* New Haven, Conn., Hill House Press, 1960.

Jansen, S. E.: A treatment program for alcoholics in a mental hospital. *Quart J Stud Alcohol, 23*:315-320, 1962.

Kaisar, H. F.: The varinax criterion for analytic rotation in factor analysis. *Psychometrika, 23*:187-200, 1958.

Karp, S. A., Witkin, H. A., and Goodenough, D. R.: Alcoholism and psychological differentiation: Effect of achievement of sobriety on the dependency. *Quart J Stud Alcohol, 26*:580-585, 1965.

Kapner, Elaine: Application of learning theory to the etiology and treatment of alcoholism. *Quart J Stud Alcohol, 25*:303, 1965.

Locke, B. Z., and Duvall, Henrietta J.: Alcoholism among admissions in psychiatric facilities. *Quart J Stud Alcohol, 25*:305, 1965.

MacAndrews, C.: The differentiation of male alcoholic outpatients from non-alcoholic psychiatric outpatients by means of the MMPI. *Quart J Stud Alcohol, 26*:238-246, 1965.

MacAndrews, C., and Geertsma, R. H.: A critique of alcoholism scales derived from the MMPI. *Quart J Stud Alcohol, 25*:68-76, 1964.

MacAndrews, C., and Geertsma, R. H.: An analysis of responses of alcoholic to scale 4 of the MMPI. *Quart J Stud Alcohol, 23*:267-273, 1962.

Machover, S., Puzzo, F. S., and Plumeau, Francis E.: Values in Alcoholics. *Quart J Stud Alcohol, 23*:267-273, 1962.

Mann, Marty: Personal communication, 1965.

Manson, M. G. A.: A psychometric analysis of psychopathic characteristics of alcoholics. *J Consult Psychol, 13*:111-118, 1949.

Matkom, A. J.: The alcoholic in the state mental hospital. *Quart J Stud Alcohol, 25*:499-505, 1965.

Mechanic, D.: Factors associated with attitudes favorable to rehabilitation among committed alcoholic patients. *Quart J Stud Alcohol, 23*:624-633, 1962.

Meer, B., and Ammons, A. H.: Age-sex preference patterns of alcoholics and normals. *Quart J Stud Alcohol, 24*:417-432, 1963.

Miller, Gary D.: Mind-Body Identity: Implications for Alcoholism. Paper presented at the tenth Annual Institute on Alcohol Studies, Austin, Texas, 1967.

Mindlin, D. F.: Attitudes toward alcoholism and self-differences between three alcoholic groups. *Quart J Stud Alcohol, 25*:136-141, 1964.

Moore, R. A., and Murphy, T. C.: Denial of alcoholism as an obstacle to recovery. *Quart J Stud Alcohol, 21*:51-67, 1960.

Moore, R. A., and Ramseur, Frieda: Study of the background of 100 hospitalized veterans with alcoholism. *Quart J Stud Alcohol, 21*:51-67, 1960.

Murphy, D. G.: Disease called alcoholism. *Contemp Psychol, 6*:348-350, 1961.

Pattison, E. M.: A critique of alcoholism treatment concepts with special reference to abstinence. *Quart J Stud Alcohol, 17*:49-71, 1966.

Ramsey, R., Jansen, S., and Sommer, R.: Values in alcoholics after LSD-25. *Quart J Stud Alcohol, 24*:443-449, 1963.

Reinhart, R. T.: The alcoholism treatment program at Topeka Veterans Administration Hospital. *Quart J Stud Alcohol, 26*:574-579, 1965.

Robson, R. A. H., Paulus, T., and Clarke, G. G.: An evaluation of the effect of a clinic treatment program on the rehabilitation of alcoholic patients. *Quart J Stud Alcohol, 26*:264-278, 1963.

Rosen, A. C.: A comparative study of alcoholics and psychiatric patients with the MMPI. *Quart J Stud Alcohol, 11*:253-267, 1960.

Seiden, R. H.: The use of Alcoholics Anonymous members in research on alcoholism. *Quart J Stud Alcohol, 21*:506-510, 1960.

Silkworth: In publication.

Slicer, A.: Linking local, state and federal efforts to combat alcoholism. Paper read at the National Conference on Alcoholism, Springfield, 1965.

Smart, R. B., and Storm, T.: The efficacy of LSD in the treatment of alcoholism. *Quart J Stud Alcohol, 25*:333-338, 1954.

Spern, L. G., Morrow, M. F., and Peterson, G. D.: Trends in admissions to a state hospital. *Arch Gen Psychiatry, 6*:543-549, 1965.

Storm, T., and Smart, R. G.: Dissociation: A possible explanation of some features of alcoholism and implications for its treatment. *Quart J Stud Alcohol, 22*:471-480, 1961.

Strayer, R.: Social integration of alcoholics through prolonged group therapy *Quart J Stud Alcohol, 22*:471-480, 1961.

Suggerman, A. A., Reilly, D., and Albahary, R. S.: Social competence and essential reactive distinction in alcoholism. *Arch Gen Psychiatry, 12*:352-358, 1965.

Sweney, A. B.: *F.A.P. Manual.* Lubbock, Texas, Psychometric Research Bureau, 1963.

Tiebout, H. M.: The role of psychiatry in the field of alcoholism. *Quart J Stud Alcohol, 12*:52-57, 1951.

Tiebout, H. M.: Surrender versus compliance in therapy with special reference to alcoholism. *Quart J Stud Alcohol, 14*:52-58, 1953.

Tiebout, H. M.: The age factors in surrender in alcoholism. *Quart J Stud Alcohol, 15*:510-511, 1954.

Tiebout, H. M.: Crises and surrender in treating alcoholism. *Quart J Stud Alcohol, 25*:495-497, 1965.

Tiebout, H. M.: Perspectives in alcoholism. Paper read at the National States Conference on Alcoholism, St. Louis, Mo., 1955.

U.S. Department of Health, Education, and Welfare: National Institute on Alcohol Abuse and Alcoholism, Publication (HSM) No. 72-9019, 1971.

Viaille, H. C.: *A Study on Treatment Predictions of Male Alcoholics in a State Hospital.* Doctoral Dissertation, Texas Technological College, August, 1963.

Vogel, M. D.: The relationship of personality factors to drinking patterns of alcoholics. *Quart J Stud Alcohol, 27*:394-399, 1961.

Voth, A. C.: Autokinesis and alcoholism. *Quart J Stud Alcohol, 26*:412-422, 1965.

Voth, A. C.: Group therapy with hospitalized alcoholics. *Quart J Stud Alcohol, 24*:289-304, 1963.

W., Bill: When A.A. comes of age. In *Alcoholics Anonymous Comes of Age,* New York, Alcoholics Anonymous, pp. 1-234, 1957.

Wadel, H. L.: Involving alcoholics in treatment. *Quart J Stud Alcohol, 26*:468-479, 1965.

Williams, A. F.: Self-concepts of college problem drinkers. #1. A comparison with alcoholics. *Quart J Stud Alcohol, 25*:586-594, 1965.

Wilson, Wayne M., and Helm, Stanley: An alcoholism program tailored to community needs. *Hosp Community Psychiatry, 21* (No. 12): 406-408, 1970.

Wine, D. B., and Edwards, A. E.: Intemperance: Psychological and sociological concomitants. *Quart J Stud Alcohol, 25*:77-83, 1964.

Wolff, E., and Holland, Lydia: A questionnaire follow-up of alcoholic patients. *Quart J Stud Alcohol, 25*:163-170, 1964.

Zax, M., Marsey, Ruth, and Biggs, C.: Demographic characteristics of alcoholism outpatients and the tendency to remain in treatment. *Quart J Stud Alcohol, 22*:90-115, 1961.

Chapter 10

THE DRUG ABUSE PROGRAM OF THE
TEXAS REHABILITATION COMMISSION

LARRY C. RHOADES

THE PROGRAM of Vocational Rehabilitation has been in existence to serve the handicapped citizens of Texas since 1929. Initially, the physically handicapped alone were eligible for services. In the early 1940's the mentally ill were included as eligible, and a few individual cases were served. The first thrust toward serving this group of handicapped individuals came in 1957 when joint agreements were entered into between the Division of Vocational Rehabilitation of the Texas Education Agency and the Texas Department of Hospital and Special Schools (now known as Department of Mental Health and Mental Retardation).

The 1966 amendments to the Vocational Rehabilitation Act added the alcoholic and the drug addict to the list of vocational handicapping conditions, and programs to serve the alcohol addict were developed. A vocational rehabilitation counselor was also assigned to work with narcotic addicts committed to the Clinical Research Center in Forth Worth. Training programs of the vocational type were developed at the Clinical Research Center and, to a limited degree, counselors in the field followed through providing services to the addict returning to his home community. In January 1970, drug abuse was added to the special program section of the Texas Rehabilitation Commission; and a consultant was appointed to develop the program.

The Texas Rehabilitation Commission has the sole responsibility for the *vocational* rehabilitation of the drug addict, drug abuser, and the drug dependent person who meets the criteria of eligibility. It is no longer a question of whether we will serve these handicapped individuals, rather it is a question of *how* we will serve them. The Texas Rehabilitation Commission does not actually rehabilitate the drug abuser. That process is carried out in highly specialized centers where well trained personnel are available. The Texas Rehabilitation Commission does provide vocational rehabilitation services to the individual who is psychologically, physically and habitually addicted to a drug.

PROPORTIONS OF THE PROBLEM

One of the questions most frequently asked regards the number of drug abusers in Texas. Unfortunately, there is no simple answer to the question; however, one method of estimating narcotic addiction is to project two hundred addicts for every overdose death. Thus, the fifty-six reported opiate deaths in Texas in 1971 (Texas Rehabilitation Commission, 1971) furnish a rough estimate. Utilizing this formula, one would calculate that there are 11,200 narcotic addicts in Texas. For this method of estimating to be meaningful, overdose deaths must be accurately detected. It must be recognized, however, that many drug deaths are not identified out of respect for the family.

One simple figure such as 11,200 narcotic addicts in Texas does not begin to indicate the scope of the drug abuse problem. Who uses drugs? Where are these people? What drugs are used? How are these people being reached by the State? To try to answer such questions, one must go beyond the mere number of abusers and look at the profiles of these people in some depth.

The number of narcotic overdose deaths in 1971 in Texas is important not only as a measure of addiction, but also because it shows a significant increase over the deaths in past years. In 1960, one narcotic overdose death was registered. Obviously, the growth in the problem is well illustrated.

Altogether, there were 237 drug overdose deaths in Texas in 1971. Twenty-one of the *narcotic* overdose deaths were males between the ages of fifteen and thirty-four. Six of the barbiturate overdoses were under thirty-four, and four were over forty-five years of age. If all the accidental drug deaths are broken down on the basis of age, it becomes apparent that most of those who died were young. Seven persons were between fifteen and nineteen, seventeen persons were between twenty and twenty-four, ten between twenty-five and twenty-nine, and eleven between thirty and thirty-four. All but nine of these were male. The death rate then tapers off until middle age, when it rises again, with thirteen persons over fifty-nine dying accidental drug deaths. Interestingly enough, ten of these persons were female.

TYPES OF DRUGS USED

Another aspect of the drug problem is usage among young people. Surveys have been made during the last two years to determine drug usage among university, high school, and junior high school students in Texas. These surveys differ in methodology, questions asked, and classification of drugs. Some of the surveys divide respondents into different age or grade levels, while others lump the entire sample together. But even with different methodologies, some trends in drug use can be seen.

Most surveys show that alcohol is the most commonly used drug. It was found that approximately 40 to 60 percent of high school students have used alcohol, and by the time they reach college, only 4 percent have not tried it.

percent being Anglo, 11 percent Black, and 35 percent Spanish surnamed. A significant pattern is that 60 percent of the narcotic addicts are Spanish surnamed and 15 percent are Black, but neither of these ethnic groups abuses any of the other drugs in any sizeable proportion. Anglos, however, tend to abuse a wide range of drugs. Only 26 percent of the narcotic addicts are Anglo, but the Anglos are the only ethnic group to abuse the other drugs.

Patients at the outpatient clinics tend to be young, since 68 percent are under thirty. Almost 60 percent of those who abuse marijuana and the hallucinogens are under twenty, while 45 percent of the amphetamine abusers and 56 percent of the narcotic addicts are between twenty-one and thirty. As in the state hospitals, barbiturate abusers tend to be older, with only 33 percent being under thirty.

If the characteristics of all drug abuse patients treated by the Department of Mental Health and Mental Retardation are combined, a few significant tendencies can be shown. Two-thirds of the drug abuse patients are male, and females are significant only as abusers of the barbiturates. Patients with Spanish surnames are principally abusers of heroin, while Anglos tend to abuse all drugs. Blacks in the state hospitals tend to abuse all drugs, while Blacks treated as outpatients are narcotic addicts. Drug abuse usually occurs in urban areas, and it is a phenomenon of the young, except for barbiturate abusers. Marijuana and the hallucinogens are most often abused by those under twenty; amphetamine abusers are most likely between eleven and thirty; and narcotic addicts are between twenty-one and thirty.

PARAMETERS OF THE DRUG PROBLEM AS INDICATED BY LAW ENFORCEMENT PERSONNEL IN TEXAS

The drug problem can also be measured in the field of law enforcement. The Texas Department of Public Safety in 1970 arrested 1,439 persons for drug offenses; and during the first six months of 1971, it arrested 745. Of these, 841 of the arrests in 1970 were for sale or possession of marijuana, and 415 of the arrests in 1971 were for the same offense.

The drug problem is further illustrated by the fact that in 1970, roughly 12 percent of the commitments (1,074 inmates to the Texas Department of Corrections), were for drug violations. The total number of inmates confined for drug convictions as of September 1971, totaled 1,819.

The mean age of inmates committed for drug offenses had decreased from thirty-six in 1964 to thirty in 1968. The ethnic distribution has also changed. In 1964, 19 percent were Anglo, 22 percent Black, and 57 percent Spanish surnamed. But by 1971, 37 percent of the drug violators were Anglo, 30 percent Black, and 33 percent Spanish surnamed. It is interesting to compare this ethnic distribution with that of the state mental hospitals, whose drug patients are 65 percent Anglo, 7 percent Black, and 29 percent Spanish surnamed, and the outpatient clinics with 54 percent Anglo, 11 percent Black, and 35 percent Spanish surnamed.

All of the figures presented in this paper come from state agency reports or school surveys, and this is probably not a true picture, since those out of contact with the establishment are excluded. Still, some basic conclusions can be drawn:

1. The drug user is not only becoming younger, but his tendency to abuse drugs is shown by the number of young overdose deaths and the commitments to the state hospitals.

2. Anglos are becoming more and more involved in drugs, from experimentation at junior high school to confinement in the state prisons.

3. Anglos and Spanish surnamed ethnic groups tend to specific patterns of drug use. The former group uses all types of drugs, while the latter primarily uses heroin.

DETERMINATION OF ELIGIBILITY FOR REHABILITATION SERVICES

In working with the drug abuser, one must acknowledge that a majority of the people in our American society take drugs; however, the fact that an individual takes drugs does not establish eligibility for the services of the Texas Rehabilitation Commission. Many people enjoy the drug "caffein" found in coffee, or the drug "nicotine" found in cigarettes, or the drug "alcohol," but these people may not be addicted.

To work with clients who are labeled drug abusers, a counselor must accept the definition which the Texas Rehabilitation Commission has outlined in the *Statewide Plan for the Drug Abuse Program* (1971):

> It appears that the most general concept that defines drug abuse is dependence. Dependence means addiction, habituation, or both. Addiction is defined as physical dependence on a drug. Habituation is a psychological desire to repeat the use of a drug intermittently or continuously because of an emotional reason (p. 1).

Thus drug abuse is defined as use of a drug for non-medical or nonscientific purposes, with potentiality of harm to the user or to society. For clarification, five types of medical-psychological abusers can be identified. The types are distinguishable as follows:

1. The experimenters	Arising from group pressure.
2. The occasional user	Arising from group usage.
3. The dependent	Arising from a psychological and physiological need.
4. The addict	Arising from fear of psychological and physiological pain: one who cannot pull away.
5. The junkie	Arising from the life of day-to-day existence only for drugs.

In order to establish eligibility for services of the Texas Rehabilitation Commission, the drug abuser must be diagnosed *medically* as having a drug abuse problem. The applicant must be involved in a recognized treatment program. Examples of recognized treatment programs are:

1. Narcotic Addict Rehabilitation Act (NARA) after-care following treatment at the Clinical Research Center (CRC) in Forth Worth, Texas.
2. MH-MR drug treatment programs.
3. Drug maintenance programs by private organizations if
   a. Food and Drug Administration (FDA) approved.
   b. State and local medical association approved.
   c. Hospital beds available for emergency use.
   d. Adequate medical after-care available.

In establishing eligibility, the drug abuser must show evidence of benefiting from the treatment program. The applicant must be able to function adequately in order to participate in the services of the Texas Rehabilitation Commission, and the applicant must be drug free or be a successful participant in a medically approved drug maintenance program.

It is not the responsibility of the Texas Rehabilitation Commission to pro-

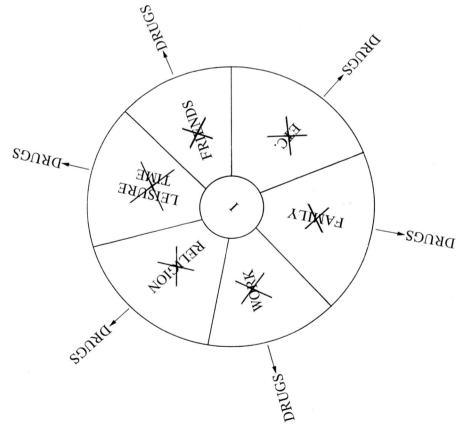

Figure 10-1. The Active Drug Abuser's World Before Rehabilitation

vide medical treatment or follow-up medical supervision to the drug abuser, but it is the responsibility of the Texas Rehabilitation Commission to provide rehabilitation services to those individuals who meet the criteria for eligibility.

In addition to establishing a disability of drug abuse, a counselor is also required to establish that a substantial handicap to employment exists, as well as a reasonable expectation that rehabilitation services will eventually render the individual fit to engage in gainful occupation.

UNIQUE FACTORS IN THE PROCESS OF
REHABILITATION OF THE DRUG ABUSER

It may be that the rehabilitation of the drug abuser differs from the rehabilitation of other disability groups of the Texas Rehabilitation Commission, in process and in objective. Traditionally, rehabilitation has been achieved by re-directing an individual into a new career or reconstructing a small segment of his world. For example, an individual with a family and home who worked as a welder experienced an accident which resulted in

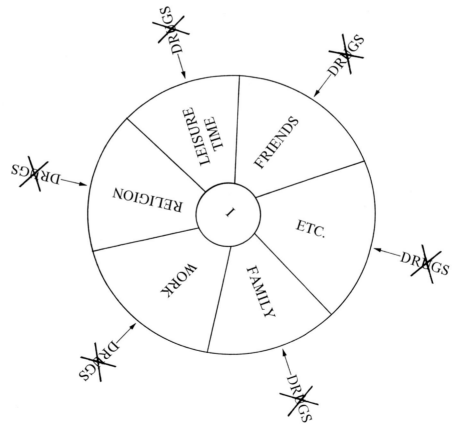

Figure 10-2. The Drug Abuser's World After Rehabilitation

the amputation of an arm and ended his capability to perform as a welder. Training for a new career was provided to rehabilitate this individual. However, rehabilitation of the drug abuser is a different matter. Normally the world of the drug abuser has totally disintegrated by the time he reaches the Texas Rehabilitation Commission. His family no longer supports him; his work experience is non-existent; his outside interest in religion, hobbies, and recreational activities has deteriorated. His entire world consists of drugs and the euphoria they provide. Thus the counselor must construct a new world in which the individual can exist and achieve a purposeful life.

No single service provided by the Texas Rehabilitation Commission will normally achieve rehabilitation of the drug abuser. Not only must the counselor strive to establish the individual in a vocational environment, but he must aid the individual in locating friends, recreational outlets, and establishing a drug-free society. Rehabilitation of the drug abuser demands a broad spectrum of services in personal, social, vocational, and recreational areas. This isolation factor is graphically presented in Figures 10-1 and 10-2.

THE REHABILITATION COUNSELOR'S CHALLENGE IN WORKING WITH THE DRUG ABUSER

It is pertinent to state at this point that there are individuals who will not respond as was planned, regardless of the rehabilitation services extended. In reality, a few individuals may even regress in the abuse of drugs because of our "help." A thin line exists here between challenge and frustration.

As a professional in the field of drug abuse, the counselor must be constantly aware of the fact that one of the most impregnable walls between the drug addict and any real assistance is the misconception that there is *one* best way to help a drug addict. Equal attention must be given to another misconception, and that is that simply because one method does not help, there is no hope. It is difficult to accept, but some drug addicts never find a workable program. A counselor must always remember that a drug addict is above all a human being, and different individuals have different needs. In all efforts toward rehabilitation, this must be kept in mind.

By the time a drug addict reaches a rehabilitation counselor's office, he has probably been denounced by everyone. Now, for the first time, someone is truly interested in knowing what drugs mean to him. This attitude is vital in the rehabilitation of the drug addict. It is essential that counselors accept the drug addict as a person; yet the counselor must never let the client forget that he himself is responsible for doing something about his problem.

Acceptance, however, must not mean that a counselor permits himself to be conned or deceived. It is no service to the drug addict to pretend you believe what he is saying when you know he is lying. You, the counselor, must convince the drug addict that, rather than feeling like him, you are feeling with him, and complete honesty is necessary if you are going to attempt to help him.

It is only after this relationship has been established that concrete results may be achieved toward rehabilitation, and this, of course, can be a slow and sometimes frustrating process. One must never lose sight of the immediate goal of helping the drug addict to achieve abstinence from drugs and to receive the possibility of the rewards for this action.

In many instances, the drug addict needs you as a counselor and as a person more than he needs the services you can provide. Rehabilitation of the drug addict can be relatively inexpensive from the standpoint of purchased services, but it can be very expensive in terms of time. Yet, time spent with him can be time spent in the best way of all. The counselor can and should be the catalyst for the drug addict's recovery. Without a doubt, the counselor's attitude and behavior toward the client can be a major influence on the outcome of a case.

CHARACTERISTICS OF THE SUCCESSFUL COUNSELOR FOR THE DRUG ABUSER

However, if this type of influence is to occur, the counselor must possess certain qualifications. First and foremost, he must be motivated. With the drug addict, one can have no prejudice toward either drug abuse or the drug addict. It is common knowledge that a drug addict is often a "con artist"; because of this, he is equally adept at knowing when he is being "conned." Therefore, it is *imperative* that one at all times be completely open and honest with him. One must neither condemn nor condone his past behavior, but strive to make him realize that he alone is responsible for his future actions and that professional assistance can only be expected if he is willing to help himself in return.

There is nothing wrong in taking credit when one is successful with a client, if one is also willing to accept the failures a counselor may experience. Since honesty is expected from the clients who are being served, it must be present in the counselor evaluating himself. Certainly, all counselors would prefer to work with clients whose rehabilitation is relatively predictable, but the fact of the matter is rehabilitation of the drug addict usually progresses in spurts, slips, and stalls. It is imperative that a counselor accept the fact that he may not always be right, for in working with the drug addict, he may be wrong a good percentage of the time. A counselor must acknowledge that rehabilitation is an individual affair and each case is different. Rehabilitation of the drug abuser will certainly test the stamina and fortitude of the counselor. The counselor who proves effective will have been afforded the opportunity to earn his title, for counseling which will be in this case the most important service rendered.

It is essential that a counselor constantly recall his purpose and not become a practitioner of medicine and begin diagnosing the problem himself or wandering into areas that are not concerns of the Rehabilitation Commission for which he works. Adequate guidelines are provided in the *Rehabilita-*

tion Services Manual of each state, which will allow a counselor to function successfully. A counselor must recognize that he is a professional person and that, to be effective, he does not need to dress and act like the drug abuser to establish rapport. The purpose, again, is to aid the drug abuser in re-establishing himself in a meaningful and supporting role in society.

REFERENCES

Maxwell, J.C.: Profile of Drug Abusers in Texas. Community Assistance Series No. 4. Austin, State (Texas) Program on Drug Abuse, 1972.

Texas Rehabilitation Commission: *Rehabilitation Services Manual*. Austin, Texas Rehabilitation Commission, May 1, 1971.

Texas Rehabilitation Commission: *Statewide Plan for the Drug Abuse Program*. Austin, Texas Rehabilitation Commission, 1971.

Chapter 11

THE EFFECTS OF MOOD ALTERING DRUGS: PLEASURES AND PITFALLS

PAUL L. ROSENBERG

INTRODUCTION

WE LIVE in an age where a nation of young people has been cast adrift, cut off from their elders, to search alone for meaning in a world that often does not make sense. The normal rites of passage have been ruptured. Our children no longer seem able to use the old cultural norms as a yardstick. These valuable traditions, which tie us so richly to the world, are being stripped of their meaning by the increasing speed of social change. Without a cultural inheritance, a young person is forced to grope for direction at a time in his life when his adolescent attachment to utopian goals and his desperate struggle for independence cloud his ability to make mature judgments. In this confusing market-place of growing up are many drugs, some old, some new, which are able to profoundly affect the depth, intensity, and meaning of our experience of reality and of ourselves.

Nursed by the impersonality of the television set, taught to hide behind the masks of conformity that have become caskets for many of their parents, our young people have been cut off from experiencing their own integralness by the blast of our mass culture. Affluence can have an emptiness as profound as that of a ghetto. People at all levels are starving, searching desperately for anything that allows them the chance to feel better. Drugs, like alcohol, often appear to offer a way out. Drugs can increase one's sensitivity to feelings or they can depress one's internal experience of one's self. They can alter the boredom and plainness that is so much of life. But the more you depend on a pill to feel alive, the less you can feel yourself. The drug becomes a device for stimulation, like masturbation, which gets you away from the real thing. Suddenly, the drug takes over; you become automatized by the need for artificial assistance which diminishes your control over your own world. Reality is not heightened sensitivity. In the confusing search for something real, people often mistake more intense experience for the deeper realities of intimacy and communication. We must avoid trying to frighten people away from the world of drugs. Rather we must illuminate the problems that drugs create. Then we must trust our youth to explore, experiment and eventually

192

choose their own way, which is indeed the process of growth and maturation.

Drugs are not good or bad. They cannot be eliminated from the American scene. We must face the reality that they are here to stay. This means that we must avoid trying to educate our youth to resist all drugs as evil. In a world where drugs are ubiquitous, we must rely on the ability of youth to choose for themselves, for we cannot protect them. When presenting the facts about drugs and their effects, we must be very careful to point out why drugs are so popular, acknowledging their pleasures as well as their pitfalls. Thus the viewpoint we present will be realistic and will help to make sense out of the confusion of the drug scene. Our children are desperate for someone they can trust. In focusing on the negative aspects of the world of drugs, in an attempt to protect by fear, we alienate the very ones we want to help. It is only with humility and honesty that we can help to convey the kind of information about drugs that will help others find their own way in the difficult world of growing up today.

HALLUCINOGENS

LSD (Lysergic Acid Diethylamide)

LSD is chemically derived from ergot alkaloids. These compounds are found in a fungus of the genus *claviceps,* that occasionally infected wheat in Central Europe. When bread was prepared from this grain, there were outbreaks of ergot poisoning with temporary psychotic behavior. Albert Hoffman, a Swiss chemist, who synthesized LSD in 1937, accidentally ingested some in 1943 and discovered its ability to produce severe distortions of consciousness. LSD remained relatively unknown in the United States until 1959 when a religious group on the West Coast began using it for the induction of mystical states.

Timothy Leary's work at Harvard on LSD began in the early 1960's. Previously, he had been an outstanding psychologist whose personality evaluation procedures are still widely used. His LSD research broke the normal boundaries of academic propriety and led to his expulsion from Harvard. He helped to promulgate the widespread use of LSD, providing many with guidelines on how to handle this powerful psychedelic drug. Concomitantly, the use of marijuana and other drugs increased dramatically, particularly among the white, middle-class. LSD was felt to be a kind of salvation. Adolescents of many ages headed for San Francisco's Haight-Ashbury in the summer of 1967 when the vision of salvation peaked in the world of flower children. Initially, the love culture seemed possible. But soon the pressures of too many mouths to feed and too much hostility turned the once peaceful hippy scene into a dangerous, desolate ghetto. And now many began to demonstrate the poor judgment and mental disorganization that can result from the excessive use of LSD. The drug that "turned on" so many people could also destroy, both by horrifyingly bad trips and gradual mental deterioration. It is fortunate that of the many millions of Americans who have experimented with LSD, only a few appear to have been seriously damaged by it.

The Acid Experience

An LSD trip can be of a magical or mystical nature, giving one's environment the quality of paradise or it can turn the world into a raging, terrifying inferno. Not only are there altered perceptual effects, but the very meaning of our existence can be called into question. A single LSD trip can totally alter one's direction in life.

The intensity of LSD experience is dose related. The drug produces hypersuggestibility. Thus, one's emotional state when taking the drug, as well as the environment or setting in which the drug is used, is extremely important in determining what kind of trip one has. You can never be sure where you are going. LSD is always a voyage into the unknown. Sometimes a trip begins slowly, with gradual changes in one's perceptual awareness. The intensity of color seems to radiate with greater vividness. The whole world may seem enriched. At other times the experience may start with an explosive force and drop into a mystical, magical, delusional world, where reality changes swiftly. Perceptal alterations, which are usually predominant, involve distortion and changes in perspective rather than true hallucinatory phenomena. At higher doses, hallucinations are more common. Synesthesias, where one sense seems to flow into another, often are reported. Music may seem to touch your body. Depth perception may alter. A plaster wall may seem like mountainous terrain and solid objects may appear to undulate to the rhythm of the music. Sexual orgasms may be experienced in multiple modes.

The ability to estimate the passage of time is altered. With the rapid flow of experimental events, the individual on LSD feels a great deal of time must have passed. Five minutes may seem like hours. Thought processes are loosened during and often following the LSD experience. Association may become more fanciful and one's judgment is seriously impaired by magical, illogical thinking. Ego integration may dissolve, causing extreme panic states. Part of traveling safely with LSD involves being able to tolerate new states of ego disorientation without fear. One needs the ability to stay calm, while feeling a loss of connection to the body and normal ego boundaries.

Beyond the usual acid trip is the possibility of religious experience. Mystical states occur spontaneously and have been reported since Biblical times. LSD sessions occasionally have similar, if not identical, transcendental qualities. People describe seeing the Godhead or the golden radiance of God. Usually the experience is related to one's religious background and is remembered as a deeply moving religious event.

Panics and "Bummers"

The increased intensity with which LSD allows us to voyage into our innermost feelings also can carry us to the depths of terror. Frequently during an LSD trip, there are brief periods when one feels afraid. If the response to this fear is running away or increased anxiety, one can create a terrifying and overwhelming crisis. For those who have taken LSD numerous times, the first encounter with the extreme terror of an LSD "bummer" frequently motivates them to stop taking the drug permanently.

Panic experiences of ego disorganization are sometimes somaticized; it is as if one is dead, that the rest of the world is dead, that one's body is coming apart, or magically bleeding to death. "Bummers" are experienced both interpersonally and intrapersonally. In a group, the heightened suggestibility of the LSD state may cause one to feel that unrelated movements of others are meant as signs of an impending attack. The paranoia may grow rapidly until it involves everything. Feelings of depersonalization or unreality become overwhelming. The more one fights or flees from the paranoia, the more frantic and intense it becomes. Suddenly there does not seem to be any hope. Out of this desperation comes the frantic terror and panic of an LSD "bummer." Often people are severely shaken and are left with intense anxiety for weeks following a bad trip. A person can often be talked down from a "bummer" by an experienced guide. Getting an individual to focus on his breathing helps to orient him and reassure him that his body is still intact. One can remind him that he is taking a drug which accounts for the experience he is having. The firm, commanding, reassuring voice of an experienced guide, helping the individual to understand what is happening, is enough to bring most people down. When someone cannot be talked down in such a manner, any of the major antipsychotic tranquilizers are rapidly effective. Some researchers have suggested that the use of tranquilizers may increase the likelihood of flashbacks.

Changes in Direction

One's conception of what is important in life is developed in our early years, matures in adolescence and usually remains stable throughout our adult life. These assumptions are rarely thought about and remain as unconscious determinants of what we want and of how we behave. LSD can cause rapid and major changes in these basic feelings which can alter totally the way a person chooses to live. To illustrate this, let us briefly review two case histories.

Tom, when brought into a county hospital by his parents, was a nineteen year old young man who had been going to college. For the past year and a half he had been taking LSD during weekly beer parties on the beach with his fraternity brothers. He continued to go to school, did better than average work and lived at home. His parents were unaware of the fact that he was taking LSD. His lifestyle remained unchanged. Approximately six months before he was brought to the hospital, he was picked up while hitchhiking by a group of hippies. He accompanied them to their commune where he took LSD. On his first trip with this familial group, he experienced profound new sensations. Their caring and sensitive relationships gave him his first deep awareness that he wanted more intimacy than he had known previously. When he returned home, he quit college which he now saw as a useless waste of time. He gave away his clothes and refused to wear shoes. His parents felt desperate as he was planning to leave home permanently to join his hippy friends.

His family never had a great deal of internal cohesiveness. They were relatively stable but rarely related emotionally. Tom had never had any of the important experiences at home that he was able to have in his new relationships. Though he was unrealistic, he was not psychotic. He had changed his values so enormously that he could no longer remain within the sphere of his earlier upbringing.

In another case, a young "straight" salesman took LSD for the first time with his girl friend. During his first and only trip, this isolated young man experienced such tremendous warmth and tenderness from his girl friend that he was overwhelmed by previously unknown feelings of love and affection. He decided that his past way of life no longer made sense. After the trip, he quit his job and went to work for a community organization which assisted young people who were having problems with drugs.

Such enormous changes in lifestyles do not always occur. Less pronounced changes are more common. Some individuals attempt to maintain their LSD heightened level of awareness after their trip. This leads to bizarre or unusual behavior, expressing their dissatisfaction with normal, comparatively mundane reality. In their search to reestablish the beatific vision experienced on LSD, some may temporarily lose their ability to make appropriate judgments. They act as if the world had been transformed and they may place untenable demands on the people around them. They may ask, "Why? Why do I need a car, or new clothes, when simple things are really enough?" This is indeed simplistic thinking, but one cannot challenge it with ordinary logic. For unless a person wants to work for certain values, one cannot force these values on him. People are very willing to give up a job or a way of life for a vision of something that seems much more important.

This has happened to many. It may be one of the reasons for the dramatic change of values we see in the counter-culture. And perhaps, in the long run, we might be wise to consider where the mad rush of progress is taking us; whether the natural pleasures of seeing the world in fresh, simple ways are not sometimes missed by our sophisticated, appliance-using society.

Flashbacks and Psychoses

The dangerous consequences of post-LSD reactions are rare. Considering the tremendous power of the LSD experience this is quite fortunate. Yet for the few who go through the terrors of repeated flashbacks or who become psychotic, an LSD trip can spell disaster. Most people recover from these sequelae, but some will remain in our state hospitals for long periods of time.

Flashbacks occur when unresolved psychic trauma is partially brought to awareness but incompletely dealt with during a trip. It is like opening Pandora's box just a bit and not being able to seal it tight again. Later, some event jars the box just enough to open it briefly. With the dread contents exposed to awareness, even in the unconscious mind, the disorientation of the LSD state flashes back suddenly. Eventually one's psychological defenses return and normal reality is reestablished. Flashbacks can be treated by psychotherapy, by repeated use of LSD in a treatment setting or by major tranquilizers. Insight-oriented psychotherapy is the treatment of choice but may take a number of years. Flashbacks frequently cease spontaneously. Flashbacks can occur with full-blown psychotic hallucinatory effects or they may appear as only mild perceptual changes. Marijuana and other drugs can precipitate them as can emotional experiences and anxiety. Other post-LSD reactions include depression, chronic anxiety states, prolonged visual effects, and paranoia.

Psychotic reactions requiring hospitalization are a consequence of using LSD in only a very small percentage of cases. Such individuals most frequently have schizophrenic decompensations or, more rarely, prolonged hallucinosis. Usually such psychotic states resolve slowly with therapy. LSD is most likely to cause psychotic reactions in individuals who have rigid defenses which are crucial to their stability or who have had previous schizophrenic illness. Well integrated individuals almost never have any of these prolonged disastrous effects, despite the fact that they too can have frightening LSD "bummers".

One syndrome that is similar to an LSD flashback is the repeated experience of being "stoned" (i.e. confused, anxious and disoriented), which occurs in some individuals who have rigid defenses against their angry and destructive impulses. If they have any drug experience, from LSD to marijuana, which loosens their defensive control of their enormous anger, they become unable to tolerate even the mildest of anxiety-producing or threatening situations. They feel "stoned" or dazed as they attempt to control their unacceptable feelings. It is much the same feeling of overwhelming confusion and disorientation that normal individuals might have briefly in reaction to a catastrophe. This feeling of being "stoned" is persistent and may last with variable intensity for years. It is aggravated by the omnipotently demanding, passive-aggressive personality style that is most frequently seen in this syndrome. Psychotherapy for this condition is often prolonged and difficult.

It is a wonder that so many severely disturbed people who have taken LSD and other psychedelics have not become more bizarre or disturbed. Perhaps the accepting, loosely structured, undemanding quality of the underground community allows disorganized individuals to function without drawing attention to themselves. It is not clear why LSD will increase the mental disability of some individuals and not others.

Physiologic Considerations

LSD is one of the most potent chemicals known. Merely 25 micrograms of this drug can cause a change in one's inner awareness. Usually, doses range from 100 to 500 micrograms, although intake of up to two to four thousand micrograms has been reported. The trip lasts from six to twelve hours with its peak occurring during the first two to four hours. For most people, tolerance will begin to develop after a single dose and may take four to eight days to wear off. Cross tolerance exists between most psychedelics including LSD, mescaline and psilocybin. Experiments have shown that these drugs cannot be distinguished experientially even by experienced users.

LSD has many sympathomimetic effects, most pronounced of which is pupillary dilation of up to six millimeters. Minor elevation in blood pressure and temperature occur, as well as muscular weakness, numbness, tremulousness, tachycardia and mild hyperglycemia. The nonspecific stress of the LSD state produces increased adrenocortical steroids. Eosinophilia and leukocytosis also can be observed. Electroencephalographic tracings show diminished amplitude and low voltage fast waves with increased desynchrony. Periods of dreaming during sleep are prolonged for the 24 to 48 hours following an LSD experience.

The mode of action of LSD remains speculative. Naturally occurring neurologically active amines such as serotonin and norepinephrine show chemical structures similar to most of the psychoactive drugs. Hallucinogenic agents may compete with and block or possibly facilitate synaptic transmissions.

LSD has been involved in a great controversy involving possible chromosomal damage. Unfortunately, these studies have utilized subjects who have had multi-drug exposure. Nevertheless, there is clear-cut evidence that LSD does increase the number of chromosomal breaks and crossovers. Chromosomal changes appear three times more frequently in LSD users than in control groups. These changes are similar to those induced by radiation, viruses, and other mutagens. There is evidence suggesting that LSD can cross the placenta, increasing the chromosomal changes in the fetus. However, from the epidemiological point of view, LSD only rarely has been implicated in congenital birth defects. The effects on germ cells still have to be evaluated. We can conclude only that we do not know the consequences of the chromosomal changes that are observed with LSD use. We must proceed with caution until adequate data is available.

Clinical Uses

Research work on LSD remains in its infancy. A number of studies already have shown some promise for LSD as a therapeutic agent. Patients on the verge of death after a protracted and painful illness, such as cancer, usually experience a great deal of anxiety and terror. With proper preparation, an LSD session can substantially change their perspective on their impending death. Most feel more accepting about the inevitability of death. Additionally, LSD has been shown to decrease pain in chronically ill cancer patients and to increase the effectiveness of opiates.

LSD has proven to be of some value in the treatment of alcoholics. More than half of the alcoholics treated with one to three high dose sessions of LSD have shown improvement. Reports from Eastern and Western Europe and the United States suggest that LSD may be a useful adjunct in insight-oriented psychotherapy. Combined with regular therapy sessions, LSD experiences inhibit ego defenses and allow for the recall of primitive fantasies and traumatic memories not usually available to the conscious mind. LSD enhances emotional abreactions. Reports from psychoanayltic researchers using LSD suggest that even the earliest of traumas, the pain of being born, has somatic traces which can be re-experienced. Claims have been made for the value of LSD in treating both schizophrenia and neurotic patients. These experiments bear further study of LSD could well become an important addition to the armamentarium of psychotherapeutic drugs.

OTHER HALLUCINOGENS

Mescaline (3, 4, 5 - Trimethoxyphenylethylamine)

Mescaline, one of the alkaloids present in the peyote cactus which grows in the Sonoran deserts of the American Southwest and Mexico, has long been used by Indians as a part of religious rituals. In these ceremonies the adult men of the tribe sit through the night after chewing peyote buttons, having visions and singing peyote songs.

Mescaline, the active alkaloid of peyote, is chemically related to epinephrine. It was studied in the early 1950's and received much popular attention. Peyote has an intensely bitter taste and often causes nausea and vomiting. Trips on peyote tend to last 12 to 24 hours while mescaline lasts 6 to 8 hours. Many drug users feel that mescaline produces a psychedelic experience that has more colorful, gentler somatic qualities than LSD, and is less likely to be terrifying. In contradiction, research work has shown that people are unable to differentiate between the effects of most psychedelics.

Psilocybin and Psilocin (Dimethyl-4-phosphoryltryptamine and dimethyl-4-hydroxyltryptamine)

The psychoactive alkaloids found in the Mexican mushroom, *psilocybe mexicana heim,* are also used by Indians in Mexico to produce religious visions. Psilocin is slightly more potent than psilocybin. Both produce states indistinguishable from LSD, but have a duration of approximately 3 to 6 hours. They are rarely, if ever, available on the street, although preparations of other substances are frequently sold as psilocybin.

DMT (dimethoxytryptamine) and DET (diethyltryptamine)

DMT often has been called the businessman's acid trip as it produces rapid hallucinogenic effects which last 10 to 30 minutes. It is inactive when taken orally. Usually people smoke DMT either by heating the crystals and inhaling the vapors or by dipping marijuana into a solution of DMT. It has a strong, acrid metallic odor. It can be sniffed or injected. Intramuscular injections can cause a tight, choking sensation in the chest and brief periods of unconsciousness followed by intense hallucinations. DMT occurs in the seeds of *Piptadenia peregrina* which are used in South America to make *Cohoba* snuff. DMT has autonomic effects similar to LSD. DET is a synthetic preparation with psychoactive properties resembling DMT.

Lysergic Acid Amide

The wild American morning glory has four species which produce seeds containing lysergic acid amide and isolysergic acid amide. The potency varies with each batch of seeds. The seeds are pulverized and taken orally, often producing a lethargic, dreamy state with frequent nausea and vomiting. Hallucinations occur at high doses close to the point where ergot toxicity is observed.

STP (2, 5, dimethoxy-4-methylamphetamine)

STP is a synthetic hallucinogen that recently has come directly from the experimental laboratory into street use. It was alleged to precipitate frequent "bummers" and last one or two days. However, larger than normal amounts were used, probably accounting for these misconceptions. It is thought to be about as potent as psilocybin.

The Peace Pill—PCP

PCP is an animal tranquilizer known as phencyclidine (Sernyl). First making its appearance in the summer of 1967 as "the peace pill" in San Francisco, PCP received a lot of attention and was known to cause frequent bad trips. Some find it enjoyable at first, but there have been repeated reports of acute paranoia and "bummers." Known as "angel dust," it is sprayed on marijuana or parsley and sold as an hallucinogen. It usually produces a greater disorganization of the thought process than LSD. Feelings of unreality are also common. It can be identified frequently by the heavy chemical odor that lingers in the air when it is smoked. A cheap chemical, which apparently is easily obtained, it is frequently sold as LSD, mescaline, or THC. At times it may be added to other drugs to boost their effect. The quality and potency of drugs obtained on the street are always unknown. Strychnine and other poisons have been found both alone and as contaminants of such drugs.

Marijuana and Hashish

Marijuana is the common name given to the dried leaves and flowers of the hemp plant, *cannabis sativa*. Hashish is made from the dried resins of the same plant, or the Indian variety, *cannabis indicus*. Hashish is more potent but contains the same active chemical, tetrahydracarbaminol (THC). It can be classified as an hallucinogen since, in adequate amounts, THC produces hallucinations.

Historical Considerations

Cannabis indicus has been used in India for centuries for religious, pleasurable, and medicinal purposes. In 1839, W. B. O'Shaughnessey published an article, "On the Preparations of the Indian Hemp," which first introduced the therapeutic possibilities of cannabis into Western medicine. O'Shaughnessey had been serving with the British Army in India. He suggested that hemp might be useful in producing analgesia, as an anticonvulsant, and as a muscle relaxant. His report generated a great deal of attention. By 1860 the Ohio State Medical Society's committee on *cannabis indicus* reported success in treating pain, childbirth, coughs, psychoses, and insomnia using this new drug. In 1889, E. A. Birch reported in *Lancet* that Indian hemp could be used in treating opiate addiction. A year later, in 1890, J. R. Reynolds reported in *Lancet* on thirty years of clinical experience using cannabis. He observed that *Cannabis* was useful as a sedative and was valuable for various neuralgias, migraine headache, and numerous nervous conditions including depression. He warned against overdose, noting the necessity to titrate the quantity given to each patient. Even the great American physician, William Osler, in his 1916 edition of his textbook of medicine, wrote concerning migraine headaches. *"Cannabis indicus* is probably the most satisfactory remedy."

Indian hemp was used extensively by physicians throughout the latter half of the nineteenth and early part of the twentieth centuries. Hemp was a frequent component of over-the-counter nerve and cough cures. In 1937 the marijuana tax act put an end to the common use of cannabis for medicinal purposes. This occurred over the objections of the American Medical Association who protested that it was a useful drug.

Since the 1920's, the use and distribution of marijuana through the fringe or criminal element of our society has given it a reputation for being associated with criminal behavior and violent crimes. The La Guardia report and many recent studies have disproved this association. Yet there remains a widespread misconception that the use of marijuana presages a moral degeneration and eventual addiction to heroin.

Why Do People Like Marijuana?

The tremendously rapid increase in the use of marijuana throughout all levels of our culture is surely the most striking drug phenomenon of the past decade. Studies have shown that from 50 to 80 percent of our college students have used or use marijuana. Of course, only a few use it daily. Yet more and more people seem to find it an enjoyable and relaxing pastime. One young man describes his feelings this way, "The thing about it is that it makes me feel whole; grass is like a wholeness where you can still function but still have that all-in-one enjoyable feeling." Many have found that marijuana is a valuable tranquilizer. It can take away the feeling of emptiness and insecurity. It can create a delicious timelessness in which the mind seems more awake and the world particularly vibrant and meaningful.

During one's first encounter with marijuana, some individuals experience nothing out of the ordinary. Anxiety about smoking grass for the first time can completely shut off the effects of the drug at moderate dosage. For others, the intensity of the new perceptions can be overwhelming. The changes in time and spatial dimension, the clarity and depth of feeling that are often reached are profound experiences. Marijuana and hashish are usually smoked but they can also be taken in the form of an alcohol extract or, more frequently, mixed in foods such as brownies or cookies.

Usually marijuana is used as a means to foster social communication, much as alcohol is used socially. By passing a "joint" around and turning on together, an immediate camaraderie is established, particularly since smoking marijuana is still illegal. Under these circumstances people often find it easier to relate and be involved. As people become more intoxicated, they tend to become increasingly withdrawn into their fantasies and reveries, thus cutting down on interpersonal communication. When alone, people tend to use the drug to decrease anxiety, to speed up their mental processes and to enjoy its somatic effects. The ability of the marijuana high to ameliorate feelings of anxiety, emotional pain and loneliness perhaps best explains why so many repeatedly turn to this drug experience. Marijuana is liked because it helps in feeling better; it is replacing alcohol as the drug of choice of today's young people.

Physiological Effects

The ability of marijuana to produce psychological and physiological effects varies with its THC content. The percentage of THC usually present in marijuana available on the streets is less than 1 percent. Panic, hallucinatory and dissociative reactions can occur when more potent preparations are available.

Initially, the drug causes drowsiness and dryness of the mouth and weakly dilates blood vessels, producing injected conjunctiva. Tachycardias, slight decreases in blood pressure, and pupillary dilation are common. Transient hypoglycemia often causes a craving for sweets. This hypoglycemic response disappears with more chronic use. At higher doses there is a diffuse depressant effect on the central nervous system. A dreamy, lethargic state occurs where inhibitions are decreased. Impairment of immediate memory, increased suggestibility, shortened attention span, fragmentation of thought, synesthesias, altered sense perceptions and moderate ataxia are all aspects of the "high" of marijuana intoxication. This hypnagogic state has qualities similar to the sedative experiences during the induction of anesthesia as well as the psychedelic experience with LSD. Coordination studies in driving automobiles have demonstrated that intoxication with moderate doses of marijuana does not impair driving skills. Higher drug levels cause difficulties with attention and perception that make driving hazardous.

Partial tolerance develops with chronic marijuana use. Tolerant individuals often find their "high" periods shortened with fewer perceptual changes. However, the timeless, tranquilizing and comforting qualities usually remain. Tolerance disappears from 3 to 5 days after drug use stops. Marijuana is not addicting. Severe psychological dependence results when individuals depend on grass to relieve their anxiety and frustrations. But there are no problems in withdrawing from marijuana. Only occasional heavy users have periods of restlessness and anxiety. Most people use it in their spare time to induce a mild euphoria. With this kind of use, psychological dependence usually does not become a problem. Morning hangovers are infrequently encountered. Yet some individuals may have these regularly. They report fatigue, lethargy, mild to moderate confusion and dissociative feelings. No fatalities have been reported from an overdose of marijuana. The drug, when smoked, is automatically self-titrated. If the user becomes excessively intoxicated, he finds himself unable to continue smoking and thus discontinues his drug intake.

Psychological Changes

During a marijuana high, one experiences a rapid flow of thoughts and associations. Often one is able to hear or feel impulses from different parts of one's self that are normally repressed. The vicious, silly, childish, or self-disapproving voices within may be clearly heard. Often one takes the role of a spectator looking at one's own feelings and reactions. There is a general enhancement of the prevailing mood. Hostile or angry feelings are usually modified or lost entirely. An individual who is "stoned" may be aware of the intensity with which he is able to perceive the external reality. There is a change in the quality of reality, as if the veil of one's anxieties were lifted and perceptions were sharpened. Alternately, one may feel cut off and fragmented, producing severe paranoia.

The marijuana high can be focused both externally or internally. One can go from the internal to the external experience rapidly. Frequently, people state that they have had to respond to external reality such as a knock on the door or being stopped by a policeman. They note that they can appropriately orient themselves except when extremely intoxicated. This control is an unusual quality of marijuana intoxication.

It often has been stated that marijuana acts as an aphrodisiac. Basically, this is true, although it does not appear to be in itself a sexual stimulant. Instead, the aphrodisiac qualities of marijuana seem to be due to its ability to remove inhibitions and allow one to focus intensely on the pleasures of sexual sensations.

The syndrome of the heavy marijuana abuser is only beginning to be understood. He tends to be an individual who feels very inadequate and uses intellectual defenses to avoid his painful feelings. The prolonged use of marijuana creates a kind of distance from the world. One observes what is happening rather than participating with feelings and reactions. This withdrawal includes a loss of interest in others as well as a lessened concern for the propriety of social norms. The chronic marijuana user has a sluggish, even flowing, almost mechanized walk that can be identified by a keen observer. He tends to neglect his body and there is a loss of general alertness. He seems to be far away and often demonstrates clearly confused or loosened thought processes. Delusional or obsessional ideation may be present. No longer does it seem meaningful to hold a job or complete school. This lack of involvement has been called the amotivation syndrome. Most of these symptoms are reversible when the individual stops abusing marijuana.

Adverse Reactions

Varying degrees of mild paranoid or fragmented feelings are commonly reported. These disappear as the drug wears off and require no treatment. Acute and chronic psychoses develop only rarely; they develop most frequently in rigid, schizoid individuals. These may require long term psychotherapy and tranquilizers. In chronic psychoses, particularly with marginal but functioning individuals, it may be difficult to get them to give up using marijuana. They have come to rely on its tranquilizing effects and do not connect their disorganization with the use of the drug.

STIMULANTS

Amphetamines

Amphetamines are a class of drugs which act as stimulants of the central nervous system. Their use and abuse extends through all levels of our culture, from the truck driver who takes a "bennie" to stay alert on the road to the housewife who needs her morning diet pill to keep up with the rapid pace of everyday life. It is little wonder that the youth subculture have adopted amphetamines as a frequently used, though less frequently abused, form of stimulation.

Amphetamines were prepared first in 1887 but did not become clinically available until 1930 when the sympathomimetic effects of amphetamines began to be compared to those of epinephrine. They were not used frequently until the second World War. There are a number of amphetamines including amphetamine (Benzedrine®), dextro-amphetamine (Dexedrine®), methamphetamine (Desoxyn® or Methadrine®). Combinations such as Obetrol® are used to decrease the unwanted side-effects of nervousness and irritability.

Pharmacological Effects

Amphetamines function as a stimulant of both the motor and sensory aspects of the central nervous system. They produce an alert, awake feeling of confidence and potency and facilitate task-oriented behavior for from 4 to 6 hours. Amphetamines stimulate heart function with the heart rate increasing proportionately to the dose of the drug. Increased irritability and increased perception of auditory stimuli are also dose-related. At high doses, toxic psychoses develop with visual and auditory illusions, delusions and hallucinations having extremely paranoid characteristics. Sexual interest often is increased on the intellectual level but the physical ability to perform may be reduced.

The pharmacological evidence suggests that amphetamines act through multiple pathways involving catecholamine metabolism, monamine oxidase inhibition and by direct intrinsic effect. The dose of amphetamines needed to produce toxic psychotic effects varies tremendously. Chronic oral or intravenous use of 100 to 500 mg per day usually precipitates psychosis but individuals have tolerated well over 1,000 mg per day without toxic signs. While not addicting, amphetamines are extremely habituating, producing profound psychological dependence. Withdrawal from the drug produces tenseness, tremors and anxiety culminating in moderate to extreme depression. People develop rapid tolerance to the effects of amphetamines so that the drug no longer remains effective unless the dose is constantly increased. With large repeated doses taken intravenously damage and loss of brain cells occurs. It is surprising, however, that despite tremendously heavy amphetamine abuse, most individuals ultimately show only minimal functional brain damage. There are recent reports of a new syndrome where inflammation and damage to blood vessels are seen in association with intravenous amphetamine abuse. There is a significant increase in cerebrovascular accidents (strokes) in these patients.

The rate of metabolism of amphetamines is relatively slow. Usually the body takes 2 or 3 days to eliminate a single dose of the drug. Much is excreted unchanged in the urine which facilitates detection when a question of toxicity arises.

Amphetamine Syndromes

The mildest form of amphetamine abuse has been common through all levels of society, from students to housewives. It is usually iatrogenic and consists of the daily use of low dosages of amphetamines from 10 to 60 mg per day. Physicians have been in the practice of prescribing amphetamines for weight gain and other symptoms of depression. Amphetamines reverse mild depression for a time, but due to the rapid tolerance that develops, individuals who begin using moderate or low doses of the drug soon find that this does not meet their needs. Slowly, they must increase the amount they take to get the same kind of effect. Many overlook the basic euphoria and sense of powerfulness that goes along with amphetamine use, believing instead that they are taking the amphetamines for weight reduction, or because the doctor prescribed it. As increasing amounts are used, insomnia often results. Fatigued in the morning, they again have to increase their intake to get through the next day. As they begin taking higher and higher doses, suspicious feelings erupt into their consciousness. They believe that people are against them. Numerous frightening perceptual experiences occur which are interpreted in a paranoid manner. There is a tremendous lability of affect with great and frantic mood swings. Thus, the physician who prescribes amphetamines freely can unwittingly convert a patient's mild depression into a toxic psychosis. At best, he can help his patient become habituated to amphetamines rather than dealing with their underlying depressed feelings.

Intravenous use of amphetamines is relatively rare. It is restricted to a very small group of individuals whose feelings of inadequacy are so extreme that they leave the individual with a total sense of powerlessness. The experience of an injection of intravenous amphetamines gives such an individual an incredible sense of power and potency. They rapidly become habituated. Usually the drug is taken in "runs," lasting several days, in which the person does not sleep, rarely eats, and takes the drug as frequently as possible, usually every 2 to 6 hours. As the drug is injected, the user experiences a sudden euphoria (a flash or a rush) which is felt as an explosive orgasmic aliveness of the body and mind. It is an extremely pleasurable sensation to feel alive when your normal state of existence is one of helplessness and apathy. Most users feel that their intellectual functioning is dramatically increased. Some write great poetic pieces, songs or long drafts of manifestos to save the world.

Usually, amphetamine abusers take this drug intravenously in small groups. Often, after the initial rush there is a great deal of talkative communication and activity. As the abuse continues, this activity takes more bizarre and paranoid forms. One "speed freak" couple had strings throughout their apartment forming a kind of spiderweb on which they would hang pictures of various objects. Their paranoia caused them to lock their door with six different locks. Like other habitual users, they tolerated a great deal of filth in the "pad" and took very poor care of their bodies.

When amphetamine abusers appear for help, they often are either acutely paranoid or seriously depressed after a long run. They may be suffering from vitamin deficiency and malnutrition. It is both this neglect and the physiological damage to the body and brain that is responsible for the well known slogan "Speed Kills."

Treatment Considerations

Toxic psychosis with hallucinations require the use of antipsychotic drugs. Panic reactions or anxiety attacks can usually be treated with sedatives or minor tranquilizers such as Valium®. Usually, amphetamine abusers have not had sufficient nutrition for a long time and require vitamins and a well balanced diet. The depression that follows abuse of amphetamines is best treated with regular exercise and rest. Amphetamine abusers are extremely difficult to rehabilitate because of their severe personality problems. Until they can develop a sense of competence and usefulness, they frequently return to amphetamines as a way out of their intolerable emotional world.

Cocaine

Cocaine is a potent stimulant. It was used by the Incas of South America as a stimulant for runners in their postal system. By chewing cocoa leaves, the couriers were able to stimulate their physical abilities much as trainers today use amphetamines to push athletes or horses to greater performance. Cocaine, often called "snow," is a preferred drug by the upper-middle class drug players of today's scene.

The use of cocaine to treat morphine addiction began around 1880. Even Sigmund Freud, in 1884, recommended cocaine for neurathenia and morphinism, insisting that cocaine was non-addicting. As one story goes, Freud was apprehensive when going to social gatherings and would often take cocaine to increase his sense of well-being. This continued only briefly until he observed its addictive potential.

Physiologic Effects

Cocaine stimulates the central nervous system. It appears to potentiate sympathetic nervous functions, perhaps by inhibiting the uptake of norepinephrine at transmitter sites. It is a potent anesthetic of moist surfaces, such as the eye, mouth and throat. When repeatedly applied to mucosal surfaces, it produces severe vascular constriction resulting in local necrosis.

Cocaine is addicting but less rapidly than opiates. Its potential for creating a feeling of competence leads to psychological dependence more rapidly than physiological addiction. Although it is addicting, withdrawal symptoms in this instance are more like those of amphetamines than of heroin. They include tenseness, muscle ache, mild nausea, general somatic discomfort, anxiety, restlessness and depression. Heavy cocaine abuse, which occurs rarely, often produces severe paranoid psychoses in which the abuser frequently feels that there are small animals or bugs which he must continue to pick off his skin.

Cocaine is a well loved drug by many who enjoy its ability to induce a sense of power and excitement that is difficult to obtain even with amphetamines. The problem users have with cocaine is that its effects are very short-lasting, usually only 30 to 60 minutes. Then there is a prolonged come-down period of 3 to 6 hours during which there is mild to marked somatic discomfort.

The Use of Cocaine

Cocaine is rapidly absorbed through the nasal mucosa. Many sniff this drug, often using a dollar bill rolled up to form a narrow tube which allows them to inhale the cocaine crystals past the hairs in their outer nose. The effects are felt rapidly but without a "rush." With extended use, vasoconstriction produces damage to the nasal mucosa. Eventually, a hole in the nasal septum may occur due to the slow erosion of nasal tissue.

Intravenous use of cocaine produces a flash of sexual and physical excitement which is extremely intense. It is a fantastically pleasurable sensation. However, the flash and high are brief so that repeated doses are needed to prevent the uncomfortable come-down. For this reason, cocaine is often combined with other drugs, frequently heroin. This combination is called a "speedball." It has both the stimulatory euphoric effect of cocaine while it has the softening and soothing qualities of heroin.

NARCOTICS

Smack (Heroin), A Seductive Curse

Heroin is the king of drugs. It is the seductive but miserable mistress for the many people who have to hide from the depression and anguish of their own experience of themselves. Heroin is king because it leaves you floating on a calm sea where nothing seems to matter and everything is okay. It is the "beautific" world of peaceful fantasy where your mind swims in the warm, comfortable, somatic sensation of being held, without pain, and protected from the concerns and worries that make up your life. Suddenly the emptiness disappears. The great, gaping hole that hurts, which you had to hide from everyone, is gone; the terrible gnawing inadequacy has vanished. And in its place is the power and comfort that's called confidence. No one can get to you when you keep "nodding."

Heroin is not a harmful drug. It can be taken for years with almost no physically deleterious effects. Its major side-effects are constipation and, for some men, impotence. It is the great seducer because it makes one feel so good. It is better than psychotherapy or sexuality. It creates a state unlike reality, where there is total safety. But heroin, like any narcotic or depressant, is an anesthetizer. It depresses the feeling world and erases from experience the very sensations which are needed to touch life. For many people whose pain is intense, heroin, they feel, is the only way to maintain a constructive lifestyle. Musicians and artists often have turned to heroin to avoid their agony and thus continue their productiveness. Many manage to continue in good health and remain employed for many years. Indeed, if it were not for the intense prejudice against the drug, the rapid tolerance that develops, the dangers of overdose, and for the consequences of non-sterile intravenous injections, heroin might well become the tranquilizing drug of choice for those who suffer from incapacitating anxiety. Unfortunately, the major traumatic effect of heroin is the problem of obtaining it in our society. Having to score daily, with their arms eating up countless dollars, causes the addict to be a slave to his body's craving for heroin.

On first exposure, heroin usually produces nausea. By the second or third dose, the nausea disappears. Then heroin is pure pleasure, at least for a while. Pleasant dreams and fantasies obliterate life's difficulties. Within a few days, tolerance develops so that more heroin is needed to get high. Soon, each day is spent trying to "cop" enough stuff to stay normal. Rarely, if ever, is heroin encountered whose quality and supply is good enough to really get off. The desperate slavery causes the gradual erosion of self-respect. This loss is often bespoken by the ease with which an addict will relate the one thing he hasn't done; it is with this that he retains his last glimmer of self-respect. He has lied, cheated, conned and maneuvered, but perhaps he has not stolen or she has not been a whore.

It is the economic pressure of the heroin scene that causes so many to lose their souls. As slaves in an environment where heroin is expensive and illegal, a whole generation of young addicted people are being forced by their society and their addiction to become criminals. It is an unfortunate sign of our culture's callousness that so many of us look on sick, dependent, disordered addicts as evil degenerates.

The English experience of giving drug users carefully supervised maintenance programs of heroin has proved that heroin itself is not necessarily a detrimental drug. They have shown that narcotic addicts can be stabilized with the official administration of this drug. Americans are beginning to experiment with methadone maintenance which is proving enormously successful.

Whether we like the moral consequences or not, we must consider the fact that there are large numbers of people in our country who feel so desperate that they go out of their way, often destroying their entire lives, to take heroin. Normal habits are essential to our functioning. We get into the habit of getting up early to get to work on time. Habits are hard to break. Once someone has become habituated to living in a world where pain is not confronted and experienced, it may be impossible for him to return to the often uncomfortable realities of life. Perhaps we must learn to accept the continuing need for maintenance therapy as a necessary compromise.

A Habit Is Getting Off

With a rope, tie, belt or old nylon stocking you stop the circulation from your shaking, sweating arm. You decide which of your well scarred veins you have a chance of hitting; then you slip in the needle attached to the eyedropper with the rubber bulb on the end. Releasing the pressure lightly from the bulb you anxiously look for the red glob of blood in the bottom of the dropper which means you've got a "register." You've got to be sure you're in the vein before you inject the stuff. If you miss, you get another abscess. The sickness hurts in your bones, your nose is running, and you hurt so much you almost wish you were dead. With a slow push it's in and within a few seconds you're beginning to feel normal again. Your dilated pupils become very small. Your confidence is back; you're all right for a few hours before the sickness begins to come again.

Most addicts rarely get high from heroin. Their increasing tolerance to the drug usually prevents them from getting enough to get them off. Their shooting just prevents them from feeling sick. Most addicts could withdraw in 5 to 10 days if they really wanted to. This rarely happens because of their fear of being sick, as well as their lack of commitment of getting clean. Most have become so accustomed to using heroin to avoid problems and have so little to look forward to, that they really do not want to give up the relief of their addiction. Moreover, today's street heroin is so diluted that most addicts are addicted to minimal amounts of heroin and have, objectively speaking, mild withdrawal problems.

The variability in the quality of street junk exists in all types of drugs. If an addict scores a few bags of "pure shit," he can accidentally overdose himself causing severe respiratory depression and death. The variety of substances used to cut junk, which then get injected intravenously, add to the dangers of heroin abuse.

It is important to understand that there are many kinds of heroin addicts. In today's drug world we are seeing more of the young addicts whose heroin experiences are recent (under two years). Such an addict usually has a greater chance of returning to the social world he came from, not having burned the many bridges that the chronic, long-term addict has already destroyed. The young addict of today is occasionally able to give up heroin with relative ease. He has a non-addicted lifestyle he has not completely forgotten.

It is hoped that the rehabilitative process will take into consideration the relatively new phenomenon of today's "young addict." There is a need for withdrawal and support facilities for young people who can return to a non-addicted way of life. The more severely addicted or chronic addict usually needs long-term maintenance therapy. Occasionally, after year's of rehabilitation, a stress-producing situation may trigger an addict's need for heroin. Habits return with lightning speed. Just shooting a day or two is enough to revive the intense need for heroin that initially took 2 to 3 weeks to develop. An important part of treating addiction is to provide addicts with withdrawal assistance when they have reverted to heroin in a period of stress. We must be willing to help the addict in times of crisis, offering him the kind of support that will enable him to find better ways of handling stressful feelings.

DEPRESSANTS

The Red Devils

Barbiturates, particularly secobarbitol (Seconol® or reds), are frequently abused drugs, particularly in the ghettos. They offer a similar kind of relief to that of heroin. They depress feelings so that you do not have to know how hard it is to be alive. When you come from a ghetto, you are depressed most of the time. Even though you may stagger around with slurred speech and slowed thought processes, it may still feel better than being aware of how unpleasant life can be. Besides, when you are "stoned," you do not notice how poorly coordinated you are.

Reds are readily available in ghettos and relatively easily obtainable by adolescents at all socio-economic levels. They are sold in rolls and can be bought at almost any school in the country, particularly in urban areas. They are addicting and can be very dangerous.

Accidental overdose or suicide can occur, particularly in individuals who take sleeping pills and have developed a tolerance to the sedative effects of the barbiturates. With their sensorium clouded by the drug, not yet to the point of unconsciousness, depressed and sleepless people have continued to take sleeping medications until lethal doses have been ingested. Alcohol, which potentiates the effects of barbiturates, sometimes contribute to this process.

Withdrawal from barbiturates can be extremely dangerous. Even with the most painful withdrawal, from heroin, death is not a serious risk. In withdrawing from barbiturates, the body becomes tremulous. As time passes, there is hypotension, fever, vomiting, uncontrolled tremors, and eventually grand mal convulsions, delirium and hypothermia. The probability of grand mal seizures increases with the amount of the drug taken daily. Since withdrawal from barbiturates represents a potentially life-threatening situation, it is essential that this be done under medical supervision. Usually doctors withdraw an individual by decreasing their maintenance levels by approximately ten percent every day or two. Convulsions can occur up to one or even two weeks after sudden withdrawal. This sometimes occurs to individuals in jail who have been separated from their source of drugs. Unfortunately, medically supervised barbiturate withdrawal is rarely, if ever, available in our local jails.

Research has shown that barbiturates change the normal EEG patterns during sleep, reducing the usual amount of rapid eye movement (REM) time. Dreams, which are important in maintaining emotional equilibrium, occur during the REM phase of sleep. Thus, barbiturates may help to create emotional tension. With non-barbiturate sedatives available, perhaps the excessive use and availability of barbiturates will decrease.

INHALANTS

Among the very young, children of elementary or junior high school age, there remains the intermittent fads of the inhalation of very toxic substances. These include glues, gasolines, and aerosols. All of them are very dangerous, potentially causing damage to numerous body organs.

Airplane Glue, Plastic and Rubber Cement

When these substances are inhaled initially, the effects often are similar to those of early alcohol intoxication, including lightheadedness, euphoria, giddiness and exhilaration. Occasionally, vivid colorful hallucinations occur which may last up to 20 or 30 minutes. Other reactions include loss of muscular control, slurred speech, blurred vision, drowsiness, stupor, and gross mental disorientation. In some cases, coma and death have occurred.

The main ingredient in these products is toluene. This organic solvent and others like it are extremely dangerous when repeatedly inhaled. Damage occurs to the brain and central nervous system, as well as to the liver and kidneys. Depression of the blood-forming elements in the bone marrow has been reported. Although this substance is not addicting, the body rapidly develops a tolerance to toluene. Repeated or regular use of organic solvents can produce severe or permanent damage.

Gasoline, Paint Thinner, Solvents, Kerosene and Lighter Fluid

These hydrocarbons are very toxic, producing distortions similar to that of alcohol intoxication. In addition, ringing or buzzing in the ears and reverberation of sound are common. Prolonged use of these drugs can cause seizures, delirium, hallucinations, coma and in some cases, death.

Aerosol Sprays

Widely used on the American scene, aerosol sprays pour out everything from whipped cream to oven cleaners. They contain propellants which, when inhaled, cause pronounced effects. These usually last only 5 to 10 minutes and include dizziness, uncontrolled laughter and varied hallucinations. Since it is often difficult to separate the propellant from the spray, concomitant inhaling of deodorants or paint often produces long term damage. Freon, when inhaled too rapidly, can freeze the larynx causing edema and death by suffocation.

Asthmador

The belladonna alkaloids can be extremely valuable in pharmaceutical agents, as well as being extremely dangerous or deadly hallucinogenic drugs. Old fashioned asthma preparations, such as asthmador, contain belladonna and in many places are still available over-the-counter. An asthmador trip is usually a tremendously frightening, overwhelming experience. There have been reports of an asthmador trip lasting as much as seven or eight days with periods of blindness and extreme confusion.

CONCLUSION

Those involved in drug rehabilitation are necessarily caught in a double bind. As they represent our society's orthodox view that sees all illegal drugs as "bad," they must present a limited orientation. On the other hand, rehabilitation specialists often realize that they lose the trust of their clients if they take an attitude which morally disapproves of all drugs. It may be difficult to be non-judgmental. Our roles as counselors is to help people differentiate between harmful drug abuse and tolerable drug use. The final decision must rest with the individual.

Chapter 12

CLINICAL AND COUNSELING PROBLEMS IN DRUG DEPENDENCE

CHARLES L. BOWDEN AND JAMES F. MADDUX

IN THE FOLLOWING pages we will discuss the approaches to handling common clinical problems in the treatment and counseling of persons dependent on morphine-like drugs. Primarily, we will attend to issues which arise between the psychiatrist, rehabilitation counselor or other counselor and the patient or client. It will be useful before doing this to review some of the factors in initial and continued use of morphine-like drugs, as well as factors associated with relapse. Understanding these factors has importance for satisfactory handling of the pharmacological, psychological, and social problems of the patient.

The terms *narcotic drugs* and *narcotic addiction* have become ambiguous. In this chapter, we follow the current medical usage in using the more precise terms *morphine-like* drugs and *drug dependence of the morphine type*. Heroin is used illicitly more frequently than all other morphine-like drugs. The terms *heroin use* and *heroin dependence,* which appear occasionally in the following pages, therefore, include most but not all illicit morphine-type drug use.

PHASES OF DRUG DEPENDENCE

Morphine-type drug dependence represents an outcome of interacting factors among the individual, the drug, and the environment. It occurs in phases in which different constellations of factors influence the process at different times.

Predisposition

Although users of morphine-type drugs vary in personality and in problems of living, most appear to suffer from chronic and severe emotional distress existing prior to the drug use. Furthermore, most apparently acquired only a low tolerance for pain or discomfort of any kind. A delinquent orientation in many, especially in those who became heroin users, made it easy to use an illegal drug. The majority try alcohol and marijuana before they first use heroin.

213

First Use

First use of heroin usually occurs before the age of twenty. Curiosity seems an important factor in the first use. Drug-using peers often encourage first use. Proselytism influences not only the first use, but also continued use, and relapse after abstinence. Many heroin users subtly encourage heroin use among relatives, friends, and ex-addicts. By bringing another person into drug use, a user reduces the possibility that the other person may look with contempt upon him and thus make him aware of his sense of shame and guilt. He effectively fights his ambivalent wish to get off drugs by having one more example that it can't be done. The need for this can be understood if we recognize that the addict tried to protect himself from responsibility for his own failures, which cannot easily be rationalized. He also makes a contact for possibly obtaining heroin. Easy availability of the drug facilitates the first use as well as continued use.

The first intravenous injection of heroin induces nausea and sometimes vomiting. The nausea and vomiting are reported as unpleasant, but emotional effects called the "high" prompt the person to repeat the experience. The drug-induced euphoria is not described as exhilaration and excitement but as tranquility, confidence, and serenity. The drug-induced serenity apparently has strong attraction for the individual with chronic dysphoria.

Symptomatic Use

Following the initial use and the discovery that the drug replaces distress with serenity, the person goes through a phase in which he uses the drug primarily for relief of unpleasant emotions. Surprisingly, even in high risk areas, there is a great deal of ignorance and misinformation about drugs and their effects. Examples are the frequent belief that snorting (sniffing) heroin will not result in addiction, and that meperidine is not a narcotic. The emotional states for which relief is sought vary, but the following occur frequently.

1. **Depression.** Depression appears in two related forms. First, the person views his world and the people in it with feelings of mistrust, of futility, of hopelessness, of being deserted, and with no expectation of getting fair, helpful, or considerate treatment from anyone. Second, he holds himself in low esteem with chronic feelings of guilt, shame, and inadequacy. Early family disruption, lack of role models for successful function through legitimate pursuits, poor educational and vocational skills, unsatisfactory work habits and poor language usage (bad grammar, marked accent, poor vocabulary) serve as background conditions for both forms of depression. Depressive episodes are often precipitated by loss of a love object, vocational failure, or monetary loss.

2. **Anxiety.** The chronic heroin user has little tolerance for anxiety and uses the drug to reduce this unpleasant feeling. Some persons use heroin to assuage anxiety arising from feelings of depersonalization or loss of ego

control. Often they are persons who cannot cope adequately with angry feelings. Less frequently, heroin is used to abort unpleasant drug-induced anxiety, particularly that induced by hallucinogens and amphetamines.

3. **Anger.** Anger is often felt along with depression and anxiety. Some heroin users take the drug primarily to control chronic anger or episodic rage, or both.

4. **Interpersonal inhibition.** Some persons hope that heroin use will magically help them achieve interpersonal closeness which is otherwise difficult because of anxiety or other unpleasant emotional states. Some male users say they began heroin use because it relaxed them and made it easier to talk to girls. Others feel they must use the drug to achieve or maintain approval by an individual or group.

5. **Pain.** Although unpleasant emotional states prompt symptomatic use of morphine-like drugs in most instances, bodily pain prompts drug use in some cases. Bodily pain sometimes represents a somatic response to chronic emotional disturbance.

6. **Pleasure.** Usually among young persons with serious emotional problems who are polydrug abusers, heroin may be taken to achieve a fantasied narcissistic, mystical or transcendental experience.

Compulsive Use

With regular daily use of a morphine-like drug, physical dependence develops, and the threat of abstinence distress provides a powerful new reinforcer of continued use.

All of the factors influencing initial use continue in the phase of compulsive use but they become relatively less important. Repeated use of heroin to ward off real or anticipated abstinence symptoms develops a strongly conditioned response. For example, the client who has experienced increased tension, body aches and pains, depression, rhinorrhea, nausea, etc., while withdrawing from narcotics may experience one or more of these from different sources and may then experience narcotic craving. This is an automatic association with what in the past has relieved the dysphoria. The individual usually does not realize that the current source of his trouble has nothing to do with physiologic abstinence symptoms.

Other conditioned responses further complicate the complex of factors which influence continued use. The person who has experienced withdrawal symptoms may, when experiencing increased tension for some non-drug reason, develop, because of conditioned association, the full gamut of withdrawal symptoms. Environmental stimuli previously paired with heroin euphoria or abstinence symptoms can set off conditioned abstinence symptoms and stimulate drug-seeking behavior. These conditioned responses occur without conscious awareness of the individual and may prompt relapse despite his strenuous and sincere efforts to abstain. Although these operant and classic conditioned reflexes occur in both man and laboratory animals, what sets man apart in that they are tied in with conscious, symbolic phenomena and emotional responses such as shame and guilt.

Another important factor in continued addiction is the sense of hopelessness which many addicts have. In many persons this undoubtedly is an extension of a pre-existing attitude, but the time-consuming career of an addict, especially if he begins during adolescence, does not allow for much in the way of maturation, psychologically, socially, or vocationally. His hopelessness is furthered by the failures he has had in trying to quit heroin use and by generally remaining in a social environment which reinforces his view that few succeed in overcoming their drug dependence.

This sense of hopelessness influences him in three major areas: his attitude toward skill versus chance, toward trust versus distrust, and toward short versus long-term goals. He believes that skills do not matter. He believes failures are due to his own incompetence, and is thus led to rely more on others. But he is distrustful of others and feels oppressed by authority, with which he does not know how to effectively deal. He tends to blame others when things go wrong. Nevertheless, he couples this with a feeling of guilt over not adequately handling his responsibilities. Long-range goals (such as staying out of trouble) have met mainly with frustration and failure. Thus he tends to seek rewards in the present. Heroin readily and effortlessly fits into the above by providing an instantaneous freedom from painful object relationships, relieves his emotion of guilt, and provides instant euphoria. Heroin use also may provide some atonement for his sense of guilt—he is punishing himself by using a drug which could kill him, thus appeasing his conscience.

Intermission and Relapse

Most chronic users of morphine-like drugs make efforts to overcome their drug dependence. Although follow-up studies have shown that nearly all chronic heroin users who are withdrawn from drugs will return to drug use if followed for five years or longer, it is also true that nearly all chronic heroin users have periods of abstinence. The relapse to drug use seems to occur in part as a conditioned response—certain conditions evoke unpleasant emotional or physical states which have in the past repeatedly been relieved by drugs; these states again prompt drug use. Follow-up studies have found a significant proportion, 25 percent or more, of chronic heroin-users to be abstaining from drug use at the time of follow-up.

Termination of Drug Dependence

Some chronic users of morphine-like drugs achieve periods of abstinence extending five years or longer. Permanent or lifetime "cure" is not considered useful terminology. First, an individual who dies after a week or two of abstinence might be considered as having achieved a lifetime "cure," even though his "cure" was very brief. Second, it seems probable that some vestiges of the physiological and psychological changes accompanying morphine-type dependence remain for many years. Like the person who has once experienced sexual orgasm, the person who has once experienced morphine-type dependence is probably never the same as he was before the experience. Nonetheless, with passage of years a gradual recovery from the effects of drug dependence seems to occur, and the individual seems to learn emotional and behavioral responses which replace the drug-seeking habit.

THE COUNSELING INTERACTION

Motivation for Treatment

Why do persons seek treatment? Many of the reasons are obvious, but the question is important because an understanding of the major motive forces in the individual will facilitate treatment process and outcome. At this point we are not able to distinguish "good" from "bad" motives. Existing scanty evidence suggests that fear of external threats, such as loss of medical license or return to prison are among the more effective motivating factors. Some grow tired of the hustle for money and drugs, of evading the law, and of facing repeated incarceration. Others are influenced by the death of addicted acquaintances. Family pressure is often a major factor. Physical debility, which often accompanies addiction, may push the person into treatment. Poor quality heroin or relative unavailability of drugs also can be determining factors. An individual may come for detoxification to reduce his physical dependence so that he can regain euphoria from heroin with smaller and less expensive doses. In the case of methadone maintenance, some addicts desire it simply as a readily available, cheap, legal supply of the stuff they have convinced themselves their lives revolve around.

The above reasons for coming into treatment foretell some common factors associated with success. Unavailability of drugs and a related factor, staying away from addicts and old haunts associated with one's drug use, are generally important. Threats of external action are probably effective in part because the act of setting limits implies caring—caring enough to say "no" beyond a certain point. Several characteristics, subsumed under the heading of maturity, seem important. Breaking away from child-like dependence on parents, developing gratifying work skills, providing for one's financial needs, being able to have close relationships with others—especially one's spouse—learning to tolerate a certain degree of pain, anxiety, failure and depression, are examples. Will power—an elusive sense of intentionality, staying with a task until its completion—is important in its own right.

Of what usefulness are the above to the rehabilitation professional working with the addict? First, these and similar data give the rehabilitation counselor a framework in which to understand the vicissitudes of the drug dependence experience. This also is important because the severity and chronicity of drug dependence can be frustrating and defeating to a rehabilitation worker who is unable to understand why his own and his client's best efforts often end in failure.

Another reason for understanding the factors influencing drug dependence is that much of it can be usefully communicated to the client, even though some of it, such as the conditioned phenomena of abstinence, may discourage the addict. If a client is aware of the inevitability of some yearning for heroin, rooted in the conditioned responses and memories of the effects of heroin, and is aware that these yearnings often cause a person to feel powerless and guilty of fantasied wrongs, he is in a better position to prevent untoward consequences of those yearnings. If he knows that he cannot eliminate these tendencies, but that he can become cognizant of such reaction patterns, the conditions that set them off and their early manifestations, he can have conscious input into the course of action he takes, knowing that his impulse to use heroin is certain to diminish or pass.

Attitude of the Counselor to the Client

Before discussing some specific problems in management, some remarks about the rehabilitation counselor's general behavior are in order. First of all, an attitude of detached optimism is usually warranted. Whatever one's attitude, it should be expressed primarily in behavior, not statements.

The term "detached optimism" is important. Frequently an inexperienced, zealous person begins clinical work with addicts and overidentifies with them, accepting many of their rationalizations, accepting too uncritically their view that it is society that is bad, and extends himself to do things for the addict. This behavior is unfortunate for several reasons. However bad society may be, it is still the individual's decision that he can't live without drugs. To do things for him, rather than help him to do things for himself, keeps him in a dependent position and implicitly carries the message that he is incapable of being responsible for his own affairs. Although in many ways he may be incapable, this is best dealt with more candidly, vis-a-vis the particular problems he has. Lastly, overidentification can lead to undue personal responsibility for patient's failures, with resultant disillusionment. Sometimes because of overidentification the worker develops a deep-seated, though sometimes masked, scorn, and dislike for addicts. Detachment, then, does not mean a lack of concern, but avoiding an inappropriate personalizing of one's clinical role—what would fall under the term "counter-transference" in psychoanalysis. Optimism is important because it is justified. Many persons, clinical staff, rehabilitation counselors and addicted clients alike, have unreasonably pessimistic views of the long-term rehabilitative prospects of the addict.

Some workers do their best to relate to the addict in his own jargon. We advise against this approach. It is of course important to understand what a person means, to be willing to use words and phrases with emotional impact and relevance, but as an effort to be "with it," to use a lingua franca, the approach has shortcomings. It is almost impossible to keep up with changes in street language usage, and, since that argot is not the one primarily used by the rehabilitation worker, he tends to appear counterfeit to the drug abuser.

In some ways, the effort is inimical to the goals of treatment, one of which is to help the person live in a straight, non-drug-using society. In part that means helping him put aside street lingo, develop better language skills and, perhaps most important and most difficult, feel comfortable using those skills. The treatment relationship, in this area as in so many others, provides a model experience wherein the addict can learn and try out such differences from his usual role function. To deprive him of that opportunity is anti-therapeutic and also can suggest a condescension toward the client—that the counselor uses argot because the client could not understand "proper" usage. A similar issue is names. If you expect the client to refer to you as "Dr. Smith" or "Miss Jones," it is belittling to call him "Jake," "Flash," or "Pablo." If, on the other hand, you wish clients to refer to you by first name, reciprocal usage is appropriate. The important point is to assiduously avoid those behaviors that suggest condescension toward and devaluation of the individual. Similarly, your non-verbal behavior can convey these messages. Punctuality in keeping appointments and responsibility in promptly carrying out whatever obligations you set for yourself are telling to the client about your seriousness of purpose and your concern for him. The reverse is obviously true.

Role Modeling

It is clear from the above that the rehabilitation counselor can be an important role model for the client. This can certainly be done in such areas as language usage, punctuality, responsibility, name usage, candor, including information about one's own behavior, and a willingness to "rub elbows" with someone different from one's self. The advantages are multifold. The addict may eventually take on, though usually belatedly, as his own, some of the values and behavior you have shown. The experience of seeing you open to criticism may be especially meaningful to a person who habitually uses rationalization and externalization. The experience may break down his defensive cultural stereotype of the cops and the robbers, wherein he presumes that you were born with a silver spoon in your mouth, had all the breaks, or are in some ways totally unlike him. There are dangers in such openness, primarily that he may wish to make you the focus of treatment which is more fun and certainly less painful than focusing upon himself.

Gross cultural differences between the clinician and the rehabilitation counselor and the addict make this difficult. It is in this area that the use of ex-addicts has the greatest benefit. The addict cannot rationalize that what the ex-addict staff person says or does is irrelevant because he is such a "different breed of cat," in fact the person, by virtue of his past addiction, shares many habits of experiences in common with the client. The same holds to varying degrees in having similar ethnic, religious, sexed, and socio-economic grouped staff work with drug abusers.

The Hidden Meaning of Language

We have talked about how the rehabilitation counselor reveals his attitude through the use of jargon and names. A special related problem is the concealed hopelessness and disparagement in the words used by the drug dependent person—and too often by others—to refer to himself: "junky," "hooked," "an addict." These terms have an air of despair and finality about them. In few medical disorders is the person identified with the disease. We speak of the "narcotic addict," but of the patient with pneumonia, not the pneumoniac. This language usage tends to come about when the disorder is viewed as prolonged and unremitting. But as has been earlier discussed, there are reasons for greater optimism and the insidious lapsing into such usage by staff or clients needs to be guarded against.

Reality Focus

The major treatment focus should be on the present. It is more emotionally charged, and the drug dependent cannot so easily rationalize or deny what has recently been observed or what he is currently doing. It is important that the counselor know the totality of the client's behavior, so that he does not sequester, for example, antisocial behavior to obtain the love and approval he desires from the client. This is of course easier to accomplish in an inpatient or therapeutic community setting than in an outpatient one. Appropriate acknowledgement of good behavior is as important as confrontation of all untoward behavior.

The continued interpretation of reality to the client has other aspects. These are the harsh facts about the high mortality rates among persons who use heroin, the frequency of serious physical disorders, the frequent overdependence on family, the legal risks, and the high proportion of time spent incarcerated. We have already discussed the importance of the individual's understanding the physiologic and long-term conditioned effects of drug dependence. This is not to say that a lot of knowledge will cure the person, but that such information is almost never harmful to treatment goals, and it frequently gives him a greater sense of understanding and thus more power to deal with what he is up against. This kind of confrontation can be particularly helpful when fitted into the reasons which caused or sustained the person's drug use.

Reality confrontation can sometimes be effective in special situations. This is particularly so when greater professional experience in rehabilitation makes such confrontation easier. A client who comes in with an unrealistic plan, often including the belief that he needs no further treatment help and will have no further problems, can sometimes be told (or reminded) in a calm but direct way that he will begin to lie to you, to himself, that he will start to use heroin, that he will again steal from his wife, that this time she will likely leave him for good, and that he will probably again end up in jail, where he has spent six of the past eight years. In effect, you are telling him what he already knows, but tries to avoid through denial, through rationalization and through getting a caring, authoritative person to accept his delusional thinking out of sympathy or love (i.e., to wish beyond his real fate). The way in which one can utilize confrontation will be a function of three variables: (1) one's own "style" (a combination of character structure and training), (2) the situation, and (3) the personality of the patient. The objectivity of the confrontation makes it very difficult for the person to hang onto his projective defenses—i.e., to externalize his conflict and blame you.

Dealing With Pessimism

Most heroin users feel pessimistic about their chances of success. As we have noted, there are understandable bases for such pessimism. The following are important ways of counteracting it.

Many clients lack the rudiments of education and social skills necessary to live comfortably in a technological society. It is important to be able to figure interest rates, to prepare a budget or income tax return, to read and understand a credit contract, to understand a technical instruction manual, to know how to utilize city public services—from welfare to the library. Education to insure these basic skills is essential. In the area of role function, it is important to know how to apply for a job, what proper employee responsibility consists of, what good child-rearing practices are. It is good to encourage interest in political issues. Generally it is best to pick issues that are immediately relevant to the individual, possibly black power or brown power, creative writing, sports, or whatever the individual case may suggest.

Self dependence vocationally and financially is important. It increases self-esteem, and esteem of others. It helps provide good usage of time which is so important in a disorder where boredom is a danger. Self dependency increases anxiety, by placing the person in an existential situation. The anxiety often motivates him to discuss issues which either were not present or which he could easily rationalize or repress previously. Lastly, it impels him to think, plan and act toward the future, thus inclining him away from his present-oriented life style.

Often a patient will react to the anxiety of trying, or to his real or fantasied failure, by prematurely giving up. A variant is to find the clinician at fault, and accuse him of thinking of the person as "just a junky." Usually a concerned confrontation of the patient with what he is doing in his habitual way can be effective here.

Another side of pessimism is the drug abuser's wish to deny his fears and his limitations and aim unrealistically high. Instead of getting a job in a cleaning plant, he wishes to start by obtaining a 200,000 dollar loan to buy his own plant. The variations are endless. Unrealistic wishing should not be supported, even passively. Confrontation may result in angry indignation at the counselor for "wanting the client to fail." Often there is no good way to handle such problems. Group confrontation is usually more effective, the client finding it harder to denigrate the views of a half-dozen persons. But such patients are often the ones most unwilling to participate in a therapy group. It is important to understand that such wishes often arise out of a frantic sense of hopelessness, and the counselor should try to turn the person's interests toward activities where it is believed he has a good chance of success.

Values

In his effort to establish rapport, a counselor will sometimes ostensibly approve or condone antisocial values of the client. We consider this ill-advised: the counselor pretends to have values not his own, or he has been corrupted by the client. On the other hand, the counselor may feel that he must reform the client, not only in his overt behavior, but in his orality as well. In our conception of rehabilitation, the counselor neither pretends to adopt nor tries to demolish the values of the patient; his task is a more complicated one of providing a helping interaction which facilitates growth of coping capacity in the individual.

Nonetheless the counselor will directly or indirectly reveal his values during counseling, as these are tested by the patient. We advocate direct acknowledgement of the counselor's values whenever the client wants to know, with the proviso that interpretation may be needed if it seems that the patient is discussing the counselor's values in order to avoid discussing the patient's problems.

Specific Problems With Methadone Maintenance

Several typical problems arise with patients receiving methadone maintenance. A patient may complain of some physical problem—a lack of sleep, anxiety after work, etc.—and plead with the physician to increase his methadone "just to see whether that's what's really causing me to have all this trouble." Both because of the conditioned response to receiving more drugs and the likelihood that a greater amount of methadone would temporarily relieve many kinds of discomforts, regardless of cause, he would, if he were given the increased dosage, have reinforced his belief in the power and necessity of the drug for handling whatever ails him. Rather, such situations should be used as opportunities to explain the above to the patient, to explore with him what interpersonal or situational factors were contributing to his tension or other symptoms and discuss alternative ways of coping.

A similar misconception arises in the patient who lives more successfully than in his entire previous life, and then attributes his success to the methadone, as if it were a fuel that made him go and without which he could not function. It is important to help him realize that his successes are his, accomplished by his own efforts, and that they could have been similarly accomplished without methadone. The methadone has simply helped to provide a stable physiologic milieu for him to try to get his life together. He could probably do equally well without it, except that in the transition period to abstinence he would have significant and prolonged withdrawal symptoms and, without methadone, would have the compulsion to use heroin.

Continuing to Care

The last point we will make is often overlooked. Too often the patients who cause the most trouble or are the most dependent get the most attention. But after a person has ceased heroin use the staff shifts their attention elsewhere. This is understandable for many reasons. The heroin-using population is large. Waiting lists are sometimes long, and financial and political pressure to treat many patients exists. One reason that parole programs and methadone maintenance programs have, at least in some situations, had considerable success may be that they continue to provide a person who cares even when the patient is doing well. This is something that many of these patients have never before experienced. Not surprisingly, for reasons such as pride, many would deny the need for any support or counseling. The nature and frequency of contact may change once the person is doing well, but it should not be prematurely broken. To do so makes it psychologically harder for the person to return to discuss his mistakes or his failing to abstain from heroin. It deprives him of the support and approval, which may be not so much stated as understood, for the successes he is having.

(PART FOUR)

THE MENTALLY RETARDED

Rehabilitation Services to the Mentally Retarded

Vocational Habilitation for the Mentally Retarded

Chapter 13

REHABILITATION SERVICES TO THE MENTALLY RETARDED

FRANK B. PERDUE

INTRODUCTION

ACCORDING TO the United States Department of Labor, there are more than 5.6 million retarded persons in this country, and approximately 3.3 million are of working age. Many of these people can be trained and successfully employed, because, although mental retardation implies limited learning ability, this is not always a severe handicap. The employable mental retardates often realize that their capabilities are limited and therefore strive harder to do a better job. Moreover, they usually do not aspire to higher skilled jobs and often perform lower-level jobs better than average workers. In fact, federal officials estimate that between 60 and 75 percent of the retardates can be taught the minimum skills needed for jobs as messengers, warehousemen, stock clerks, gardeners, laborers, clerks, millhands, restaurant workers, maids, cleaning women, and so forth (Kelly and Simon, 1969).

There are approximately 307,000 mental retardates in Texas today according to the *Texas Plan to Combat Mental Retardation* (1966). Many of these have vocational potential to the extent that they may be self-sufficient. Some may be able to be employed but need some type of supervision during after-working-hours. Some may never be able to be employed outside a sheltered workshop.

The vocational rehabilitation counselor is charged with the responsibility of providing every resource through the Texas Rehabilitation Commission and/or community to enable the retardate to achieve his maximum vocational potential. The counselor's biggest responsibility, therefore, is to help the retardate to develop his personal and social maturity through a variety of experiences, projects, and programs now available in the state.

This chapter is expressly designed to be used as a reference for vocational rehabilitation counselors working with the mentally retarded. The purpose is to give an overview of the services available to the retardate. Parents, lay people and professionals may find it useful as a resource. The primary concern, however, is to show how the retarded can be habilitated.

History and Philosophy

Vocational Rehabilitation came into being as a result of World War I. Shortly after the war, in 1919, the National Congress established a Vocational Rehabilitation Program for Veterans and, in 1920, followed this with a law to provide rehabilitation services for the civilian disabled. The law provided funds to the states, in the form of grants, to carry out rehabilitation services. Federal legislation was accepted by the 41st Texas Legislature in 1929, and the State Board of Education was designated to administer the program.

The early legislation did not provide for the rehabilitation of the mentally retarded; therefore, little or nothing was done toward the rehabilitation of the mentally retarded until 1943. At this time, the Federal Congress amended the 1920 Act (Public Law 113), thus expanding the program of Vocational Rehabilitation to include the mentally handicapped.

Again, in 1954, Congress amended the Act to provide increased grants to the states for special and improved services to the handicapped (Public Law 565). This particular law paved the way for establishment of special facilities to study the problems of rehabilitation of handicapped individuals.

In 1955, the Texas Legislature enacted the *Mentally Retarded Persons Act,* which did many things toward bringing the movement of vocational rehabilitation of the mentally retarded into the limelight. One important phase of this legislation was that 50,000 dollars was earmarked for services to the mentally retarded. This act did not give an extra 50,000 dollars to the Vocational Rehabilitation program for the mentally retarded, it merely took 50,000 dollars of existing Vocational Rehabilitation funds and certified them to be spent on specific services for the mentally retarded.

The director of Vocational Rehabilitation, in 1957, realized the necessity for initiating a plan for counselors to work specifically with the mentally retarded, to experiment with them, and to learn as much as possible about how rehabilitation for mentally retarded should be done.

In September of 1957, a supervisor for services to the mentally retarded, along with three field counselors, was appointed. The counselors were located in areas where there was a concentration of population. This initiated the Texas Program for the rehabilitation of the mentally retarded.

Prior to the appointment of the special counselors, some rehabilitation for the mentally retarded was done by counselors working in the general program. Some successes were met, and a great deal of insight was gained as to the type of case service needed for this particular disability.

The newly appointed counselors, working with the mentally retarded, were highly qualified specialists who had had experience in the field of mental retardation. The director, in 1957, was very wise in giving these counselors a wide latitude, to experiment and try to determine at what levels of employment the retardates were most successful. Also this wide latitude permitted the special counselor to experiment with different degrees of mental retardation and determine to a small degree, which level of mental retardation was most susceptible to vocational rehabilitation.

Mentally retarded individuals, eligible for vocational rehabilitation services, were those within the I.Q. range of 50 to 75.

The special counselors soon learned that those retardates with I.Q.'s between 65 and 75 were the best risk, vocation-wise, and for a short time this group comprised the majority of the clients on the vocational rehabilitation counselor's caseload. As the program grew older, the type of retardate selected for vocational rehabilitation began to be determined more by performance and social adjustment than by I.Q.

Presently, counselors are placing people according to their practical ability rather than in categories established by I.Q. numbers. After all these years, counselors are saying that vocational rehabilitation is now handling many retardates that in the beginning were considered nonfeasible. This is based on knowledge of past performances of retardates that have been observed in a rehabilitation setting.

The National Association for Retarded Children sees the mentally retarded as having the same basic needs as everyone else. What is different is the manner in which they are able to obtain need fulfillment. Each retardate has to be viewed on an individual basis. The concept of individual differences when applied to the retarded enables the counselor to see that he is dealing primarily with a person with mental retardation. It gives him the opportunity to plan anew each time he accepts another retardate for services. No two retardates are alike even though they may be classed in the same group, come from the same background, and have exactly the same intelligence score one as the other (NARC, 1961).

Who Are the Mentally Retarded?

The *Texas Plan to Combat Mental Retardation* (1966), which was published as a result of the Governor's Committee on Mental Retardation Planning, defines the mentally retarded as children and adults who, as a result of inadequately developed intelligence, are significantly impaired in their ability to learn and to adapt to the society in which they live. Dr. Sam Kirk, in his book *Educating the Retarded Child* (1951), defines the mentally handicapped child as one who is diagnosed as having low intelligence, who is unable to profit sufficiently from the curriculum of the public schools, but who can be educated to become socially adequate and occupationally competent, provided special education facilities are furnished.

The Texas Education Agency, *Administrative Guide and Handbook for Special Education,* Bulletin 711 (1971), says that children who are EDUCABLE MENTALLY RETARDED are those who reveal a reduced rate of intellectual development and a level of academic achievement below that of their peer age group, as evidenced by significant deficits in all essential learning processes.

The American Association on Mental Deficiency (Heber, 1961) adopted a definition of mental retardation that is used by the Texas Rehabilitation Commission as well, that is, mental retardation refers to subaverage general intellectual functioning which originates during the developmental period and is associated with impairment in adaptive behavior. *Subaverage* refers to performance which is greater than one Standard Deviation below the population mean of the age group involved on measures of general intellectual functioning. Level of *general intellectual functioning* may be assessed by performance on one or more of the various objective tests which have been developed for that purpose. The definition specifies that the subaverage intellectual functioning must be reflected by *impairment in adaptive behavior*. Adaptive behavior refers primarily to the effectiveness of the individual in adapting to the natural and social demands of his environment. Impaired adaptive behavior may be reflected in levels of (1) maturation, (2) learning, and/or (3) social adjustment.

Rate of **maturation** refers to the rate of sequential development of self-help skills of infancy and early childhood, such as sitting, crawling, standing, walking, habit training, and interaction with age peers.

Learning ability refers to the facility with which knowledge is acquired as a function of experience. Learning difficulties are usually most manifest in the academic situation and if mild in degree may not even become apparent until the child enters school.

Social adjustment is particularly important as a qualifying condition of mental retardation at the adult level where it is assessed in terms of the degree to which the individual is able to maintain himself independently in the community and in gainful employment as well as by his ability to meet and conform to other personal and social responsibilities and standards set by the community. Within the framework of the present definition mental retardation is a term descriptive of the current status of the individual with respect to intellectual functioning, and adaptive behavior. Consequently, an individual may meet the criteria of mental retardation at one time and not at another. A person may change status as a result of changes in social standards or conditions or as a result of changes in efficiency of intellectual functioning, with level of efficiency always being determined in relation to the behavioral standards and norms for the individuals chronological age group (Heber, 1961).

The Habilitation of the Mentally Retarded
Through Texas Rehabilitation Commission Services

When the vocational rehabilitation counselor has a retardate referred to him he has the responsibility of determining eligibility for vocational rehabilitation services and then developing a suitable Plan of Habilitation. It is proposed that a person who meets the following criteria should be considered for the vocational rehabilitation program:

a. He is of working age, or will be upon completion of his rehabilitation plan of preparation for employment;

b. it has been demonstrated in competent psychological and medical examinations and evaluations that a mental impairment exists and makes it likely that the individual will be incapable of adjusting to adequate jobs;

c. it has been concluded from such competent psychological and medical examinations and evaluations that prognosis for the vocational rehabilitation of such an individual is favorable; and

d. he is lacking in adequate educational opportunity or in the other services available through vocational rehabilitation by which he may be prepared for and assisted in finding suitable employment (Hegge, 1950, p. 23).

Finding the retarded person promptly so that rehabilitation may begin before he is subjected unduly to the disintegrating effects of idleness and hopelessness, is important. Referrals come from many sources. In fact, anybody can make a referral to Vocational Rehabilitation—doctors, parents, teachers, social welfare workers, employers and many others. The most satisfactory referral source is the Special Education Department of the public school. The most work-ready people who come to us are from this source (NARC, 1961).

Once the vocational rehabilitation counselor has determined that the mental retardate is to be an accepted case and a plan of action is to be carried out, the referring agency is to be contracted and made aware of the services to be provided.

The purpose of this section is to provide a step-by-step procedure of Rehabilitation, from referral to closure, with the mentally retarded. The first step after referral is to obtain all available current information on the mental retardate. During the process of completing the application for vocational rehabilitation services, the vocational rehabilitation counselor should have the mental retardate or his parents sign a Release of Information form which will allow other agencies to provide information that will help, first of all, to establish eligibility and that will also aid the counselor in estimating the extent of disability or handicap. Information should be retrieved from schools, institutions, doctors, hospitals, or any other source.

The vocational rehabilitation counselor should obtain a general medical examination including a urinalysis. The general medical may indicate a need for a blood serology or X-ray in which case the counselor will arrange for these. If the serology is positive, the counselor must arrange for treatment through the County Health unit or some other source of treatment (RSM, 1972).

The general medical may indicate a specialist examination and this should be done promptly. A psychological examination should be obtained on all mentally retarded referrals. It should be used to establish eligibility along with abstracts of school records, etc., and documented in the client's case folder. The psychological examination should be comprehensive and should not only include the I.Q. score, but assess social functioning as well as adaptive behavior. The counselor should furnish the examining psychologist with as much background information as possible prior to the examination.

Establishing Mental Retardation as a Disability

The Texas Rehabilitation Commission has determined in its Manual of Policy that in cases of mental retardation, the disability will be established on the basis of *functional ability,* with the help of the following guidelines.

1. A valid individual test of intelligence with an IQ of 50-85. For those clients scoring 70-85 it is important to note that a measured intelligence quotient in and of itself is insufficient diagnostic evidence of the existence of mental retardation, and that the presence of maladaptive behavior and deficit educational functioning . . . is particularly important in determining disability. Therefore an individual with a 70-85 IQ may or may not be classified as mentally retarded, since many people in this borderline area may neither experience any particular problems of adjustment nor demonstrate any evidence of maladaptive behavior.
2. Assessment of social functioning and evaluation of behavior indicating inadequate personal and social functioning and maladaptive behavior. When the assessment of social functioning and educational progress cannot be provided by the school, the Counselor and school staff will review the cumulative school record of the student and make a determination of the social functioning and educational achievement. The results of this determination will be documented in the case record and summarized in the vocational rehabilitation plan when it is written.
3. Assessment of educational progress and achievement indicating inadequate levels of educational achievement (Sec. 02-3, p. 1).

In cases where the I.Q. is below 50, consideration of an individual's vocational potential will be determined by the counselor and justification for his decision will be made in the case file (Texas Rehabilitation Commission, 1972).

Determination of Personal and Social Adjustment

When studying the client's vocational assets and liabilities, the vocational rehabilitation counselor must evaluate the extent of the vocational handicap and determine a plan of action. A big part of this evaluation must deal with the personal and social adjustment of the retardate through observed behavior, his attitude toward social elements in his environment, the degree and nature of acceptance of the client by the community, and sociological data from the client's home and family.

PLANNING SERVICES

1. **Counseling and Guidance.** The vocational rehabilitation counselor needs to be sure that the retardate and his parents/guardian are involved in the counseling process. A great deal of support should come from the parents as the Plan progresses. The vocational rehabilitation counselor has the additional responsibility of informing the parents of the progress or lack of progress. Counseling and guidance make up the continuous service which ties all other parts of the rehabilitation process into an organized plan. This

service begins at the first interview and runs through to satisfactory placement and adjustment on a job. Counseling helps the retarded person to understand his assets and liabilities, the causes of his present problems and the steps necessary to correct these difficulties. It plays an important role in the selection of a specific job goal by relating the client's abilities to job requirements and job oportunities in the community.

2. **Training** for a job is one means of preparing for suitable employment. It may include personal adjustment training, prevocational, vocational and supplementary instruction. Training is provided either to prepare the retarded person for a job or to make him more advantageously employable through added skills and capacities. Regardless of the type of training involved, it must be directed toward eventual employment. Many of the mentally retarded unable to immediately meet competitive employment standards in the open labor market may secure such training through a sheltered workshop program. The counselor should acquaint himself with the labor laws and policies established by the Wage and Hour Division of the United States Department of Labor.

3. **Evaluation.** Medical diagnosis and other examinations, which may include not only a basic physical examination, but specialist examinations such as psychological evaluation and laboratory examinations; the extent of the applicant's retardation is discovered, his eligibility for services and his ability to meet the physical demands of work are determined. The type of job he can do best is ascertained by interview and tests of aptitudes, interests, and by a review of his education, work experiences, home conditions, family attitudes, and other factors that can be determined by the use of a sheltered workshop. Out of this comes a unified rehabilitation plan and a job goal. The client and his family take part in both, and his desires are given full consideration.

4. **Physical Restoration.** Since many retardates are multiply handicapped, the reduction of physically disabling conditions is in keeping with good rehabilitation practice and essential to total rehabilitation of the client. The physical restoration of an individual may include any type of medical or allied service which will aid in eliminating or substantially reducing his disability as a job handicap. Included are medical, surgical services, hospitalization, and artificial devices of all types such as prosthetic limbs, wheelchairs, and hearing aids.

5. **Other services** provided during the rehabilitation process are such things as *room and board, transportation, training materials, occupational tools* and *equipment,* and *occupational licenses* when necessary.

6. **Job Placement.** Placement in employment is the culmination of all the aforementioned steps. It should make the best use of the individual's ability and take into consideration his disability, his temperament, as well as providing for his future development. Every person accepted for services by

Vocational Rehabilitation is entitled to our most sincere efforts at placement.

7. **Follow-up.** For a reasonable time, follow-up on an individual's job performance is necessary. He may need further service—that is, additional counseling, medical, surgical and psychiatric care—or he may require supplemental job training. Of great importance is to keep in mind the individual's social and adult educational needs as they relate to his vocational rehabilitation success.

The Rehabilitation Plan

All vocational rehabilitation counselors are required to develop a Vocational Rehabilitation Plan for the client which will be comprehensive enough to provide the kinds of services needed to eventually result in employment for the client. Essentially, there are three things necessary in the narrative part, that is:

1. how the client's disability represents a vocational handicap;
2. the basis for arriving at the vocational objective; and
3. a justification of planned services as a means of attaining the vocational objective.

Factors to Consider in Predicting
Employment Success of the Mentally Retarded

"How do we predict social and vocational outcomes for the retarded?" In an attempt to answer this question, the Research Utilization Branch, Division of Research and Demonstrations, Office of Research and Demonstrations, Social and Rehabilitation Service, Department of Health, Education, and Welfare (Washington, D.C.) surveyed the literature, producing an annotated bibliography of 569 items, then analyzed the materials in an attempt to dredge out the main findings and their significance for the practitioner (R and D, 1970).

Counselors need to hold firmly in mind that follow-up studies have consistently found a high proportion of the adult retarded achieving satisfactory adjustment in a variety of areas. They should therefore raise their expectations for the retarded.

There are many criteria of success and failure for the retarded, each with its own determiners. Even "vocational success" may have several meanings. The counselor should therefore use broad criteria in evaluating the retarded, lest he reject clients who ought to be accepted.

In making practical decisions and predictions regarding a client, the good counselor will not depend on individual measures of personal and behavioral traits. He will be wise to use assessment data more as a measure of present status than of future performance.

Where early retardation has been related to adverse social and cultural factors, the movement from instability to stability may take a period of years. Failure at any point, or even a succession of failures, should not in itself lead the counselor to terminate services.

The counselor will therefore need repeated assessments as his client progresses, and must avoid premature conclusions.

The counselor needs to remember that intelligence tests cannot be used with any precision in predicting success of the retarded nor even as a sure basis for classifying them educationally. In general, a recent Wechsler Performance score seems to predict their adult occupational success better than other intellectual measures.

The counselor should know that manual dexterity and social maturity, as measured by the Purdue Pegboard Test and the Vineland Social Maturity Scale, are useful in predicting work efficiency and social competence of the retarded in training situations. However, their usefulness has been validated only for the small industry type of workshop.

There is no reliable way to predict success or failure on the basis of personality measures, even though it is agreed that personality greatly affects adult adjustment of the retarded. The counselor can expect help from projective techniques as well as from objective measures of motivation and social sensitivity in assessing present status, but these have little long-range validity.

The value of psychological measures used to assess the retarded depends greatly on the experience of the psychologist in interpreting the client's responses. Counselors and psychologists therefore need broad, extensive experience in working with the mentally retarded.

The application of selection ratios and cutting scores in determining the eligibility of a retarded applicant for services is not warranted by the validity or reliability of available measuring instruments. Such devices may be quite inaccurate, and often tend to eliminate the client who needs services the most.

Even if a counselor could have complete knowledge of a retarded client, he would still have to bear in mind that final outcome depends not only on the individual but also in great measure on effective environmental intervention and societal accommodation.

A number of studies have demonstrated that mildly retarded persons move upward and become stable socially and vocationally over a period of time.

Resources in Texas Available for the Mentally Retarded

Listed below are some six resources available for the mentally retarded that every vocational rehabilitation counselor should use. A brief description will be given.

1. FEDERAL EMPLOYMENT OF THE MENTALLY RETARDED under Schedule A authority. Since 1964, the United States government has allowed the vocational rehabilitation counselor to certify the mentally retarded for employment in lieu of his having to take Civil Service examinations. The counselor must work closely with the federal coordinator at all federal installations and

must provide him with a letter of certification.

2. NATIONAL ASSOCIATION FOR RETARDED CHILDREN—On-The-Job Training Project. The On-the-Job Training Project, funded by the United States Department of Labor and administered by the National Association for Retarded Children (NARC), encourages business to provide job opportunities for the mentally retarded. NARC assists a business in pointing out occupational areas where retardates can alleviate manpower shortages. In addition, NARC will reimburse an employer one-half of the entry wage for the first four critical weeks of employment and one-fourth of the entry wage for the second four weeks of employment.

The NARC Project and an employer enter into an agreement whereby the employer agrees to hire a mentally retarded person at the same pay rate that he would hire a non-retarded employee. For providing a retardate with an on-the-job training opportunity, the NARC Project agrees to reimburse the employer the specified portion of the training costs, as indicated.

All potential trainees are screened and certified to be work-ready prior to referral to the employer. Certification of being work-ready means that the retarded individual can adequately perform in a normal work environment and has had some training for the specific job assignment. The NARC Project works closely with the employer and the potential trainee in evaluating the requirements of the work situation and the trainee's needs and abilities. The employer has absolute right of selection. Trainees selected are considered regular employees from the start. The employer also has absolute right of trainee termination.

AFL-CIO and other labor unions have indicated their interest in this program. They have expressed their desire to assist in its implementation where possible.

3. HALFWAY HOUSES. The halfway house is a transitional living facility which provides the essentials of community living, such as room, board, evening and night-time supervision, and recreational activities. Such service should enable a person with an employment handicap to move from dependent status to an independent status.

4. DENTON STATE SCHOOL, RICHMOND STATE SCHOOL, AND VERNON CENTER PROJECTS. The purpose of the Richmond and Denton State School Projects and Vernon Center is to offer residential facilities and personal, social, and work adjustment training to mentally retarded young men and women who evidence potential for independent living and employment. These retardates may have demonstrated an inability to make satisfactory competitive work adjustments, or they may merely come from communities lacking sufficient vocational outlets for their specialized needs. The Projects also serve as an evaluation facility to aid the field counselors in determining feasibility and to establish realistic goals for their clients.

5. REGIONAL REHABILITATION CENTERS. This program is intended to fill a gap in services and, in this sense, is supplemental to programs available

in the home community. The basic design of this program is to provide in-depth vocational evaluation and work adjustment training. In order to accomplish these established objectives, the client will be enrolled in a number of job sampling activities through which a determination will be made as to the client's relative vocational strengths and weaknesses.

Four State Schools have joined with the Texas Rehabilitation Commission in providing this residential program. The ultimate goal of this training is to maximize vocational strengths to the extent that the client can be integrated into competitive employment in the community.

6. EXTENDED LIVING SERVICES. As a result of the passage of House Bill 287 during the 61st Legislature, the Texas Rehabilitation Commission was charged with the following responsibility of supplying extended rehabilitation services to the mentally retarded who are not eligible for vocational services under laws and regulations in effect at the date of enactment of this legislation. Included in this responsibility is the provision of extended sheltered workshop employment opportunity, as well as extended community residence services, for the mentally retarded. Listed below are the objectives to extended living services:

a. To provide extended sheltered workshop employment opportunities to the severely mentally retarded who are otherwise ineligible for Vocational Rehabilitation sponsorship. It is anticipated that this service will help the retardates function to their optimum capacity in regards to productivity.

b. To provide extended community living services to the severely mentally retarded who are otherwise ineligible for Vocational Rehabilitation services. By living away from their homes, it is expected that the participants will develop a great deal of self respect and will feel less dependent upon others.

c. To demonstrate how services provided for under House Bill 287, 61st Legislature, can be of benefit to the severely retarded.

As soon as funds become available, this program will be implemented statewide (in Texas) and will be an excellent resource for the more severely retarded.

THE COOPERATIVE SCHOOL PROGRAM

The Cooperative Program, which was initiated on a statewide basis in February 1962, was a new and somewhat unique experience for Vocational Rehabilitation (Texas Education Agency, 1971).

Prior to the Cooperative Program, there was little effort put forth in rehabilitating the mentally retarded in our general population. Before this time, the main effort toward rehabilitation in this field was centered around the State Schools for the mentally retarded.

All of the services offered in the Cooperative Program have been available for a long time.

Example: The public schools were educating the mentally retarded long before the Cooperative Program. The Division of Special Education carried on its function in cooperation with the public school before the Cooperative Program.

The Vocational Rehabilitation Division had policies covering the vocational rehabilitation of the mentally retarded years before the advent of this program.

Although all three agencies were carrying on programs with the same goals, they were not working together. Before the beginning of the Cooperative Program, Vocational Rehabilitation served only a handful of mentally retarded clients through the General Rehabilitation program.

In 1962, the Division of Special Education and Vocational Rehabilitation, Texas Education Agency, launched a new program—the Cooperative Rehabilitation Plan. This program enabled local school districts, through a cooperative agreement with the Texas Education Agency, to provide an organized and systematic basis for vocational rehabilitation services to all eligible handicapped youth enrolled in special education classes in a public school. Vocational rehabilitation services to the blind and partially sighted are provided through the State Commission for the Blind (Region V, 1969).

Requirements

As a result of Senate Bill 230, (61st Legislature) and the *Administrative Guide and Handbook for Special Education,* the cooperative school-work program shall now include all educationally handicapped students whose impairments constitute a vocational and/or employment handicap. The program shall include the mentally retarded, physically handicapped, emotionally disturbed, minimally brain-injured, and those with language and/or learning disabilities of an extent to render them incapable of functioning in a normal work-training situation.

The program for the educable mentally retarded permits each pupil to make progress at his own rate of development without comparison to theoretical norms or to members of his group, and has as its major goal community work adjustment. In lieu of the twelve traditional grades of the public school, the students will complete the levels of educational development and be eligible for graduation, with a diploma, from his high school. The program is free of an expected annual promotion or retention of the pupil. The objectives are the attainment of physical competencies, personal and social competencies, and vocational competencies through a program of functional experiences.

A student who is of employable age and who may have potential to adjust to a work situation in the community is assigned to the senior high school program, on-job-training level. On-job-training may be done at work stations in the school in vocational training classes or in the community and/or with a prospective employer. A student may be scheduled in on-job-training for a part of a day or for a full day. The amount of time per day and the length of time spent in on-job-training are determined by the individual needs and abilities of the students.

Emphasis is on vocational evaluation planning and suitable job training, with specific attention being given to personal and social adjustment on and off the job and to skills needed for daily living in the home, on the job, and during leisure hours. Efforts are made to assist the student to adjust to the work world, to learn a particular job, to develop work skills and to become a productive employee.

The teacher and the vocational adjustment coordinator may refer a handicapped student to the rehabilitation counselor to receive the services of the cooperative program. The rehabilitation counselor will evaluate the school records and determine the eligibility of the student for enrollment as a client of the Texas Rehabilitation Commission.

When a student has successfully completed on-job-training and is of employable age, and has acquired marketable work skills, he is ready to be assigned to the employment level of the program.

At the employment level, emphasis is placed on getting and holding a job, on maintaining acceptable behavior patterns, and on becoming a more productive employee. He is given assistance in solving the problems which he may encounter in community placement.

He may be employed full time and never attend classes at school, or he may be employed for part of the day and attend school part of the day. He will be supervised and receive assistance with encountered problems in both instances.

If he is unable to adjust to community employment even marginally, upon professional evaluation he may be terminated from the school program at age twenty-one.

Criteria for Graduation

When a student has proven himself capable of holding a job for at least one semester and has demonstrated acceptable behavior patterns, he has completed the educational developmental levels and is ready for school graduation and receives a diploma.

A Regular diploma shall be awarded a student who completes his prescribed educational program, including one semester of successful community work experience. He must be within the same chronological age range, or older, of the graduating class.

Operational Plan

Vocational Rehabilitation: The operational aspects of the program as they relate to that phase of the total program which are currently, traditionally, and legally the functions of the Texas Rehabilitation Commission will be the responsibility of the same Agency. Authorized rehabilitation services will be provided under conditions stipulated in the *State Plan* for the Texas Rehabilitation Commission.

In setting up a program of this type and scope, it is recognized that certain services to occupationally handicapped youth can legally be the responsibility of both Special Education and the Texas Rehabilitation Commission. The very nature of the problem and the common objectives made this so. It is believed the program will provide a continuous and uninterrupted service through "common areas" without duplication or encroachment of one division on the legal responsibility of the other. It should mean an enrichment of the separate programs of each division and save substantial sums of public money.

Duties of Key Personnel

A *Rehabilitation Counselor* will be assigned to specific schools to supervise rehabilitation program operations. His duties among other things shall be:

1. To accept all 16 year olds in Status 00 (referral).
2. To consult with school officials on training arrangements within the participating school districts for those services that will be without cost to the Texas Rehabilitation Commission.
3. To provide rehabilitation services, not offered within the unit, for the individual trainee when extended services are needed.
4. To receive and evaluate, from the public schools, all records pertaining to those individuals accepted for rehabilitation services.
5. To initiate and conduct joint conferences with the vocational adjustment coordinator and school staff in screening applicants and providing services.
6. To approve all job training. He shall evaluate training facilities, make training arrangements and agreements, advise with the trainer and vocational adjustment coordinator when indicated.
7. To approve all expenditures for client services.
8. To approve all individual rehabilitation plans for clients accepted for rehabilitation services.
9. To supervise the vocational adjustment coordinator's work with rehabilitation clients.
10. To maintain individual case records of rehabilitation clients.

A *Vocational Adjustment Coordinator* will be assigned full time to each participating unit. His duties are as follows:

1. To administer vocational rehabilitation services under the direction and in cooperation with the rehabilitation counselor assigned to the local school district.
2. To maintain class records and reports required of all special education teachers.
3. To participate in joint conferences with the vocational rehabilitation counselor and school staff in referral of applicants enrolled in regular school program for rehabilitation services.

4. To be responsible for securing job training stations and supervision of on-the-job training under the direction of the rehabilitation counselor, and act as liaison person between the local community and the Texas Rehabilitation Commission.

5. To formulate reports of successes and failures with the vocational rehabilitation counselor, using this information to adjust program of services and to evaluate program operation.

6. To act as consultant to the rehabilitation counselor in all instances concerning clients.

7. To attend to classroom responsibilities—at least one hour per day.

8. To schedule parent conferences with rehabilitation counselor.

A survey was made to determine the types of jobs to which educable retarded youth were assigned for on-the-job training. It was based on the first year operation of the Texas statewide Cooperative Program of Special Education-Vocational Rehabilitation in the public schools. Data received from 60 percent of the participating school districts provided information concerning 436 pupils who were assigned to 99 different jobs. The jobs were distributed among ten categories and one miscellaneous group. Findings of this study suggest diverse job training opportunities for educable retarded youth.

The results of this study indicate that there is little limitation of opportunity for job training for retarded youth as far as the type of jobs is concerned. Although a large percentage of pupils are sometimes assigned to one or two specific jobs in a field, there are many other jobs for which these youths may be trained (Strickland, 1964).

The Vocational Rehabilitation Counselor of the Mentally Retarded

Since it is highly necessary that the person doing the counseling should maintain an eclectic point of view, it is important that he should have made an attempt to provide himself with an appropriate background. He must carefully avoid the possibility that he will have either a limited or a biased point of view. Because of the importance and difficulty of the problem, any person dealing with the mentally retarded should have adequately prepared himself in a number of fields. Basic preparation for the counselor, however, should be in the field of psychology since all behavior is psychological.

It is a fundamental principle of psychology that man never gets beyond his experiences and is, therefore, the product of all the experiences which he has had up to and including the situation at the time of observation. What frequently and inaccurately in the laymen's language may be called native intelligence or natural ability along certain lines, is but the accumulation of the effects of formal education and informal experiences. Very few persons without psychological training can be relied upon to have so profited by their informal experiences that they are competent enough to understand the behavior of man. All counselors dealing with the mentally retarded, or any other individual for that matter, should have had the opportunity of acquiring through university training a rich background in psychology. In addition the counselor should have fundamental information related to the fields of education, job requirements, vocational placement, and family living, and should know his community and all its resources (Yepsen, 1950).

In dealing with the mentally retarded we have a group wherein there is a fine margin between success and failure; therefore, we must expect as many hidden assets to help a doubtful case to succeed against our expectations as we must be prepared to find developing in the training period hidden liabilities which were not apparent at the time we determined feasibility. In other words, in working with the mentally retarded, whether of school age or older, the rehabilitation counselor must not be discouraged by his errors in judgment any more than he has come to expect in his work with other individuals.

COUNSELING THE MENTALLY RETARDED

Dr. Lloyd N. Yepsen (1950), in his chapter "Counseling the Mentally Retarded," has stated that *counseling* is a word used to describe the interpersonal relationship which takes place when one or more persons seek to influence the behavior and attitudes of another person or persons. In the application of the principles of counseling to the influence and control of the mentally retarded, it is not necessary to abandon the basic techniques which are effective with any other group of individuals. However, there is likely to be a different emphasis upon the basic techniques because of the type of person whose behavior and attitudes it is desirable to change.

The mentally retarded individual is fundamentally the same as the so-called *normal* person, only operating at a lower level of intelligence. As a result, the degree of self-sufficiency is at a much lower economic and social level— sometimes precariously so mainly because of the enlightened attitudes and behavior of society in general. The potential *normalcy* of the mentally retarded cannot and must not be overlooked. There are still many people who have not entirely divested themselves of the idea that the physically or mentally handicapped person is qualitatively different from others in the *normal* group. Whatever differences may appear to be qualitative, in reality, only quantitative. There are differences in degree but not in kind.

Dr. Yepsen further states that counseling is based upon the understanding that the behavior of man is modifiable. The counselor also has as his goals not only the acquired use of tools and new methods but particularly the favorable modification of attitudes and general adjustability.

It would be a rather dreary outlook if it were not possible to modify human behavior. Some untrained persons who are working with the mentally retarded hold to the belief that, although it is possible to change the behavior of the average individual, the behavior of the mentally handicapped cannot be changed. They argue that the behavior of the mentally retarded—unwholesome, dependent and non-social as it may be—is the only type of behavior of which they are capable. Such an attitude is not only erroneous but is inimical to the best interests of the individual and contrary to the welfare of society. Ample research has shown that the mentally retarded person *is* modifiable and, therefore, susceptible to counseling.

Experienced professional workers in this field well know that the large number of mentally retarded persons in the community have not reached their full potential because they (1) have not been understood, (2) have not been adequately prepared for life, and (3) have not been given appropriate vocational training. Such negative conditions for personal development have placed a severe burden upon society and especially upon all who are concerned about the problem. Much of the social and economic ineffectiveness of the mentally retarded person is tragically unnecessary. Adequate counseling can serve to increase his effectiveness in all areas of his activities so that he may become self-supporting and an asset to society. However, the counselor must realize that he is dealing with an intellectually limited individual and be prepared to work with greater patience, in smaller steps, and with a greater number of contacts (Yepsen, 1950).

In reviewing the range of responsibility—toward client, family, community —along with the many ramifications of retardation, the counselor, already burdened with a heavy caseload and other duties, might very well react negatively to the additional work load projected here. This is understandable. Certainly, measures should be taken to keep counselors' caseloads within manageable proportions. Moreover, the duties outlined here should not be perceived as being directed at the counselor alone. The task of rehabilitating the retarded individual, vocationally and socially, must be undertaken by the full array of health, educational, and welfare services in the community.

In many instances the counselor will have the primary responsibility for planning the client's program. The scope of his study of the client, the family and the community should include an appraisal of resources as well as needs. Even when the community does not have highly developed clinical and welfare services, the counselor is not without assistance or the possibility of recruiting others to contribute help. For example, the counselor should consider soliciting the aid of churches, recreation agencies, parent organizations, service clubs, veterans' organizations, chambers of commerce, and other groups and individuals, to provide services which are beyond his time or professional role but which have a bearing on rehabilitating the mentally retarded client.

In coming to a decision of how and when to counsel, the experienced counselor will first evaluate himself by weighing his own professional training, experiences, biases, and capabilities. As for the extent to which he should carry the counseling, he should do as much as is necessary to bring about *the desired rehabilitation results,* but *no more.* When pathological conditions —physical, emotional or social—appear to be present, referral to the required specialized resource is urged as early as possible.

In circumstances where adequate supervisory resources are not available, the counselor should apply for supplementary resources to obtain the needed assistance pertinent to counseling. He must, therefore, be alert to the range of services which can be made available to him at the local, state, regional, and national levels. He should determine available provisions for purchasing consultation within his organization. The counselor should consider other disciplines as possible sources of help in advancing his competencies in counseling and in knowledge of retardation. He is urged to keep abreast of the literature and to attend conferences, institutes and courses related to both the fields of rehabilitation and of retardation.

The counseling process for mentally retarded clients is essentially the same as for all disabled persons. They are amenable to and can profit from counseling. As with all developmental disabilities, lifelong experiences of failure and rejection often create particularly difficult rehabilitation problems which can only be resolved through personal counseling.

The intellectual limitations of the retarded client, and particularly his deficit in verbal communication, do necessitate modifications in usual counseling techniques and require the utilization of a wider range of approaches. The counselor must be particularly aware, in the case of the mildly retarded, of the fact that many derive from socially and economically deprived environments in which they have acquired motivations, attitudes, and a social value system antithetical to work. In the case of the more severely retarded who are about equally distributed through all economic levels, there is more likely to be a serious discrepancy between the aspirations and values held by the parents and the clients' potentials for achievements. Resources for enabling retarded individuals to achieve vocational and social self-sufficiency are advancing markedly (United States Department of Health, Education, and Welfare, 1963).

REFERENCES

Governor's Advisory Committee on Mental Retardation Planning, and the Governor's Interagency Committee on Mental Retardation Planning: *The Texas Plan to Combat Mental Retardation*. Austin, Texas, State Printing Office, June, 1966.

Heber, Rick: *A Manual on Terminology and Classification in Mental Retardation*, 2nd ed. Washington, D.C., American Association of Mental Deficiency, 1961.

Hegge, Thorlief: Psychological aspects of the mentally retarded. In Di Michael, S. G., (Ed.), *Vocational Rehabilitation of the Mentally Retarded*. Washington, D.C., Government Printing Office, 1950.

Kelly, James M., and Simon, Alex J.: *The Mentally Handicapped as Workers—A Survey of Company Experience*. New York, American Management Association, 1969.

Kirk, Samuel A. and Johnson, G. Orville: *Educating the Retarded Child*. Cambridge, Mass., Riverside Press, 1951.

National Association for Retarded Children, Inc.: *The Mentally Retarded and*

Their Vocational Rehabilitation—A Resource Handbook, William A. Frawnkel, Consultant. New York, National Association for Retarded Children, 1961.

Predicting Success for Mentally Retarded Adults. *Research and Demonstrations, BRIEF.* Vol. 4, no. 1, August 14, 1970.

Region V Education Services Center: *Guidelines for a Cooperative School Program.* Beaumont, Texas, Region V Education Service Center, 1969.

Rehabilitation Research and Training Center Staff: *Annual Progress Report of the Rehabilitation Research and Training Center in Mental Retardation.* Windel L. Dickerson, Project Director. Austin, University of Texas Press, 1969.

Smith, Robert M.: *Clinical Teaching: Methods of Instruction for the Retarded.* New York, McGraw-Hill, 1968.

Strickland, Conwell G.: Job training placement for retarded youth. Reprinted from *Exceptional Children,* Vol. 31, no. 2, pp. 83-86, October 1964.

Texas Education Agency: *Administrative Guide and Handbook for Special Education.* Bulletin 711. Austin, Texas Education Agency, March 1971.

Texas Education Agency, Texas Rehabilitation Commission, and Special Education Programs of the Independent School Districts of Texas: Plan for Rehabilitation of Handicapped Students through the Cooperative Program between the Division of Special Education of the Texas Education Agency, the Texas Rehabilitation Commission and the Special Education Program of the Independent School Districts of Texas. Revised, Austin, 1971 (Mimeographed).

Texas Rehabilitation Commission: *Rehabilitation Services Manual.* Austin, Texas Rehabilitation Commission, February 1972.

United States Department of Health, Education, and Welfare (Division of International Activities), Social and Rehabilitation Services: *The Use of a Group Approach in the Rehabilitation of Severely Retarded Adolescents in Agriculture in Israel* (E. Chigier, Chief Investigator). Tel Aviv, Israel, Israel Association for Rehabilitation of Mentally Handicapped, October 1970.

United States Department of Health, Education, and Welfare (Vocational Rehabilitation Administration): *Special Problems in Vocational Rehabilitation of the Mentally Retarded.* Madison, Wisc., U.S. Department of Health, Education, and Welfare, November 1963.

Vocational Rehabilitation for the Young Mentally Retarded Adult in the State of Texas. Austin, Texas Education Agency Press, 1962.

Yepsen, Lloyd N.: Counseling the mentally retarded. In Di Michael, Salvatore G. (Ed.), *Vocational Rehabilitation of the Mentally Retarded.* Washington, D.C., Government Printing Office, 1950.

Chapter 14

VOCATIONAL HABILITATION FOR THE MENTALLY RETARDED*

JOHN W. GLADDEN

THROUGHOUT HISTORY there have been those individuals who, because of some accident of birth or failure in development, never achieve normal mental and social maturity. Until the last two hundred years, attitudes toward these unfortunates were a function of the prevailing mysticism or religion of the times. Thus, during some periods, they were viewed as creatures of scorn, products of the devil, and persons to be avoided. At other times, they were accorded the respect due "children of God" and worshipped as such. It was only at the close of the eighteenth century that interest in and efforts for them were demonstrated with any consistency, organization or discipline.

The study of those that we now call "mentally retarded" essentially began in France about 1790. Two physicians, Dr. H. Itard and Dr. E. Seguin, were the first to attempt any systematic work with the retarded; and each gained international recognition for his efforts. Itard's endeavors are thoroughly described elsewhere (Itard, 1932) and are recommended reading for the serious student even today. Dr. Seguin was responsible for the establishment of the first public institution in the world for the retarded about 1794 in Paris and later was invited to the United States where he worked with them for the remainder of his life. He also was largely responsible for establishing the first institution in the United States in 1848.

Dr. Seguin worked over fifty years in the area of institutional care of the mentally retarded. His teaching procedures, which he referred to as the "physiological-sense training method," were the origins of today's Montessori methods. Seguin's efforts were directed toward keeping retarded children at home and in public schools. He conceived of institutions as places where the retarded could be brought for short-term help and training so that they might gain the proficiencies that would permit them to live at home and attend public schools. His concepts of training included very few ingredients of custodial care. Dr. Seguin ruled over what might be called the "Golden

---

*Special appreciation is here expressed to Erie Dell Adams, M.D. for suggestions and assistance with the medical classification system.

Era" of mental retardation and was recognized as the outstanding authority in his field.

A complex combination of phenomena conspired to defeat the efforts of Seguin and to imprison the retarded in the attitudinal confines where they remained for over one half of a century. Binet and Simon (1905) developed a test of intelligence, making it simpler to "diagnose" the retarded, and, thus, simpler to produce larger numbers of them, each one needing help. Early in its development the age of science spawned misadventures in the field of genetics, particularly case history type studies tracing apparent familial tendencies toward retardation and crime. One such study was especially devastating inasmuch as it "convincingly demonstrated" how retardation, crime, and other undesirable traits are genetically transmitted (Goddard, 1912):

> When Martin Sr., of good family, was a boy of fifteen, his father dies, leaving him without parental care or oversight . . . The young man joined one of the numerous military companies that were formed to protect the country at the beginning of the Revolution. At one of the taverns he met a feeble-minded girl by whom he became the father of a feeble-minded son . . . This illegitimate boy was named Martin Kallikak, Jr., . . . and from him came four hundred and eighty descendants. One hundred and forty-three of these, we have conclusive proof, were or are feeble-minded, while only forty-six have been found normal . . . thirty-six have been illegitimate . . . thirty-three sexually immoral persons . . . twenty-four confirmed alcoholics . . . three epileptics . . . three were criminal . . . eight kept houses of ill fame.

In a surprisingly brief time the public outlook toward the retarded changed from one of concern and care to one of fear and hostility. The retarded became objects of scorn, and there evolved a public and professional consensus that they should be locked up and/or exterminated. Institutions became places of incarceration rather than training. Ideas of small group living, architectural aesthetics, and individuality gave way to concepts permitting the maximum number of persons in the minimum available space. No attempts were made to help the retarded at home, or to return them home from the institutions. As more and more retardates were found, more institutions were required; and in a five-year period, 1925-1930, there was over a 300 percent increase in the number of institutions for the mentally retarded. The life span of the institutionalized retarded was kept to less than twenty years.

Parents of retarded children became ashamed of their offspring. The children most often were hidden from public view or put away in institutions to be forgotten. Fantasies were concocted concerning post-natal accidents to explain the cause of a child's retardation, thereby eschewing the need for a scientific explanation and, also, avoiding the stigma of what would appear to be "God's punishment for the sins of the parents." It was not until after World War II that the plight of the mentally retarded was discovered by the public. Although many significant advances have occurred in the last three decades in the areas of diagnosis, etiology, special education, and treatment of the mentally retarded, tremendous needs for advancement remain. The state of knowledge in the field of mental retardation significantly lags behind similar fields of study; and public opinion is best characterized as ridden with apathy, mythology, superstition and ignorance.

The preceding brief history of mental retardation has been presented here to partially explain why knowledge and efforts in this field are so unremarkable. During the more than 170 years that the professional and lay public have been studying the retarded, a majority of that time has been devoted to punitive and isolative ends rather than to remediation and prevention. As the reader will note in the remainder of this chapter, the definition of mental retardation is incomplete; the major causes are not known, the "cures" have yet to be discovered; and methods of treatment and training are just beginning to be developed.

SCOPE OF THE PROBLEM

A panel of distinguished citizens appointed by President Kennedy in the fall of 1961, reported the following information to the American public (President's Panel, 1962):

> An estimated 3 percent of the population, or 5.4 million children and adults in the United States are afflicted, some severely, most only mildly . . . an estimated 126,000 babies born each year will be regarded as mentally retarded at some time in their lives. Mental retardation ranks as a major national health, social, and economic problem:
>
> It afflicts twice as many individuals as blindness, polio, cerebral palsy, and rheumatic heart disease combined. Only four significant disabling conditions— mental illness, cardiac disease, arthritis, and cancer—have a higher prevalence but they tend to come late in life while mental retardation comes early. Over 200,000 adults and children, largely from the severe and profound mentally retarded groups, are cared for in residential institutions, mostly at public expense.
>
> The nation is denied several billion dollars of economic output because of the underachievement, underproduction, and/or the complete incapabilities of the mentally retarded.
>
> Mental retardation does not respect station in life or geography. The more severe cases of mental retardation are likely to be associated with organic defects.
>
> Strikingly high concentrations of mental retardation in specific sections of metropolitan communities also point to a strong correlation between economic status and intellectual development.
>
> Prevalence of mental retardation tends to be heavily associated with lack of prenatal care, prematurity, and high infant death rates. Women who do not have prenatal care are approximately three times as likely to give birth to premature babies as are women who receive adequate prenatal care, and very small premature babies are ten times more likely to be mentally retarded than are children of normal birth.

Although the Panel's findings are now more than a decade old, only numerical adjustments with regard to population growth are necessary to render the data current. Thus we now estimate a total of more than 6 million retarded in the United States, based upon 3 percent of the 1970 population.

As will be discussed at length later, it is possible to identify precisely an extensive array of causal factors, usually diseases or injuries which result in organic pathology. However, these factors are identifiable in only 15 to 25 percent of cases of retardation. Presently in 75 to 85 percent of the cases, it is not possible to specify the cause(s). The majority is comprised mainly of the highest level retarded who show no gross abnormality of the brain.

There is persuasive evidence that children born of mothers receiving little prenatal care are tremendously more prone to retardation than are children of mothers receiving adequate care. Likewise, low socio-economic families, neighborhoods, or geographical regions produce the majority of the retarded. It therefore would appear that both physiological and psychological deprivations play important roles in the etiologies of mental retardation.

In discussing prevention and/or amelioration, one must remember that mental retardation is a complex phenomenon which results from a wide variety of causes, mostly incompletely understood or unknown. A significant number of bio-medical factors may be treated with success, permitting the arresting of certain conditions and the prevention of others. Non-physical or psychological factors quite often are the eventuation of complicated social, cultural and economic situations which do not lend themselves readily or easily to manipulation.

DEFINITIONAL CONSIDERATIONS

Due primarily to unresolved theoretical issues concerning the nature of "intelligence," no single definition of the term "mental retardation" has been developed which satisfies all concerned. To review and resolve all of the controversies surrounding these terms is not the purpose of this chapter, especially when excellent expositions exist elsewhere (e.g., Robinson and Robinson, 1965), particularly in several of the eminent contributions to the present volume. However, an attempt will be made to provide the reader with an appreciation of the theoretical complications in the field and an understanding of the nature of the definitional dilemma. For a variety of theoretical and practical reasons, it would appear that the term "intelligence" and "mental retardation" are definitionally interrelated. The understanding and utility of the term "mental retardation" would depend upon the utility and acceptability of the term "intelligence." There is no universally accepted definition of "intelligence."

Intelligence

Psychologists and others long have acknowledged the merits of an "operational definition" of intelligence (Boring, 1923) but, paradoxically, have not developed one that is compatible with a theoretical system, sufficiently predictive for practical or non-laboratory settings, and generally acceptable to the consumer, i.e., the non-psychologist. The following paragraphs briefly describe a few of the definitional detriments, but by no means are an exhaustive catalogue of the problems.

Theoretical and experimental endeavors with respect to the concept of "intelligence" are best characterized by their diversity. Since 1921, when more than a dozen eminent theorists submitted their notions of "what intelligence is" to the *Journal of Educational Psychology* and found little agreement among themselves, there have been only a few definitional commonalities present in the literature. Most writers have indicated that at least one or more of the following are basic to the concept of intelligence: (1) the rate and/or ease of learning; (2) the amount learned; and (3) the capacity to cope or adjust to environmental standards. Great differences remain with regard to whether intelligence primarily is a function of heredity or of the environment, whether it is to a large or to a small extent affected by cultural factors, whether it can be measured independently of personality or emotional factors, whether intelligence should be defined in terms of "potential" or observed levels, and whether intelligence is stable and transitional, or variable and situational.

The heredity-environment controversy raged early in the twentieth century (cf. McNemar, 1940; Skeels *et al.,* 1938; Watson, 1925). Fortunately, only a few extremists for each position remain, and most theorists agree that there is an interaction between genetics and environment which sets the limits of intellectual growth and the variations within these limits.

It is difficult to ignore the data which indicate that intelligence is quite sensitive to, and may be depressed by, cultural factors which are not indices of ability (e.g., Macland, Sarason, and Gladwin, 1958; Anastasi, 1964). For example, a child may be reared in a culture that makes demands of him which are totally different from demands he might have received in a second culture. If the child were evaluated according to his ability to meet the demands of the second culture, where he had no opportunity to learn and/or practice certain things, he probably would be found to be substandard. In an extreme example, the cultural effects would be recognized by all observers. Unfortunately, in most cases the observer does not take the time or does not have the skill or information to fully take into account the cultural factors.

Another controversy concerning intelligence exists in regard to its relationship with personality and/or emotional facets. One position holds that "intelligence" and "emotions" are indelibly intertwined and have meaning only in relationship to each other. A second school of thought feels that it is both possible and necessary to treat the two as separate and distinct concepts. Interestingly, the Stanford-Binet tests of Intelligence were derived from a philosophy that sought to evaluate intelligence, as being independent of personality, while the Wechsler tests are based upon a view of intelligence that encompasses personality factors.

A major point of contention for theorists revolves around the issue of whether to conceptualize intelligence in terms of "potential," i.e., the highest possible for an individual, or in terms of the present and observed. A re-phrasing of the issue would be, "Is intelligence what it is now or what it might be?" Jastak (1949) is an eloquent spokesman for those that define intelligence as what might or could be, i.e., potential. The weakness of this position is found when one attempts to measure potential: *if potential is what could be, but what is not, how does one measure something that is not, that has not yet occurred?* Writers have pointed out the danger of inferring from a response that has occurred to a response that might occur (e.g., Rotter, 1954).

The final debatable point to be considered concerns the permanence or stability of intelligence and is closely related to the controversies already discussed. This last controversy grows, in part, from the inherent relationship between the concept and the methods used to assess it. One theoretical position holds that intelligence is relatively fixed and permanent and usually may be altered only downwardly. The second school of thought is that intelligence, like most behavioral concepts, is situation specific; and its variability is a function of changing environmental features.

The preceding paragraphs are not intended as a comprehensive consideration of the problems inherent in developing a definition of "intelligence." Rather they are designed to show, with calculated brevity, only *some* of the factors that are responsible for the lack of a definition of intelligence. Without a comprehensive and comprehendable definition of "intelligence," it follows that a definition of "mental retardation" will be lacking. In the following paragraphs, a select sample of such definitions will be considered; and finally, the definition that currently enjoys widest use will be discussed.

Mental Retardation

In light of the definitional problems with "intelligence," it is easily understandable that definitions of "mental retardation" reflect, at best, an unstable truce or working compromise with the theoretical. One approach has been to define the mentally retarded as those with measured intelligence below a certain level, generally an Intelligence Quotient (I.Q.) less than 70. This approach is widely used, and often has been incorporated into State Laws for diagnostic reasons; and yet, at the same time, it has been perhaps the most readily and easily criticized. However, because of the nearly fifty years of widespread use of standardized intelligence tests and in the absence of other equally popular and easily utilized techniques, this approval still is widely seen. For purposes of communication, and with full recognition of the faults of such an approach, definition by IQ classification will be utilized later in this chapter in the discussion of classification and diagnosis.

A second definitional approach is that of Tredgold (1937) who states that mental retardation, or "amnetia," is "a state of incomplete mental development of such a kind and degree that the individual is incapable of adapting himself to the normal environment of his fellows in such a way as to maintain existence independent of supervision, control, or external support." As can be seen, the major criticism within this definition is social adequacy, a concept that most probably is specific to adults, rather than children, and one which might fluctuate considerably, depending upon the beholder, and his definition of the "normal environment." One of the requirements of a good definition is that it specify both *what is* and *what is not* of the matter being defined. Tredgold's definition particularly has trouble in that the small children, the blind, the psychotic, and other persons as well as the retarded are "incapable of adapting . . . to the normal environment" (p. 4).

Kanner's is a similar approach which defines two types of mentally retarded, those who "are deficient in every sphere of mentation," and those "whose limitations are definitely related to the standards of the particular culture which surrounds them" (1957, p. 55). This approach also seems specific to adults and is more conversational in direction than scientific.

Not all theorists have directed their definition toward the adult and/or the I.Q. For example Doll (1941) says,

> If we look to the substantial work in this field prior to the recent abuses of mental tests in the diagnosis of mental deficiency, we observe that six criteria by statement of implication have been generally considered essential to an adequate definition of the concept. They are (1) social incompetence, (2) due to mental subnormality, (3) which has been developmentally arrested, (4) which obtains at maturity, (5) is of constitutional origin, and (6) is essentially incurable (p. 215).

Strong arguments have been presented against each of the six criteria. Taken individually, the first four criteria are criticizable; but when viewed as a whole, they have found strong supporters. Cantor (1955) has argued convincingly against the inclusion of the term "essentially incurable" within a definition of mental retardation on the basis of the lack of logic in doing so. One could be certain that a condition is incurable only after there is absolutely no possibility of a cure, *or,* after death. The belief, "once retarded, always retarded" is slowly giving way to a more optimistic view.

The American Association on Mental Deficiency (AAMD) published a new definition in its manual on classification and terminology (Heber, 1961). This definition has been widely accepted, probably more to facilitate communication than anything else. The AAMD definition is developmental in approval and avoids many of the problems besetting other definitions. It relies upon measured behavior but does not talk about a specific I.Q. score cut-off, nor does it utilize the concept of "potential." This definition does not require permanency of retardation but rather permits the designation of mental retardation without subscripts of "primary" or "secondary." The AAMD definition reads: "Mental retardation refers to subaverage general intellectual functioning which originates during the developmental period and is associated with impairment in adaptive behavior." The manual goes on to define carefully each element of the definition:

Subaverage refers to performance which is greater than one Standard Deviation below the population mean of the age group involved or the measures of *general intellectual functioning*. Level of general intellectual functioning may be assessed by performance on one or more of the various objective tests which have been developed for that purpose. Though the upper age limit of the developmental period cannot be precisely specified it may be regarded, for practical purposes, as being approximately sixteen years. This criterion is in accord with the traditional concept of mental retardation with respect to age and serves to distinguish mental retardation from other disorders of human behavior.

The definition specifies that the subaverage intellectual functioning must be reflected by *impairment in adaptive behavior*. Adaptive behavior refers primarily to the effectiveness of the individual in adapting to the natural and social demands of his environment. Impaired adaptive behavior may be reflected in: (1) maturation, (2) learning, and/or (3) social adjustment.

Rate of *maturation* refers to the rate of sequential development of self-help skills of infancy and early childhood such as sitting, crawling, standing, walking, talking, habit training, and interaction with age peers. In the first few years of life adaptive behavior is assessed almost completely in terms of these and other manifestations of sensory-motor development.

Learning ability refers to the facility with which knowledge is acquired as a function of experience. Learning difficulties are usually most manifest in the academic situation and if mild in degree may not even become apparent until the child enters school. Impaired learning ability is, therefore, particularly important as a qualifying condition of mental retardation during the school years.

Social adjustment is particularly important as a qualifying condition of mental retardation at the adult level when it is assessed in terms of the degree to which the individual is able to maintain himself independently in the community and in gainful employment as well as by his ability to meet and conform to other personal and social responsibilities and standards set by the community. During the pre-school and school-age years social adjustment is reflected in large measure, in the level and manner in which the child relates to parents, other adults, and age peers . . .

Within the framework of the present definition mental retardation is a term descriptive of the *current* status of the individual with respect to intellectual functioning and adaptive behavior. Consequently, an individual may meet the criteria of mental retardation at one time and not at another. A person may change status as a result of changes in social standards or conditions or as a result of changes in efficiency of intellectual functioning, with level of efficiency always being determined in relation to the behavioral standard and norms for the individual's chronological age group (Heber, 1961, pp. 3-4).

The AAMD definition encompasses a much larger group of individuals than would have been considered retarded heretofore. It accepts as subaverage anyone scoring more than one standard deviation below the mean of the standardization group or general population. Since the appearance of this definition general practice has been to continue viewing the retarded as the more severely impaired and to not include or emphasize those in the marginal or borderline areas of intelligence.

The AAMD definition has many shortcomings, especially when applied to rigorous, scientific criteria, but has sufficient advantages over other definitional approaches to be the definition of choice.

CLASSIFICATION OF MENTAL RETARDATION

For extensive and detailed classification systems within the field of mental retardation, the reader is referred to other sources (e.g., Dunn, 1963; Heber, 1961; Sarason, 1958; and Robinson and Robinson, 1965). Traditionally classification systems have been in medical, behavioral, and educational contexts. A brief presentation of one of each of these systems follows.

Medical Class of Mental Retardation

The most popular and widely used medical classification system is found in AAMD's *Manual on Terminology and Classification in Mental Retardation* (Heber, 1961). This system of classification outlines eight genetic etiologic categories, into which any cases of mental retardation may be classified. A brief description of each of these categories follows:

1. Diseases and conditions due to infection. This includes both prenatal infection, such as that due to German measles and congenital syphilis, and postnatal cerebral infections such as encephalitis or meningitis.
2. Diseases and conditions due to intoxication. This includes those cases resulting from cerebral damage due to serums, drugs, and all toxic agents such as carbon monoxide, lead, arsenic, etc. The parental Rh incompatibility cases also would be classified here.
3. Diseases with conditions due to trauma or physical agent. Within this category are those instances of injury to the brain during both prenatal periods resulting from mechanical or physical agents.
4. Diseases and conditions due to disorder of metabolism, growth, or nutrition. Within this category are the disorders due to faulty metabolism of fats, carbohydrates, and protein, and nutritional deficiencies. Examples of these disorders are the cerebral lipoidoses, phenylketonuria, galactosemia, hypothyroidism and gargoylism. Many of these disorders are visually obvious and/or otherwise easily diagnosed, and may be arrested if treated early enough. It is known that many if not all of these may be genetically determined.
5. Diseases and conditions due to new growths. This category includes those disorders resulting from new growths in the brain, e.g., neurofibromatosis, trigeminal cerebral angiomatosis (whose major characteristic is the "port wine stain"), and tuberous sclerosis. Some of these also may be of genetic origin.
6. Diseases and conditions due to (unknown) prenatal influence. This category is used when no definitive causal factor is specified but when it can be established that the etiology existed at or prior to birth. Examples are anencephaly, proencephaly, acrocephaly, hydrocephaly, macrocephaly, microcephaly, mongolism or Down's syndrome, and the Laurence-Moon-Biedl syndrome. At least one of these conditions, Down's syndrome, is associated with chromosomal aberrations. A small number of cases of Down's syndrome, those associated with chromosomal translocation or mosaicism, are thought to be hereditary.
7. Diseases and conditions due to unknown or uncertain cause with the structural reactions manifest. The postnatal conditions are presumed to be hereditary or familial, but of unknown cause. This category differs from the previous one in that those conditions are known to have existed at or before birth, while these have an onset after birth.
8. Diseases and conditions due to uncertain (or presumed psychologic) cause with the functional reaction alone manifest. Classification into this category occurs when mental retardation appears without any detectable indication of physical pathology to account for the retardation. Extreme diagnostic caution

is required for this classification because all physiologic and anatomic possibilities must first be negated, and this is difficult to do with certainty in our present state of knowledge. It is within this category that the greatest numbers of mentally retarded fall. Herein are found the cultural-familial type of retardation and retardation due to environmental deprivation, retardation associated with emotional disturbance, and retardation associated with major personality disorders.

Individuals falling within the first seven of the categories listed above are those with particular and specifiable and diagnosable syndromes. They tend to be the more severely retarded but constitute a definite minority of those considered to be mentally retarded. Those individuals falling into category eight tend to look and act more "normal," and comprise the vast majority of the mentally retarded.

In the past some writers have drawn a distinction between the *mentally retarded* and the *mentally deficient.* According to such a dichotomy, the first seven classifications above would refer to the mentally deficient, e.g., those with organic deficits which permanently reduce intelligence. Category eight would contain the mentally retarded. For a wide variety of reasons, such a distinction is no longer widely used.

A classification system based upon etiology has many obvious advantages, most of them associated with simplicity and neatness. The simplicity is tremendously misleading in that only in extraordinarily rare cases do complex human beings lend themselves to "pigeon-holing." Never is it easy to label a deficit as entirely due to physiology rather than life experiences, or vice versa. For these and other reasons, other classification systems should be considered as supplemental to etiologic classification.

Measured Intelligence and Adaptive Behavioral Classification

As was mentioned previously, the AAMD *Manual in Terminology and Classification* developed a definition of mental retardation based upon two major interdependent dimensions: *measured intelligence and adaptive behavior.* Classification by each of these is briefly described below.

Measured intelligence, or *current* intellectual functioning is obtained from objective, standardized psychometric instruments. Measured intelligence is divided into five levels on the basis of the Standard Deviation units of the

TABLE 14-I

STANDARD DEVIATION RANGES AND I.Q. SCORES
FOR THE LEVELS OF MEASURED INTELLIGENCE

Level of Deviation in Measured Intelligence	Range of Level of Standard Deviation Units	Level of Measured Intelligence According to Descriptive Terminology	I.Q. Ranges	
			S-B[1]	W-B[2]
-1	-1.01 to -2.00	Borderline Retarded	83-68	84-70
-2	-2.01 to -3.00	Mild Retarded	67-52	69-55
-3	-3.01 to -4.00	Moderate Retarded	51-36	54-40
-4	-4.01 to -5.00	Severe Retarded	35-20	
-5	← -5.00	Profound Retarded	←20	

[1]S-B refers to Stanford-Binet Intelligence tests, forms L and M.
[2]W-B refers to Wechsler Adult Intelligence Scale and Wechsler Intelligence Scale for Children.

testing instruments. Taking some liberty with data presented in the 1961 AAMD Manual (pp. 58 and 59), the preceding table depicts the Standard Deviation ranges and corresponding I.Q. scores for each of the five levels of Measured Intelligence.

Misuse of the Measured Intelligence Classification System is tempting because of the apparent ease of assignment. Utility of the system would be much improved if all examiners were of equal skill and all testing instruments of the same, known level of reliability and precision. Obviously neither of

TABLE 14-II

SLOAN-BIRCH ADAPTIVE BEHAVIOR CHART

	PRE-SCHOOL AGE 0-5 *Maturation and Development*	SCHOOL AGE 6-20 *Training and Education*	ADULT 21 and up *Social and Vocational Adequacy*
Level I	Gross retardation; minimal capacity for functioning in sensori-motor areas; needs nursing care.	Some motor development present; cannot profit from training in self help; needs total care.	Some motor and speech development; totally incapable of self-maintenance; needs complete care and supervision.
Level II	Poor motor development; speech is minimal; generally unable to profit from training in self-help; little or no communication skills.	Can talk or learn to communicate; can be trained in elemental health habits; cannot learn functional academic skills; profits from systematic habit training. ("Trainable")	Can contribute partially to self-support under complete supervision; can develop self-protection skills to a minimal useful level in controlled environment.
Level III	Can talk or learn to communicate; poor social awareness; fair motor development; may profit from self-help; can be managed with moderate supervision.	Can learn functional academic skills to approximately 4th grade level by late teens if given special education. ("Educable")	Capable of self-maintenance in unskilled or semi-skilled occupation; needs supervision and guidance when under mild social or economic stress.
Level IV	Can develop social and communication skills; minimal retardation in sensori-motor areas; rarely distinguished from normal until later age.	Can learn academic skills to approximately 6th grade level by late teens. Cannot learn general high school subjects. Need special education particularly at secondary school age levels. ("Educable")	Capable of social and vocational adequacy with proper education and training. Frequently needs supervision and guidance under serious social or economic stress.

these factors exist, so use of the system should be approached with caution and prudence. An additional consideration has to do with the waste of assigning one number or range of numbers—i.e., an I.Q. score—to represent the complexities of a human being. As in the case of any labeling, it is highly probable that more information is lost than is gained.

As indicated earlier, *adaptive behavior* loosely refers to the degree to which an individual copes with, masters, and/or survives in his environment. More specifically, "it has two major facets: (1) the degree to which the individual is able to function and maintain himself independently, and (2) the degree to which he meets satisfactorily the culturally-imposed demands of personal and social responsibility" (Heber, 1961, p. 61).

Precise measures of adaptive behavior are now being developed, but behaviors presently referred to in the following classificatory system are global, descriptive and may be described as samples. Exactly what is adaptive in terms of behavior depends in part both upon the chronological age of an individual and his level of ability. Sloan and Birch (1955) have presented the preceding table, Table 14-11, to illustrate different levels of Adaptive Behavior at each of three age groupings.

Educational Classification of Mental Retardation

Within the educational context, the favored classification system is based largely upon I.Q. scores but corresponds only roughly to other I.Q. based classifications. A relatively large number of terms, which frequently are synonymous with each other and used interchangeably, generate a good deal more heat than light. These terms include "mentally handicapped", "educable", "moron", "imbecile", "trainable", "mentally defective", "ament", etc. Perhaps the most consistent terms are "educable", "trainable", and "custodial". Translated rather freely into corresponding I.Q. score ranges, the "custodial level" is from zero to approximately twenty-five, the "trainable level" is from about twenty-five to around fifty, and the "educable level" is between fifty and seventy or seventy-five. This is very similar to the old "idiot", "imbecile", "moron" system in which the "idiot level" is from zero to about twenty or twenty-five, the "imbecile level" is from around twenty or twenty-five to forty or forty-five, and the "moron level" is from around forty to over seventy.

Cruikshank (1958) has published a set of terms that seems popular and that has been used with some consistency in recent years. He refers to those with I.Q.'s between eighty and ninety-five as "slow learners". The "mentally handicapped" would be those with I.Q.'s between fifty-five or sixty and eighty. The "mentally deficient" would be those with I.Q.'s between thirty and fifty-five or sixty. The "custodial" would have I.Q.'s below thirty.

Within Cruikshank's system the "slow learner" probably would be kept in the regular classroom, but probably would not achieve total independence and self respect as an adult. The "mentally handicapped" correspond to the "educable retarded," while the "mentally deficient" correspond roughly to the "trainable retarded" level. Cruikshank has shifted I.Q. levels upward in his "reclassification", but has neither radically revised an existing classification system nor created a brand new one.

It is unfortunate that the educational classification system relies so heavily upon the I.Q. score, and equally unfortunate that educators still tend to hope that a complex human being may be described in essence by one number, range of numbers or label.

As one may readily observe there is no universally accepted system of classification. Medical, behavioral, and educational systems, when used in isolation, are flaw-laden and of questionable utility. However, the prudent person who is willing to use a coalition of efforts, who does not expect "something for nothing" and who will acknowledge his end result as less than perfect, may with effort find what he is seeking with regard to classification.

HABILITATION FOR THE MENTALLY RETARDED

Vocational rehabilitation is a unique attempt by a concerned society to return to its disabled members a sense of personal dignity and respect as a result of the products of their labors and/or talents. The process is designed to restore to the disabled the opportunities to participate and communicate with others as equals. Usually both within the rehabilitation process and with the person being rehabilitated is found the motivation to achieve independence, productivity, and self-sufficiency. The term *rehabilitate* implies returning to one what he has lost and allowing the regaining or re-achieving of a role, position or status within a given domain.

With respect to the mentally retarded, vocational efforts are *habilitative* rather than *rehabilitative* in thrust. One begins at the beginning with vocational training for the retarded, not with attempting to restore what was lost. For the most part, the retarded have been treated as needing something that was lost all of their lives; and yet it is not that they have lost something, but that they merely have failed to gain it. The retarded person, unlike the adult victim of a physical injury, will not have memories of the rewards of self-sufficiency. He, rather, has known mostly failure and has little knowledge of what it is that may be realized in the habilitation process.

The population explosion and the gigantic strides in technology have produced a society that seriously overtaxes its resources. The numbers of retarded have increased correspondingly with the general population; and due to antibiotics, there now are more adult retarded than ever before in history. For the types of jobs that the retarded do well, there is keener and keener competition. Automation has eliminated thousands of these kinds of jobs. In spite of all of the preceding factors, the vocational outlook for the retarded is not necessarily dim.

General Misconceptions About the Mentally Retarded

There are a number of misconceptions about the mentally retarded and their "rehabilitative potential" that should be corrected. For example, quite often the retarded are thought to be mentally ill and are feared and avoided because of their emotional instability. There are definite differences between mental retardation and mental illness, with the latter being associated with emotional instability. Actually, the mentally retarded might be expected to be much more unstable than they are in fact, considering their reduced abilities to cope with a frustrating and demanding environment. Clarke and Clarke (1958) have published information in their excellent book that indicates a higher percentage of major and minor emotional disturbances in the retarded than in normal individuals, but the evidence is somewhat subjective in nature and far from definitive. Suffice to say, some of the retarded may be mentally ill, but all of the retarded are not emotionally disturbed; and fear of emotional disturbance should not lead to an avoidance of the retarded.

A second misconception that should be corrected is that the mentally retarded are dangerous and/or delinquent. There is little or no reliably demonstrated relationship between mental retardation and crime or delinquency. The retarded may "fall in with the gang" and be easily led, but most brushes with the law occur because a retarded youngster is either lost or has dropped out of school because of an inability to meet the academic demand placed upon him.

Perhaps the major misconception about the vocational potential of the mentally retarded is that they are helpless and unemployable. It does not take much exposure to even the most severely retarded to observe that improvement in the person's behavior is possible. It has become popular, justifiably so, to believe that the major detriment to progress by the retarded is the lack of imagination on the part of the rest of us. Ample evidence demonstrating the employability of the retarded has been available for several decades (cf. DiMichael, 1952).

Another misconception that does great injustice to the mentally retarded is the notion that they are ideally suited for routine, repetitive tasks that would be too boring for their normal peers. On a purely theoretical basis one certainly might build a good case in support of this notion, but in actuality, the mentally retarded appear to become just as bored in monotonous work situations as anyone else. It is true that the severely retarded may be conditioned to an incentive system which partially may yield sustained performance with routine work activities. However, it would be foolish to develop a vocational plan for the retarded that was built upon this popular misconception.

A final fairly common misconception is that the most difficult part of the habilitation process with the retarded is finding employers and positions that are suited to them. This notion is grossly untrue. The quantity of jobs that could be performed by the retarded and the quality of work they can do is staggering (e.g., see Engel, 1952). Given a chance, most retarded will provide a level of work that is surprising. However, most of the problems faced by the mentally retarded are not task-related, but, rather, occur in non-work related areas such as leisure time, transportation, etc. In simple terms, finding a job for the retarded person is the easiest part and only the beginning of the habilitation process.

The Habilitation Process
in Work with the Mentally Retarded

The habilitation process with the retarded has fundamental differences from the rehabilitation process of most other disabled persons. For example, the physically handicapped person typically will not require the intensive supervision of his living quarters, bill paying, religious activities, marital interests, etc., that will be necessary for the retarded. One might argue convincingly that all persons need instruction in sex education and family planning, but there can be no doubt that these are an absolute *must* for the retarded client. A physically handicapped person who has been vocationally restored might well be expected to manage his own courtship, marriage, etc., but to take these things for granted with most of the mentally retarded is to defeat the habilitation process. The habilitation plan must be comprehensive with regard to *all spheres of life* for the mentally retarded. By necessity, it will begin early, be more comprehensive, and last longer than the typical plan or process.

Not only will the retarded individual need individualized training and counseling, but his employer and parents also will require much attention and effort. Because almost all children are their parents' most precious possession, and because impaired children usually are even more precious, in a great many cases one will find that retarded individuals have been *overly protected* by the parents. Parents may not be inclined to *turn loose* or let go of their retarded child, and thereby, unintentionally, impede his vocational habilitation. When the child is a girl, because of a fear of pregnancy, and/or social disease, parents typically are even more reluctant to let go. However, criticism of these parental attitudes is only unproductive. The habilitation process must, in these cases, include training and counseling for the parents, directed toward gaining parental assistance in seeking a measure of vocational, social, and economic independence for their offspring.

Employers often eschew the retarded worker for both specifiable and unspecified reasons. It is known that some employers doubt the ability of the retarded because they fear the retarded *cannot hold up their end*. Other employers feel, somewhat justifiably, that the retarded will warrant a good deal more supervision and management than the normal person and thus become an employment liability. Still other employers fear for the health and safety of the retarded and have legitimate concerns regarding accident or workman's compensation type of insurance. These, and other similar concerns, do merit attention and may not be avoided as considerations in vocational planning.

The unspecifiable reasons for not employing the retarded must also be considered. Some employers simply fear or avoid the retarded because the retarded *don't look right* or *make me feel uncomfortable*. Psychotherapeutic efforts should not be attempted with these employers if they do not respond to reason and logic. The vocational habilitation plans and processes must take all of the above factors into account and develop methods for overcoming them or finding alternatives to them.

It cannot be disputed that minimum wage laws have been an asset to this country, but they have seriously affected the employability of many of the retarded whose actual production may not be worth the minimum wage. Special "exemptions" from minimum wage laws are available through the U.S. Department of Labor, and these exemptions are quite appealing to potential employers and significantly increase the employability of the mentally retarded.

The Role of Sheltered Workshops
in the Habilitation of the Mentally Retarded

No discussion of vocational habilitation for the mentally retarded would be complete without considering sheltered workshops. Excellent discussions of sheltered workshops are available elsewhere (Dubrow, 1967; Frawnkel, 1967; and Redkey, 1967), and only a general review will be presented herein. The term "sheltered workshop" is, at best, generic, and refers to a wide variety of things, some of which are, and some of which are not, workshops. The following paragraphs describe three settings which might justifiably be called workshops.

The **transitional workshop** is a work center that has as its main goal the work-training of handicapped people. The production and marketing of goods is secondary in objective and usually is conducted for training purposes and to assist in paying the overhead costs of the workshop. The training and especially the movement of handicapped people through the workshop are the true measure of its value. It is designed to teach, train, and prepare the handicapped for vocational placement elsewhere.

The benefits of the transitional shop to the handicapped are immense. The workers are permitted to learn their physical and mental capacities and preferences for work. The transitional workshop usually is not production-oriented and, therefore, may require a subsidy to continue operation. Inasmuch as the goal is vocational restoration or habilitation, transitional shops frequently have a financial base of support within the community.

The **extended employment workshop** has been called also the "terminal workshop." This type of workshop typically must be production-oriented, but has as employees those handicapped who simply cannot be placed in industry for one or more reasons. This workshop relates wages directly to production and typically procures contracts from governmental and industrial concerns as sources of revenue.

Although the extended employment workshop is production-oriented, it typically also requires a community subsidy. The philosophy that "having a partially sufficient employee is better than a totally dependent person" is easily defended, and most communities are willing to provide the subsidy. Workers are periodically evaluated to insure that those who are capable are moved to jobs outside the workshop.

The third type of workshop is not a workshop in the sense that the preceding two are. The **activity center** has as its major goal socialization or recreational activities that may secondarily generate some income. The activity center is designed as a place where the more severely handicapped may engage for a part of each day in recreational endeavors with their peers. These endeavors are purposeful, that is designed to accomplish something, and usually produce limited income. Typically, participants in the activity centers are not paid wages, and any revenue generated goes to pay for the expenses of the center.

It is very wise for extended employment workshops and activity centers to maintain a close liaison. Quite often, there will be movement from one to another, as participants of each improve and/or degenerate.

Ideally, each of the three types of workshops would be available for the mentally retarded. Generally, due to labor and wage-and-hour laws, it is not possible to combine elements of all three under one roof. The three types of workshops in conjunction with the availability of jobs within the private sector will tremendously foster the habilitation process for the mentally retarded.

SOCIAL FACTORS OF HABILITATION

Although the major concern of this section is the vocational habilitation of the retarded, it would be negligent to ignore the social aspects of the process. The major premise of the remainder of this section is that "the vocational success of the adult retarded is largely dependent upon his social competence." Within this perspective, one of the less important aspects of vocational success for the adult retarded is vocational ability.

The dangers and problems of independent living offer great impediments for the mentally retarded. The unsupervised retarded will have had little experience in contacting physicians, dentists, attorneys, etc. Likewise, his appetite for current events will be so little that he is likely to be unaware of such things as changes in transportation schedules and a great many other things indirectly related to his work. All of this is not to say that the retarded cannot be prepared for independent living, but the odds are not in their favor. Training for independent living ideally would take place during adolescence or young adulthood, and should be an integral part of the habilitation plan and process. Charles (1957) has shown the increase in probability of success for the retarded, for example, who have attended special classes.

Ideally, the retarded would receive a schedule of social training that would be graduated from totally dependent to near or totally independent living. The first phase of training would be in the home or institution and would be directed toward self-help skills, safety skills, communication, etc. The second phase of training might be in a "quarter-way" facility where both vocational and home living skills would be taught, stressing the importance of cooperative efforts in home living. Next might be "half-way house" living for a brief period (up to three months) during which more and more independence and responsibility would be given to the client. Finally, the retarded would go to group sheltered living or independent living, depending upon the social competence of each individual. Group sheltered living involves a small number of residents living together cooperatively with only a minimum of supervision.

Only a few comprehensive vocational habilitation programs are available now to met the needs of the mentally retarded. Perhaps as more and more retarded earn their way in our culture, society will cast off the existing barriers and make room for the mentally retarded as responsible citizens.

REFERENCES

Anastasi, A.: *Fields of Applied Psychology.* New York, McGraw-Hill, 1964.

Benda, C. E.: Psychopathology of childhood. In Carmichael, L. (Ed.), *Manual of Child Psychology* (2nd ed.). New York, Wiley, pp. 1115-1161, 1954.

Binet, A. and Simon, T.: Méthodes nouvelles pour le diagnostic du niveau intellectuel des anormaux. *Année Psychologique, 11*:191-244, 1905.

Boring, E. G.: Intelligence as the tests test it. *New Republic, 6*:35-37, June, 1923.

Cantor, G. N.: On the incurability of mental deficiency. *Amer J Ment Defic, 60*:362-365, 1955.

Charles, D. C.: Adult adjustment of some deficient American children (II) *Amer J Ment Defic, 62*:300-304, 1957.

Clarke, Ann M. and Clarke, A. D. B. (Eds.): *Mental Deficiency: The Changing Outlook.* New York, Free Press, 1958.

Cruikshank, W. M. and Johnson, G. O. (Eds.): *Education of Exceptional Children and Youth.* Englewood Cliffs, N.J., Prentice-Hall, 1958.

DiMichael, S. G. (Ed.): Vocational rehabilitation of the mentally retarded. *Amer J Ment Defic, 57*:169-337, 1952.

Doll, E. A.: The essentials of an inclusive concept of mental deficiency. *Amer J Ment Defic, 46*:214-219, 1941.

Dubrow, M.: Sheltered workshops for the mentally retarded as an educational and vocational experience. In Meyer, E. L. (Ed.), *Planning Community Services for the Mentally Retarded,* Scranton, Pa., International Textbook Co., pp. 237-242, 1967.

Engel, Anna M.: Employment of the mentally retarded. *Amer J Ment Defic, 57*: 243-267, 1952.

Fraenkel, W. A.: Starting a sheltered workshop. In Meyer, E. L. (Ed.), *Planning*

Community Services for the Mentally Retarded, Scranton, Pa., International Textbook Co., pp. 190-196, 1967.

Goddard, H. H.: *The Kallikak Family.* New York, Macmillan, 1912.

Heber, R. F.: A manual on terminology and classification in mental retardation *Amer J Ment Defic,* Monogr. suppl., 1961.

Itard, J. M. G.: *The Wild Boy of Aveyron* (Trans. by G. and Muriel Humphrey). New York, Appleton-Century-Crofts, 1932.

Jastak, J. A.: A rigorous criterion of feeblemindedness. *J Abnorm Soc Psychol, 44*:367-378, 1949.

Kanner, L.: *Child Psychiatry* (3rd ed.). Springfield, Thomas, 1957.

McNemar, Q. A.: A critical examination of the University of Iowa studies of environmental influences upon the I.Q. *Psychol Bull, 37*:63-92, 1940.

Macland, R. L., Sarason, S. B. and Gladwin, T.: *Mental Subnormality.* New York, Basic Books, 1958.

Meyer, E. L., (Ed.): *Planning Community Services for the Mentally Retarded.* Scranton, Pa., International Textbook Co., 1967.

President's Panel on Mental Retardation: A proposed program for national action to combat mental retardation. Washington, D.C., GPO, 1962.

Redkey, H.: A way of thinking about sheltered workshops. In Meyer, E. L. (Ed.), *Planning Community Services for the Mentally Retarded,* Scranton, Pa., International Textbook Co., pp. 180-189, 1967.

Rotter, J. B.: *Social Learning and Clinical Psychology.* Englewood Cliffs, N.J., Prentice-Hall, 1954.

Skeels, H. M., Updegraff, R., Wellman, Beth L., and Williams, H. M.: A study of environmental stimulation, an orphanage preschool project. *U of Iowa Stud Child Welf, 15*:129-145, 1938.

Sloan, W. and Birch, J. W.: A rationale for degrees of retardation. *Amer J Ment Defic, 60*:258-264, 1955.

Terman, L. M. and Merrill, Maud A.: *Stanford-Binet Intelligence Scale.* Boston, Houghton-Mifflin, 1960.

Tizard, J.: Longitudinal and follow-up studies. In Clarke, Ann M., and Clarke, A. D. B. (Eds.), *Mental Deficiency: The Changing Outlook.* New York, Free Press, pp. 422-449, 1958.

Tredgold, A. F.: *A Textbook of Mental Deficiency* (6th ed.). Baltimore, Wood, 1937.

Watson, J. B.: *Behaviorism.* New York, Norton, 1925.

Wechsler, D.: *Wechsler Adult Intelligence Scale: Manual.* New York, Psychological Corp., 1955.

Windle, C.: Prognosis of mental subnormals. *Amer J Ment Defic, 66,* Monogr. suppl., 1962.

———————————

(PART FIVE)

THE VISUALLY DISABLED

VOCATIONAL REHABILITATION SERVICES
FOR THE BLIND

PSYCHOLOGICAL IMPLICATIONS OF
BLINDNESS

Chapter 15

VOCATIONAL REHABILITATION SERVICES
FOR THE BLIND

Randolph H. Greene

I N ALL FIFTY STATES and in the territorial possessions of the United States, vocational rehabilitation services are available for blind individuals. Funds for these service programs are provided through joint State and Federal appropriations. Thirty-seven states have *separate agencies* for the blind and visually impaired. In other states, services for the blind are combined with rehabilitation programs for other disability groups or they are a part of the public welfare agency. Recently the trend has been to combine all social welfare and rehabilitation services under one "umbrella" agency.

Burt L. Risley has written as follows:

> There is more than substantial justification for this separateness; there is often compelling necessity for it. This separateness obtains because of historical reason, sound theoretical principles, and practical facts.
>
> Visual disability historically has been accorded considerable attention, with the victims of this disability receiving the benefits of services which evolved in the nature of separate disciplines. In the fifth century, B.C., the Greek historian, Herodotus, noted the high degree to which opthalmology had developed as a specialized science in Egypt. And a thousand years before Herodotus visited Egypt, books had already been written about treatment of eye problems in that country.
>
> Manuscripts developed early in the histories of such religions as Judaism, Buddhism, and Christianity reflect the separate attention already being accorded to the problems of the blind at that time. In 1526 Juan Luis Vives, the Spanish humanist concerned about the mendicant status to which so many of the blind in Europe seemed relegated, presented what may well be one of the first written proposals for vocational rehabilitation of the visually disabled. Organizations of the blind were known in early Russia. Institutional care for the blind was available in ancient Egypt and in India. The guild for Japanese blind masseurs was organized in the ninth century. One of the most famous institutes for the blind in the world, L'Hôpital des Quinze-Vingts in Paris, was founded by King Louis IX on or about the year 1254. Dogs have been used to guide the blind for thousands of years.
>
> Special education of the handicapped—the prerequisite for optimum rehabilitation—began when Hauy, Klein, and Howe instituted their respective schools for the blind around the start of the nineteenth century. For the blind, systematic attempts to compensate for disability have been in progress since the Renaissance. The list could go on and on, but the pattern would be the same; activities relating to services to and rehabilitation of the handicapped most often begin because of

267

concern about the problems of blindness—a problem the treatment of which usually has been and still is approached separately from other problems in our society. Vocational rehabilitation, as it is presently known in this country, probably began in 1918 with the enactment of the Smith-Sears Veterans' Rehabilitation Act; administrators acting under the authority of that pioneer federal legislation drew upon techniques, skills, resources, methods, and facilities previously developed by those who were involved in services to the blind.

The establishment and maintenance of autonomous programs for the visually disabled is supported by a number of well established theoretical principles. One is always reluctant to generalize about the respective extent of debilitative effect as between various disabilities, for there are many variables and severity of disability will depend upon individual situations. But certainly no one who is knowledgeable about rehabilitation can dispute the seriousness of blindness—for the individual victim, for his family, and ultimately for his society. Some who are overly enthusiastic about the efficacy of those vocational rehabilitation services, with which they may be familiar, might on occasion refer to blindness as a "mere inconvenience." Such a position, of course, is hardly subscribed to by those laboring under this disability—blindness is a serious business; it is a catastrophic disability. For the visually disabled individual in a sighted world, blindness is a form of uninsulated isolation. For those who are congenitally blind, the result is perhaps even more pronounced. Blindness immobilizes, isolates, and affects the total individual. This necessarily has substantial vocational ramifications.

It is axiomatic that successful treatment of so catastrophic a disability requires total treatment of the victim. In order to effectively assist the person, there must be an integration of services and a coordination of all efforts. It is axiomatic, too, that a complex and difficult problem can best be dealt with through specialization. Blindness is a severe and complex problem, and has broad ramifications for the total personality of an individual. There are many distinct facets to this problem, but yet the problem is not hopeless and much can be done. Autonomy in services, therefore, is desirable so the professional worker can function in a creative capacity, while developing a high level of specialization . . .

There are also a number of hard facts which make practical the separation of services to the blind from programs of general rehabilitation. The crux of the matter is that, other things being equal, the visually disabled get more and better services where separate programs have been established to deal specifically with the visually disabled and this higher level of service is not accomplished at the expense of any other disability group. In 37 states at the present time, rehabilitation programs for the blind are conducted separately from the states' general vocational rehabilitation program. Of these 37 separate programs for the blind, 27 have authority to serve individuals whose primary handicap is of a visual nature, regardless of whether or not visual disability is so severe as to amount to legal blindness. Only in 13 states and 4 territories are service to the blind conducted as an integrated part of the general vocational rehabilitation program of the state.

BLINDNESS

Blindness is defined as central visual acuity of 20/200 or less in the better eye, with best correction, or a field restriction to the extent that central visual acuity in the better eye subtends an angle no greater than 20 degrees. Therefore, it is possible for blind individuals to have some residual sight. In many instances this remaining sight is useful although the partially blind individual is limited in performing activities which require average visual acuity. An individual who is blind, but who retains some residual sight is frequently referred to as *partially blind, partially sighted,* or *industrially blind.* Within the blind population it is estimated that approximately 80 percent have some useful sight, while the remaining 20 percent are totally blind or have such limited sight that it is not useful for any practical purpose. The phrase *visually impaired* is used to denote persons with impairments of vision which limit their activities, but their sight is better than the definition of legal blindness. An example would be a person with one normal eye and one blind eye; or a person with central visual acuity between 20/70 and 20/200 in the better eye with best correction.

The severity of the disability often determines the extent and the complexity of the rehabilitation services required. The blind person who has a *concomitant disability*—for example, epilepsy, mental retardation, or paresis—would usually present a more difficult rehabilitation need than an individual whose only disability is blindness. Other characteristics which are not so easily defined and which cannot be examined in a laboratory, may be as limiting as a concomitant disability. These include the blind person who does not speak English or who is not motivated to become rehabilitated, or the blind person who is so overprotected by family members that his attempt to become rehabilitated is hindered.

Attitudes which are unwholesome or which are founded on prejudicial data can become one of the strongest deterrents to successful rehabilitation. These attitudes may be those formed by the general public, by the employer who is considering a blind applicant, or by the blind person himself. The adventitiously blind person who has had normal sight prior to becoming blind may have possessed some of these unwholesome attitudes and it may be that, until he has obtained adequate knowledge about his blindness, his negative attitude can prevent successful rehabilitation. During the past twenty-five years, there has been a great improvement in public attitudes toward blindness. The improved attitudes are due to better public information, more blind people in the job market, and greater mobility within the blind population, thus enabling more members of the general public to see a blind person functioning independently. The need still exists, however, for a great amount of accurate information about blindness being made available through the public media. When the blind person becomes aware of the possibilities for successful vocational rehabilitation, and his family and associates are aware of the benefits, the payoff is positive attitude and one less deterrent to rehabilitation.

THE VOCATIONAL REHABILITATION PROCESS

The rehabilitation counselor or another member of the rehabilitation team becomes aware of a blind individual through one of many and varied **referral sources.** Through proper liaison with the medical community including hospitals, with public welfare agencies, with other social agencies within a community, with civic and service organizations, and with the United States Employment Service, the counselor will find numerous blind people being referred who can be considered for vocational rehabilitation services. After receiving referral information, the counselor arranges for an initial interview with the prospective client. Most experienced counselors find that an interview in the home of the client reveals a great amount of information which becomes important during the rehabilitation process. When a client comes to the office for the initial interview, there is no opportunity to evaluate his living conditions, his family members, and social and cultural factors which may either enhance or impede his rehabilitation.

During and following the initial interview, the counselor begins to formulate plans for the rehabilitation program. The next step is to obtain **medical information**, usually in the form of a general physical examination and a special eye examination, to determine the extent of visual impairment and the existence (or absence) of other disabling conditions. After this information is secured, the counselor must establish *eligibility*. In order to be eligible for rehabilitation services, an individual must be disabled; the disability must be a hindrance to successful employment, and there must be a reasonable likelihood that vocational rehabilitation services will enable him to become successfully employed.

Physical restoration services in the form of surgery or medical treatment for the purpose of alleviating or diminishing the disability become the primary considerations once medical reports have been received and examined. In many instances, surgery or medical treatment for the condition causing a visual impairment will restore the client's sight or improve it to the extent that he no longer has a disability. Prosthetic appliances such as low-vision aids may assist in reducing or overcoming the disability.

After all avenues for improvement of the disabling conditions have been investigated and there is no hope for improvement, both the client and the counselor must plan a *rehabilitation program*. Although *counseling* is an important part of the total vocational rehabilitation process and enters into all phases of contact with the client, it is at this stage of the rehabilitation process that perhaps the most intensive and extensive counseling becomes necessary. The client must be assisted to recognize the limitations imposed by blindness and yet must be supported and encouraged to overcome feelings of despondency. At this time, the counselor must use every possible resource to motivate the client to become involved in his rehabilitation program.

The rehabilitation center for the blind offers a valuable training opportunity assisting the blind person to adjust to the limitations of blindness and to learn methods and techniques for coping with the problem. The aim of the rehabilitation center is to assist each blind person in training to reach his *maximum level of independence* in all activities of his daily life and to *reestablish confidence* in himself. The training program in a rehabilitation center usually includes instruction in orientation and mobility, personal grooming, Braille, typing, personal management, crafts, shop, and basic communication skills. The average length of training in a specialized rehabilitation center for the blind is four months, although every program is tailored to meet the needs of each individual client. Thus, some clients may be able to complete the training program within a three-month period while others may require as long as a full year of this intensive training. While in the rehabilitation center, the client receives complete *psychological services,* including psychological counseling, group therapy, testing and interpretation of tests results. In most centers there is a program of *vocational evaluation, vocational exploration,* and *vocational counseling.* When the client completes such a training program, he should have a better concept of himself, including his strengths and his limitations, his intellectual functioning level, his vocational interests, and the possibilities open to him for vocational training.

When the client returns to his home community, the vocational rehabilitation counselor again becomes intensively involved in the rehabilitation program, and normally the client enters *vocational training.* This may be in a university, a trade school, a business college, a technical school, a sheltered workshop, or on-the-job training.

Sheltered workshops for the blind, more commonly known as lighthouses for the blind, have been established in the larger cities throughout the United States. These sheltered workshops provide jobs for blind individuals who are not capable of engaging in competitive employment, either in industry or business. While the traditional lighthouse for the blind still conducts such well-known activities as manufacturing brooms and mops and sewing products to be sold in the market, many of the more progressive lighthouses are moving into greater and greater involvement with sub-contracts. Many of these are of an industrial nature and require highly skilled individuals to operate the modern assembly-line machines. Many of the products are fabricated, assembled, and packaged as components for industrial factories.

THE PLACEMENT PROCESS

Placement is a complex subject to investigate, possibly because it is not clearly understood. It is shunned, avoided, and usually relegated to a position of insignificance, frequently pushed into the far distant recesses of the rehabilitation counselor's mind. In fact, the counselor may hope it will never again rear its ugly head. A complete search of literature will reveal a paucity of definitive studies and very few thorough investigations into this process. It is the contention of this writer that more information on placement, clearly presented with meaningful explanations, will enhance the rehabilitation counselor's understanding and thereby contribute to a more positive attitude.

Counselors offer many excuses for avoiding placement activities. These include: "When adequately trained, the client with a relatively minor disability can find his own job." "There is not enough time to devote to placement activities, since other duties keep me fully occupied." "The state employment service has the responsibility for placement, and, therefore, I do not need to become involved." "There are no clients on my caseload who are ready for employment." "Most of my clients are so severely disabled that they cannot successfully compete for jobs and, therefore, must seek sheltered workshop employment." These negative remarks illustrate the lack of appreciation and insight into placement and its vital role in the total rehabilitation process.

A Workable Placement Program

A placement program that has been developed by trial and error over a period of many years is offered here for the rehabilitation counselor who wishes to organize his activities and fulfill his responsibilities. This program requires a basic attitude of acceptance and understanding of the fact that placement activities are the responsibility of every rehabilitation counselor. Inherent is an understanding that a counselor cannot function effectively without a deep knowledge of and commitment to placement. It is essential in counseling with the client, in making recommendations to the client, and in assisting the client to achieve his vocational rehabilitation goals. Placement activities should be carefully planned, and sufficient time should be set aside so that these activities become a part of the counselor's regular routine. He should recognize that placement is the summit of the rehabilitation process and that establishing eligibility, developing a vocational plan, providing medical services, and arranging for vocational training are only steps leading to the summit. Any rehabilitation program without placement and *follow-up services* is incomplete.

It is recommended that a caseload of employers be developed. The "employer caseload" should include a minimum of thirty-five employers who are contacted routinely. Approximately thirty of these employers should have blind persons working successfully in their organizations. The counselor must exercise considerable care and skillful selection to make sure that these employers are convinced of the merits and advantages of employing individuals who are blind. Regular contact with the employer will provide continuing employment opportunities as vacancies within this organization occur due to attrition or promotion. If these employers are carefully cultivated, they will be receptive to the idea of filling these vacancies with other blind persons.

A small portion of the employer caseload will be made up of new employers who are being cultivated. Over a period of time the counselor may expend a considerable amount of effort before one of these employers can be convinced that a blind client will be an asset to his organization. However, a thorough job will insure that this new employer remains on the employer caseload for a number of years. This caseload will be continuously changing just as the client caseload is continuously changing, with new employers being added to the caseload regularly and others being deleted as necessary. In the same way that a file system is maintained on the client caseload, the counselor must keep a current file on his employers. The counselor's responsibility to his employer caseload is parallel to his responsibility to the client caseload.

Follow-up services are essential to a successful placement program, and indeed to any comprehensive rehabilitation program. The client should be contacted frequently during the early stages of his employment to assure everyone that he has been placed to the satisfaction of both himself and the employer. Frequent contacts by the counselor will keep relatively minor problems from ballooning into crises. The writer recalls an incident which will illustrate. After three weeks of operating a machine in a potato chip factory, a mentally retarded blind client was capably performing all activities and knew as much about the operation of the machine as any other employee in the company. Unfortunately, during the night shift a slight alteration in production was made, and it was necessary for the client to print the word "header" on the end of each carton as it came through his machine. The client was unable to spell the word, but fortunately the counselor was maintaining close contact through follow-up services. The counselor spent more than two hours teaching the client how to spell this difficult word and how to print it on each carton. Although learning to spell this word may seem insignificant, it became a crucial factor in what has been a successful placement.

In the above case, the employer recognized and appreciated the interest of the counselor in determining that the client was performing all duties of his particular job. The employer's knowledge that the counselor continues his interest after the client is on the job, results in more secure employment for the client. The confidence of the employer is maintained and strengthened. Concurrently, the need for intense follow-up services lessens as the client develops his skills and his confidence. Similarly, the employer's confidence in his new employee matures, and the need for the counselor's involvement diminishes. From this point, all contacts made by the counselor are to maintain this employer's position on the employer caseload.

Placement Requires Salesmanship

Possibly the careful reader has noted that some of the techniques in placement are similar to those used by the successful salesman. Certainly, the employer caseload is comparable to the salesman's file of prospective and active customers. Likewise, maximum sales are realized by the salesman who gets out of his office to make personal contacts with his customers. Good organization and personal contact are as essential to the counselor as they are to any salesman.

Most definitions of selling or salesmanship include a strong emphasis on convincing or persuading. Usually an attempt is made to persuade another person that a new idea or concept would be beneficial or that a new product should be used or a service purchased. Persuasion is as applicable in placement as it is in salesmanship. If the salesman can convince the customer of the advantages of his product, the customer will realize his need for that product. Once this need is recognized, the sale can be completed.

Can placement be approached in a similar manner? Most certainly. When the employer has been made aware of the positive attributes and abilities of a blind person—his qualities of loyalty, punctuality, regularity, and high production—he will then be ready to accept the blind person as a desirable employee.

Claude I. Shell in his article, "Selling — Another Role for the Placement Counselor" (1968), has presented a penetrating study of placement as it relates to selling. He states:

> There are three steps in this selling process for the successful counselor. First, he must sell himself. On the surface this statement appears unnecessary because it would appear obvious that he must already be convinced of the soundness of the concept that the blind can be successful employees. Such assumptions are unwarranted and dangerous. There are people in placement of the visually handicapped who are not themselves convinced that their clients can hold their own in competition with the sighted without being a drag on the employer. Such a person cannot succeed in the placement process. A second step is the selling of the client, the handicapped person. This person must be convinced that he can perform competitively in the world of work if he is going to succeed. This is no mean task, and it may require all of the professional skill of the counselor. Next, the counselor, or "salesman" by this time, must sell the employer (on) the concept that a visually handicapped person can perform in industry without being a burden on his employer. This step involves selling of the concept that the blind are employable, not that one particular blind person is suitable for one specific job. In accomplishing this, heavy reliance can be placed on the regular sales techniques, with certain necessary modifications, that are used to train salesmen in business and industry (pp. 33-34).

Examine Your Own Feelings About Blindness

Mr. Shell raises a fundamental issue which should be of concern to every rehabilitation counselor working with blind clients:

> There are people in placement of the visually handicapped who are not themselves convinced that their clients can hold their own in competition with the sighted without being a drag on the employer. Such a person cannot succeed in the placement process (p. 34).

Certainly, this statement would imply that every counselor must be introspective, examining his own attitudes and feelings about blindness.

Placement and follow-up services are fundamental and are, therefore, essential to every complete rehabilitation program. The rehabilitation counselor who is dedicated to the ideals of vocational rehabilitation recognizes the critical need for placement and incorporates it into his everyday work schedule. He fully accepts this responsibility and makes certain that each client receives the very best in placement and follow-up services. He cannot conscientiously relegate placement to a role of insignificance; nor can he delegate this responsibility.

The federal regulations governing vocational rehabilitation services, are explicit. They require that every agency recognizes its responsibility for placement and follow-up services. George A. Magers, Consultant for Guidance, Training, and Placement of the Blind, Rehabilitation Services Administration, Washington, D.C. (1966), has said:

To obtain the means with which to compete for employment in a changing labor market is the desire and the duty of all blind persons who have the capacity and ability. To provide these means is the responsibility of our society. These are the precepts underlying the philosophy of restoration and utilization of human resources so fundamental to vocational rehabilitation (p. 119).

The rehabilitation counselor who has critically examined his own feelings about blindness and who feels adequate and comfortable while working with blind clients will find himself where the action is. He will experience tremendous challenges which are intensely stimulating. When this happens, he will have answered the question, "Placement—passé or pertinent?"

SUMMARY

Blindness is a catastrophic disabling condition requiring specialized vocational rehabilitation programs, specialized techniques, specially trained rehabilitation teams, and training programs specially designed to assist the client to cope with the problems it incurs. Blindness may be a total loss of sight or a partial loss of sight, while other visual impairments may cause serious interference with the client's ability to function in his vocation. Concomitant disabilities along with blindness usually create complex rehabilitation problems which are extremely difficult to resolve. At least one other complicating factor exists due to prejudicial attitudes on the part of the general public, the client's family members, or the client himself.

The vocational rehabilitation process offers an answer to the dilemma being faced by a blind client when he can be stimulated and motivated to become involved in his own vocational rehabilitation program. There are methods of training and assisting the blind individual to learn compensatory techniques and skills which can restore his independence and his self-confidence. Specialized rehabilitation centers are available throughout the country to assist with adjustment problems and a clearer understanding of vocational interests and vocational goals.

Once the blind client has become adjusted to his disability, has gained his self-confidence, and has been vocationally trained, the placement specialist offers assistance in locating a suitable job and overcoming the initial problems encountered on the job. Follow-up services provided by the rehabilitation counselor or the placement specialist are usually offered for a short period of time until the client has become satisfactorily adjusted to his work situation, and the employer knows that he can perform all of the duties of his job, and produce at the level of his associates. At this time, the vocational rehabilitation process is complete for the blind client.

REFERENCES

Bauman, Mary K.: *Characteristics of Blind and Visually Handicapped People in Professional, Sales, and Managerial Work.* Pennsylvania Office for the Blind, 1963.
Bauman, Mary K. and Yoder, Norman M.: *Placing the Blind and Visually Handi-*

capped in Clerical, Industrial and Service Fields. Pennsylvania Office for the Blind, undated pamphlet.

Bauman, Mary K. and Yoder, Norman M.: *Placing the Blind and Visually Handicapped in Professional Occupations.* Pennsylvania Office for the Blind, 1962.

Borow, Henry: *Man in a World at Work.* Boston, Houghton Mifflin Company, 1964.

Carroll, Thomas J.: *Blindness.* Boston and Toronto, Little, Brown and Company, 1961.

Cholden, Louis S.: *A Psychiatrist Works with Blindness.* New York, American Foundation for the Blind, 1958.

Crawford, Fred L.: *Career Planning for the Blind.* New York, Farrar, Straus and Giroux, 1966.

Cutsforth, Thomas D.: *The Blind in School and Society.* American Foundation for the Blind, New York, 1951.

Farrell, Gabriel: *The Story of Blindness.* Cambridge, Harvard University Press, 1956.

Gowman, Alan G.: *The War Blind in American Social Structure.* New York, American Foundation for the Blind, 1957.

Hanson, Howard H.: Work. *Journal of Rehabilitation,* Vol. 32, no. 2 (March-April), 1970.

Magers George A.: Placement—Key to employment. *Blindness—AAWB Annual,* Washington, D. C., 1966.

McGowan, John F. and Porter, Thomas L.: *An Introduction to the Vocational Rehabilitation Process.* U. S. Government Printing Office, Washington, D. C., 1967.

Oklahoma State University: *Workshop for Placement Specialists.* Stillwater, Oklahoma, December 1965.

Risley, Burt L.: An unpublished document prepared for the National Citizens Advisory Committee on Vocational Rehabilitation. Austin, Texas, 1967.

Shell, Claude I.: Selling—Another role for the placement counselor. *The New Outlook for the Blind,* Vol. 62, no. 2, pp. 33-37, 1968.

Southern Ilinois University: *Developing Employment Opportunities for Blind Persons in Competitive Occupations,* Follow-up Seminar. New Orleans, Louisiana, December 1962.

Southern Illinois University: *Developing Employment Opportunities for Blind Persons in Competitive Occupations,* Follow-up Seminar. Austin, Texas, October 1965.

Thomason, Bruce and Barrett, Albert M.: *The Placement Process in Vocational Rehabilitation Counseling.* U. S. Government Printing Office, Washington, D. C., 1960.

Veterans Administration: *Occupations of Totally Blinded Veterans of World War II and Korea.* Washington, D. C., 1956.

Veterans Administration: *War Blinded Veterans in a Postwar Setting.* 1958.

Chapter 16

PSYCHOLOGICAL IMPLICATIONS OF BLINDNESS

James B. Caylor II

T HE FIELD OF WORK for the blind has been an organized effort on a national scale for approximately the past seventy years. During this time, many advances have been made in understanding the psychological implications of blindness, but there are still certain basic precepts which must be considered in examining this field of rehabilitation. It is clearly evident that blindness is a major disability involving social, psychological, and vocational problems; but examinations into the extent of these difficulties often appear to lose sight of the fact that "the blind" are people. As people, visually handicapped persons react to their environment in much the same manner as those in society in general (Raskin and Weller, 1953). To appreciate this fact, as simple as it sounds, is not always as uncomplicated as it may appear. However, to apply psychological reasoning in order to understand better the problems of blindness, this fact must be accepted. Although this may be a beginning, certain other information must also be considered in order to evaluate the problem adequately.

One important consideration that must be given to the problems of blindness is the pathology of the disability, with particular reference to the age of onset and the circumstances which led to the visual impairment (Raskin, 1962). A congenitally blind person (one who was born blind) has had a different developmental history than an adventitiously blinded person (one who has lost his sight after a significantly long period of possessing normal vision). Furthermore, persons who have lost their vision due to a progressively gradual condition have encountered different circumstances from those of the individual whose loss is due to a sudden traumatic cause, such as an accident. Also, there are degrees of visual loss ranging from total blindness to high partial vision.

It is the purpose of this chapter to examine the above-mentioned conditions more thoroughly and hopefully to convey to the reader some of the common problems found in adjustment to a physical disability, as well as those that may be a direct result of visual loss specifically. This investigation of the problem will also attempt to indicate some of the other circumstantial and environmental influences which are commonly found among individuals who are visually handicapped.

PATTERNS OF ADJUSTMENT

Various patterns of adjustment to blindness or visual impairment exist just as they do with other physical disabilities. Understandably, not all visually-handicapped persons achieve "adjustment," but through the assistance of various rehabilitation services, this desired factor is usually achieved. For purposes of this chapter, adjustment is defined as that stage of social, psychological, and vocational adaptation which enables an individual to function within the limits of his potential, while dealing effectively with his environment. Understanding adjustment processes must require the recognition that due to the fact that people and circumstances differ, there are no set sequences or stages that an individual must go through to achieve adjustment following onset of blindness. However, there are certain recognized components that commonly exist in the adjustment process (Cholden, 1958). The following section will deal with five of these components: denial, anxiety, contra-indicated hope for return of vision, depression, and finally, adjustment.

Denial

Beginning with the understanding that defense mechanisms are commonly used to deal with anxiety and stress, it is important to remind the reader that blindness is a major disability and as such, often creates situations of stress. Added to these particular situations are also those which life itself presents. Handicapped persons, in order to tolerate or deal with stresses, commonly use denial as a defense. This defense, as its name implies, is the person's rejection of the idea that he is handicapped or that he feels the stress that his situation produces (Harriman, 1965). In many cases where individuals are employing this defense extensively, it is not uncommon to find persons that have had both eyes enucleated to deny the fact that they have no vision. In other cases, partially-sighted individuals who are rapidly losing their remaining vision will deny the fact and often create situations in which they are embarrassed and ridiculed. Counseling attempts to deal with the extensive use of denial are often unsuccessful even though this presents a major barrier to the rehabilitation of the client. In many instances, however, the use of denial over a short period of time, and to no great degree, appears to afford the visually handicapped person the opportunity to progress through an initial stage that is necessary for him to adapt to his situation. The use of denial is not an uncommon defense in terms of humans dealing with stress. However, when it is used to deal with the stresses of a handicap, it is usually employed more commonly and to a greater degree.

Denial is also often used by the congenitally blind to deal with stresses which they encounter. It has long been realized that persons who have never had vision learn certain concepts on a verbal level but are often unable to put these into practice. Two examples of this are the use of verbal concepts on a superficial level to explain characteristics of appearance and color. Unless a congenitally blind person has had the opportunity to factually investigate an object, he may be able only to "parrot" a description of this object. For example, it is impossible for a totally blind person to examine a two-story building all at the same time as a sighted person will do; thus, he may be able to give a detailed description of the various parts of the building, but without a true realization of the total appearance.

Colors to the congenitally blind person also present such a problem. They learn and can verbalize what various colors typically represent and what colors go with other colors, but often they do not have a clear understanding of the various colors that are commonly and naturally known to a sighted individual. When confronted with specific questions concerning descriptions of appearance of objects or colors, the blind person may find himself in a dilemma and recognize his inadequacy to understand clearly these concepts. Due to this fact, he often feels stress and resorts to denial in order to compensate for his inadequacies. He may deny the importance of getting a total picture of the appearance of an object and depreciate the importance of color combinations that possibly may make his dress very inappropriate.

The blind and visually-handicapped may also resort to denial so that they may compensate or alleviate the stresses they feel about their own reaction to their blindness. Also, they may employ denial as a defense in an attempt to decrease many of the public attitudes that they feel are inappropriate and pitying toward the blind. Clients may often refuse services, such as instruction in braille and mobility training with the cane, because these skills are typically related to blindness, and to accept the need for these is to accept the fact that one is blind. Clients often choose to be dependent upon sighted individuals, even though it hurts their pride, rather than accept the realization that they are blind and need special instruction to learn compensatory skills.

Although these are just a few examples of situations where denial is used, it is a natural part of an individual's psychological makeup, unless it interferes with the client's reality of his situation, thus becoming an atypical mechanism. Professionals in the field of work for the blind should learn to detect denial as a defense mechanism and be able to determine whether it is simply being used to decrease or cope with stress, or whether its extensive use is creating a psychological problem interfering with adjustment and preventing an individual from functioning at his potential. The extensive use of denial may also be a major deterrent to the adjustment of a family whose constellation contains a newly or congenitally blinded person. However, the problems of family adjustment will be discussed in a later section in this chapter.

Anxiety

Many case studies of individuals adjusting to blindness indicate a transition from the period where various defense mechanisms are used, such as denial, into a phase where marked anxiety is easily observable. In many instances it is felt that a visually-handicapped person eventually will come to the realization that his denial is, in essence, a lie that he has been telling himself. Upon this realization, he feels a great deal of anxiety which is not only directed to his blindness, but also to his ineffectiveness in dealing with his own reactions to his handicap (Harriman, 1965). These persons often seem to feel that they are incapable of controlling their own emotions, and this adds to their basic feelings of inadequacy and lack of self-confidence. The overt results of this anxiety can be seen in almost everything the person does and generally make his life quite miserable. In this stage, he may show the symptoms of phobic and/or conversion reactions, together with many other reactions that add to his discomfort (Cholden, 1958). During this time, he may have difficulty with sleep reversal, diarrhea, acute hypertension, an oversensitive nature, bitterness and increased aggressiveness, and other reactions. He may find himself floundering in a situation in which every attempt, on his part, to relieve this anxiety only results in added problems.

In a discussion of anxiety reactions, it is important to note that not all anxiety is problem-producing, but that in many cases it can be a factor which can be directed toward productive activity. However, as in the employment of denial, when anxiety reaches the level where it becomes a definite deterrent to daily living and adjustment, then it must be dealt with. Perhaps, at this point, it is important to define the ideology of anxiety as it relates to blindness. First of all, it can be said that anxiety resulting from loss of vision is perhaps one of the earliest stages when an individual feels the full implications that his visual handicap is going to have upon his life. Anxiety can be said to be an anticipation or apprehension of danger or threat which can have its basis in internal or external experiences. Cholden (1958) indicates that the advent of blindness may be similar to the "death" of the sighted person and the "rebirth" of the blind individual. Whatever the case, loss of vision is traumatic and creates a natural situation where apprehension of threat exists. This threat may involve an extreme feeling of helplessness, a fear of being a burden to others, the threat of future financial disaster, the fear of social isolation, and other critical feelings of insecurity.

Psychological and/or rehabilitative counseling often appears to be ineffectual in alleviating these fears. However, if the level of anxiety is not severely abnormal, counseling which will aid the client in attempting to effectively deal with these fears can be offered to the client. While certain aspects of anxiety reactions, such as future employment, may involve a long-term process of counseling, the client's feelings about himself, his family, his social activities, and the fear of his environment in general can be reduced. Also, counseling may be directed to assisting the client in developing an adequate and appropriate pattern of defense mechanisms to deal with these reactions.

Another symptom of anxiety that is commonly noted is the behavior that may be termed "acting out" behavior. In this situation, the individual may exhibit actions which are atypical of his general behavior before the advent of his visual impairment. These behaviors are often characterized by an overt overcompensation to some of the insecurities and inadequacies the individual may feel. For example, a person who was shy before losing his vision suddenly exhibits marked aggressive social behavior. Another example is the person who was previously very dependent upon his wife and family and suddenly becomes extremely independent, even to the point of being aloof and obnoxious. In some instances, such as overaggressive behavior, this compensation (if channeled properly) can be a motivating and productive force. On the other hand, the previously dependent person who becomes almost totally independent may refuse the assistance he desperately needs in order to be able to function adequately and comfortably in daily living. Whatever the reaction and compensatory behaviors, however, anxiety is at the base of these problems and is a common factor in the adjustment process. Later in this chapter, anxiety reactions will be discussed as they are typically noted in the congenitally blind person.

Contra-Indicated Hope for Return of Vision

It has long been recognized in the field of rehabilitation that the presence of false hopes for return of vision is one of the greatest deterrents to adjustment (Cholden, 1958.) In many cases, these false hopes may be due to rationalization on the part of the client in an attempt to find some degree of security. Many professionals in work for the blind suggest that these false hopes stem from superficial and inadequate appraisal of their visual condition by their ophthalmologist or physician. Other cases show clearly that these feelings are due to and encouraged by the family of the client. Whatever the cause, contra-indicated hope for restoration of sight can most definitely prolong or prevent a client from undertaking the responsibility to accept his visual limitations and from taking productive steps to alleviate its handicapping consequences.

One of the symptoms of false hope that is commonly observed is a sudden dependency upon religion. While in many cases this religious fervor is honest and realistic, too often the client's faith is superficial and what may be called "pseudoreligious". In the latter situation, the client's primary religious attitudes may be based on the hope for a miracle which will return his vision. In such cases, this type of "religious" reliance is frustrating to the client and only delays his acceptance of the fact that he is now, and most probably will be in the future, a severely visually-impaired individual. Often, if vision is not miraculously returned, the client may feel that both the cause of his blindness and the absence of a cure are due to punishment from God. Moreover, the client may feel that his visual loss and its poor prognosis are the punishment for the sins of his family or perhaps of society in general. Such attitudes are difficult for the client to deal with and may add to the myriad of anxieties he already feels about his situation. In counseling, attempting to deal with such attitudes is difficult for, while the reality of the situation needs to be dealt with, the possibility of destroying hope and faith may present problems for the client from which the chances for recovery are poor.

Many case studies also indicate that the newly blinded, or those who are progressively losing their vision, often travel from ophthalmologist to ophthalmologist (or in some instances, visit other healing arts professions) trying to find some doctor who will give them a glint of hope for the return of their vision. These individuals frequently incur medical bills that place them in an extreme financial indebtedness. The unwillingness to accept a professional diagnosis, or the need to avoid the realization of blindness, also delays the acquisition of services to the client, and hence his adjustment process suffers.

Again, stark reality concerning the poor prognosis of a visual disability may create other problems which will be detrimental to the client. It is important that the client, when reality is presented, have the opportunity to receive professional counseling which will enable him to deal with the anxiety that may result. While it is hoped that the client may be able to accept this reality, the immediacy of acceptance at this point is not critical. However, if the client can be assisted in establishing a basis for later acceptance, this may, in itself, prevent peripheral problems. This is particularly important with the individual who is losing his sight progressively, for his acceptance may be as tediously gradual as the slow deterioration of his vision. Whatever the condition of the visually handicapped individual, counseling can be very beneficial in aiding a client to work through this often disappointing and frustrating phase of adjustment.

Depression

Another reaction that is commonly found in the adjustment process is depression. While depressive reactions are commonly found among all individuals, whether handicapped or not, it is, for several reasons, probably the most noticeable factor in rehabilitation. First, whether the depression is psychotic or neurotic in nature, it is usually rather simple to identify, due to its symptoms. Secondly, depression is commonly observed because it appears to be more or less expected as a reaction to a handicapping disability such as blindness (Cholden, 1958; Harriman, 1965). Since all people have experienced stages of melancholia or depression in their lives, they are somewhat familiar with the symptoms and can easily find these in others with whom they may be overempathizing. The person who has recently lost his vision is naturally expected to experience depression because of the trauma it has effected in his life.

Depressive reactions to visual disability appear to be of two types: first, the reaction that is characterized by an intense mourning of the loss of vision;

and secondly, the anger that an individual may turn toward himself as a result of his own frustration. While there are other characteristics and symptoms of depression noted, these two types appear to be almost natural and often necessary stages in adjustment. It should be noted that both types of depressive reaction mentioned above may exist separately or together in an individual, but may not always be the direct result of blindness itself. However, the deep sense of mourning a newly blinded person may feel is associated with the concept of the "death" of the sighted person and the "rebirth" of the visually-handicapped individual (Cholden, 1958). The anger an individual may turn toward himself may be due to a variety of reactions to stress, such as guilt, feelings of inadequacy, social incompetence and self-pity, among others.

In rehabilitative psychological counseling, depressive reactions are commonly encountered and can usually be dealt with effectively. However, if the depression is characterized by a deep sense of mourning, it is more difficult to cope with and often appears to be a normal reaction that the client himself must experience and deal with (Cholden, 1958). If this reaction exists over a long period of time, however, the client may need and seek assistance in order to overcome this extremely uncomfortable state. On the other hand, if the client is directing anger toward himself, this active reaction may be channeled through counseling to become a motivated force. If this anger can be directed toward alleviating or reducing the handicapping effects of blindness, then the client may find the determination to overcome his limitations.

During the stage of depression, whatever its characteristics, it often appears that the client is coming face to face with the full emotional implications his visual impairment has placed upon him. The client may, for the first time since losing his sight, become less dependent upon his defense mechanism and deal effectively with the anxieties that he feels. It is not uncommon to note, however, that a person may not be equipped to cope with his depression and once again he will rely on his defenses or seek further medical consultation. Whatever the pattern of adjustment the client experiences, depression does appear to be an integral part of an individual's psychological reaction to stress.

Acceptance

Once an individual can accept the fact that he is visually-handicapped, he can deal with his problems more effectively and realistically. This acceptance must involve the person's recognition of his limitations, as well as his abilities. Hopefully, he will learn how to take advantage of his abilities in order to compensate for his limitations and, if possible, be able to overcome many of his limitations through training. It is important at this point to distinguish between acceptance of blindness and adjustment to blindness. If an individual can honestly admit to himself that he is blind, it does not mean that he has adjusted adequately to the multivarious implications which his disability has placed upon his life. Adjustment to a disability may be described as *the point in time where an individual is capable of functioning within the limits of his potential in his personal, social, and vocational endeavors.* It is important to distinguish between acceptance and adjustment from a rehabilitation standpoint because adjustment involves the total individual and his ability to find happiness in living. This is not to say that blind persons must be happy being blind but rather that they can be happy despite the fact that they are blind. However, acceptance of the fact that a person is visually disabled is necessary before the individual can achieve adequate and ongoing adjustment.

PERSONALITY MANIFESTATIONS
WHICH COMMONLY INTERFERE WITH ADJUSTMENT

Any discussion of adjustment to blindness would be inadequate without first examining some of the personality manifestations that are commonly observed. These emotional factors often constitute the dominant problems that have to be dealt with in psychological counseling. Moreover, these problems which may or may not be a direct reaction to blindness may present a disability greater than the limitations commonly imposed by blindness. Since these problems are commonly encountered by professionals in work for the blind, this section is based on a survey done some years ago in the field (Bauman, 1950). The results of this study indicated seven areas of personality manifestation which are commonly observed. These areas are sensitivity, somatic symptoms, social competency, attitudes of distrust, feelings of inadequacy, depression, and attitudes toward blindness (Bauman, 1958).

Sensitivity

The client that presents problems involving sensitivity often has a tendency to worry frequently or seems generally unstable, to brood a great deal over minor problems, and he is easily hurt. Such persons overreact to others with little or no reason to justify their behavior. In family and social situations they are inconsistent in their behavior and make others uncomfortable by their unpredictable reactions. Newly blinded men or women exhibiting such characteristics often create conflicts that may lead to marital separation. Due to oversensitivity, blind children have poor peer relationships and often become social isolates apart from their dependency upon the family (Cholden, 1958). Sighted individuals seem to suspect this oversensitive nature when they encounter a blind or disabled person and, therefore, try to avoid those subjects that they feel might elicit an uncomfortable response.

This latter situation often creates a very superficial type of relationship which precipitates occasion for the overreaction. Thus, oversensitivity on the part of a blind person has a "snowballing" effect which leads to additional abnormal behaviors. Psychological counseling is effective in dealing with this trait through supportive approaches. The client must understand the causes and consequences of such behavior which will enable him to avoid overpersonalizing his interpretation of people and situations.

Somatic Symptoms

Somatic manifestations indicate problems that are a result of nervous tension. Such manifestations include loss of appetite, sleep reversal, fatigue, headaches, diarrhea, and others (Vital and Health Statistics, 1970) Individuals with these symptoms frequently show high anxiety rates and difficulty dealing effectively with tension and stress. Another aspect of somatic symptoms is a tendency toward hypochondriatic reactions. These tendencies indicate a high degree of insecurity and an overconcern with health. Many times the blind or visually-handicapped individual is extremely aware of the problems that his blindness has placed upon him and fears the advent of accidents or acute illness. Because of these feelings he may seek to avoid all situations which might possibly lead to further physical complications.

Often counseling can assist the client in reducing some of the basic tensions he feels, thus reducing the physical symptoms which bother him. If the person shows an extreme overconcern with his health, many of his basic insecurities may be alleviated through support and encouragement. The client whose fear of becoming hurt or ill has driven him into isolation and inactivity, may create a situation where he encounters physical difficulties due to a change in his eating, sleeping, and needed exercise activities. Also, isolation and inactivity may allow the client to slip into an introspective state in which his tensions and fears will increase. If such tendencies are present, counseling may be extremely necessary to get the client moving again toward a normal and productive existence. Rehabilitation center and teacher training may assist the client in learning those safety techniques in traveling and daily living that will give him the confidence to function within his environment.

Social Competency

Social competency involves those abilities and attitudes which enable a person to meet and talk to others with ease. Persons who lack the self-confidence and social confidence to become involved with others, particularly in group situations, encounter many difficulties in their daily living. Poor social attitudes that are a result of an individual's feelings of inadequacy due to his blindness may prevent him from functioning in many social and vocational situations. Moreover, these persons may become social isolates who are highly critical of society as a result of their own inability to establish and maintain interpersonal relationships. Many of these problems may be successfully dealt with in individual counseling, but social activities and group therapy are often the most appropriate experiences for them. In many cases, these inadequacies are not as much the fault of the development of poor social attitudes as they are a lack of social experiences on which to gain social maturity. If this latter is the case, then experience in actual group situations may be the most productive approach to adjustment (Kurzhals, 1970).

Attitudes of Distrust

Attitudes of distrust are sometimes referred to as paranoid tendencies. These attitudes involve the individual's overevaluation of himself and a suspicious nature that results when this evaluation does not agree with that of others. These individuals often feel persecuted and misunderstood, together with the idea that they have not been fairly dealt with in various situations. Since blindness imposes the restrictions of being able to observe others at all times, these tendencies are sometimes compounded. Also, communication with others often requires eye contact and the ability to see facial expressions in order to determine the way in which something is said. Blindness, as with other disabilities that impose communication restrictions, may be the cause or add to existing paranoid tendencies. While counseling can do little to remove these communication barriers, it can aid the client in understanding his own deficits and give him a realistic evaluation of his abilities. The client should also consider the fact that while some individuals treat him in a suspicious manner, this is not their intention. Rather, some social encounters which might make the blind person suspicious are actually just the result of the sighted individual's discomfort in relating to a blind person (Scott, 1969). Whatever the cause, attitudes of distrust will generally require the establishment of good rapport before a client can be confronted with his own inadequacies. Realistic but supportive counseling is often successful in alleviating this personal and social handicap.

Feelings of Inadequacy

Feelings of inadequacy are commonly found in various disability groups. Such feelings reflect a general lack of self-confidence, the inability to trust in one's own decision-making, and a general lack of ability to deal with one's own problems. Such feelings are often indicated by self-depreciating statements, the unwillingness to attempt new tasks, dependency upon others, and pessimistic attitudes toward the future. Rehabilitation counseling can offer support and encouragement to the disabled individual to get him moving in a positive direction. If the client can be psychologically assisted to gain enough motivation to become active and experience success in simple endeavors, then his ability to depend upon himself may increase. He can be assisted in better understanding his abilities and avoid the tendency to dwell on limitations. Helping the client to deal with his feelings of inadequacy as a disabled individual is crucial to the rehabilitation process and often requires immediate attention before the client will actively move toward acceptance of his disability and eventual adjustment to it.

Recurring Depression

Although depression was previously discussed as a factor in the adjustment process, it is important to note several other aspects of this factor. Depression can be regarded as a condition of morale wherein the person may feel that life is hardly worth living and wherein he becomes pessimistic about the future. Clients in a depressive state can show either guarded optimism about the future or a total lack of faith altogether. Often it is important to aid the client in dealing with his "now" problems and in avoiding, as much as possible, trying to project so much of his life into the future. If a client can be assisted to see that many of the problems he anticipates in the future can be avoided through positive action today, he may be able to avoid further encounters with depression. Activity is a good antidote for depression if this activity helps the client to feel that he is positively doing something about his problems.

Attitudes Regarding Blindness

It is important to ascertain, if possible, which of the problems a client is experiencing are due to his basic personality style and which are the direct result of his blindness. Problems related to blindness include a client's feelings about the dependency he feels, his inability to relate to others, the bumps he encounters in moving through his environment, and the attitudes he and his family may have about his disability. Such attitudes are typically negative and show the extent of the client's lack of adjustment. For example, the poorly adjusted individual will have many negative attitudes about his condition. However, as acceptance of his visual handicap occurs and progress toward adjustment is noted, these attitudes diminish. Rehabilitation counseling and training can do much in giving the client the proper perspective in terms of differentiating between the true limitations his disability imposes and those that are a psychological result of his anxieties. Counseling should emphasize the reality of the client's attitudes, with guidance and support being given to *do something* about these emotionally frustrating conditions.

CLIENT-FAMILY ADJUSTMENT

A problem that is too often noted in the rehabilitation of the blind, sometimes at the very time when the client is advancing toward adjustment to his disability, is a continued lack of adjustment on the part of the client's family. In the case of the congenitally blind child, the family's lack of adjustment may be traced to the birth of the child or even to circumstances during the period of pregnancy. In the case of the adventitiously blind, the family's lack of adjustment may occur at the time of sudden blindness as a result of an accident or problems arising from the initial diagnosis of a progressive visual deterioration. Whatever the circumstances, lack of adjustment in the family may be a deterrent to the client's adjustment. It is not uncommon to see a blind person progress beautifully through a program of training at a rehabilitation center and achieve a high degree of adjustment, only to return home to the same stifling, overprotective atmosphere he left several months earlier.

Often, a return to this environment may eradicate whatever the client has achieved through rehabilitation services.

To better understand some of the problems in client-family adjustment, it is necessary to examine some of the critical stages in this process. The following discussion deals with problems commonly encountered by the family and client in their reaction and adjustment to blindness. While this discussion begins with problems concerning the congenitally blind (Warnick, 1969), it also deals with problems commonly found in adventitious blindness.

The Family's First Realization
That the Child Is Handicapped

While there are always some doubts in the minds of parents concerning having children that might possibly have physical defects, certain conditions magnify these doubts. The possibility of known hereditary factors may cause expectant parents a great deal of anxiety about the forthcoming birth of their child. Also, certain diseases, such as rubella during the first trimester of pregnancy, can also cause extreme doubt in the minds of the parents about the general health of their child. Even at the time of birth when some physical conditions are difficult to diagnose, a mother may observe certain behaviors in her new child that add to her suspicions that the child's vision is defective. In cases of premature births, which require incubation, the possibility of retrolental fibroplasia is present. While this condition may result in an early total blindness, it can also cause initial partial loss of vision which may become more advanced in time. In this latter case, the full extent of the visual loss may not be immediately detected, but observations of the child's early behavior may suggest to the mother that something is wrong. Thus, in the situations mentioned above and in many others, the family's early realization may be the beginning of feelings of guilt and anxiety.

Adolescent and adult conditions also create this initial period of suspicion. A husband may notice that his wife has become increasingly clumsy in her daily activities. While the wife may deny the presence of any visual difficulties, the husband may begin to suspect that something is wrong. He may encourage the wife to look into these problems; or, as happens, many times, the anxiety of his suspicions will also cause him to deny and overlook these problems. However, both the husband and the wife continue to be doubtful even though they may delay seeking medical consultation. As in the case of the congenitally blind, these suspicions cause stress and begin a series of psychological reactions that are commonly seen in rehabilitation.

Impact of the Final Diagnosis

The next stage in family-client adjustment comes when a final diagnosis is made that indicates the presence of a visual disability or a condition that will eventually lead to severe visual impairment. Whether this diagnosis is made on a newly born child or an adult, the final confirmation of previous suspicions adds new anxieties. In almost all instances, this diagnosis is made by an ophthalmologist or other consulting physician, and the manner in which they present their findings to the family and client is critical (Cholden, 1958). While the family and client need to be realistically confronted with the diagnosis, it is also imperative for the doctor to appreciate the trauma of the situation. Understandably, a blunt and pessimistic explanation of the disorder can often heighten anxiety to almost unbearable limits. On the other hand, the doctor who presents false hopes or minimizes the reality of the condition only delays the critical factor of acceptance in the client and his family.

The point of final diagnosis may require the use of other consultants, such as trained professionals in the field of work for the blind and visually handicapped, in order to avoid trauma that may be disabling as the visual condition itself. The use of rehabilitation services at this point may be extremely critical with the congenitally blind, to help the parents not only deal with the anxieties they feel but to maturely accept and insure that the child still have an appropriate developmental childhood.

Separation from the Family

A very critical stress point for the child and family is the eventual need for entrance into school. Anxiety can easily result by the threat of this first separation from the family. Whether the child is entering kindergarten, public school, or a school for the blind, this may be the first time the child has been taken out of the home and away from the care of his parents. While it is not difficult for most families to admit that education is necessary, they may have a great deal of difficulty dealing with this initial threat of separation. The child is frightened by the new environment he encounters in the school, and the parents fear all types of imaginable situations where the child could be hurt. This cleavage in the dependency of the child upon his family creates anxieties that often require the consultation and guidance of experienced practitioners in the field of work for the blind.

In progressive stages with the adventitiously blind, there is also an initial threat of separation from the family constellation. The newly blinded husband may have to leave his family in order to receive rehabilitation training that will enable him to function in his future endeavors. The acquisition of special and adapted skills used by the blind often takes considerable time, and the client may be away from his wife and family for a period of months. Even though it is clearly necessary that the client be involved in this initial separation, the anxiety for him and his family is still very much present. Many clients refuse this training simply to avoid this separation, and many families discourage the client's separation to the point that he is forced to remain helpless and dependent. Careful rehabilitation counseling is extremely necessary on this point and can be one of the most critical factors in the rehabilitation of the client. Likewise, the child who is denied an education because of his and his family's anxieties concerning separation is often severely handicapped by the lack of proper developmental opportunities.

Rejection of the Blind Member by Peers

Rejection by peers is a problem that is commonly encountered but more often anticipated by blind persons and their families. Many poorly adjusted blind persons, particularly those who have been overprotected or who are bitter, lack the ability to establish good interpersonal relationships. This situation is often seen when the child enters school and has a tendency to isolate himself from his classmates. On the other hand, his behavior may be so inappropriate that his peers are uncomfortable around him, and either tease or avoid him. The newly blinded adult may feel that his blindness is a barrier between him and his friends and may therefore have extreme difficulty relating to them. He may also be so overly sensitive about his condition that he makes others feel uncomfortable around him and slowly he finds himself separated from social contacts, and in some instances, from his family. While these are situations that often do actually occur, the fear of rejection may even be a greater problem. The family of the blind child may exhibit extreme anxiety when the prospect of their child participating in social activities is mentioned. The blind person himself may anticipate such extreme difficulties in social situations that he simply chooses to avoid them. Whatever the situation, actual rejection and fear of rejection are problems that almost always have to be dealt with when the client and/or his family lack adjustment. Here again, rehabilitation counseling can offer the support, encouragement and guidance to alleviate these extremely uncomfortable situations and attitudes.

Sibling Relationships

In examining client-family adjustment, it is important to consider the attitudes of other siblings toward their blind counterpart. Brothers and sisters of a blind child can do much to influence his relationships with other children. If he is accepted as a playmate by his brothers and sisters, he will most probably learn to relate naturally to other children. However, if the siblings overprotect or neglect him, he may become isolated and withdrawn in his own playtime activities. It is not uncommon to note within a family constellation that the parents of a blind child have made an adequate adjustment and created an environment conducive to good developmental experiences, but the siblings prevent the child from learning appropriate peer group relations. Rehabilitation teachers and counselors may often have to bring this situation to the attention of the parents and offer the siblings guidance in dealing with their blind counterpart.

Even with the older adult who loses his vision, the influence of his brothers and sisters upon his adjustment is critical. They may feel the responsibility of being "their brother's keeper" and deny him the opportunity to function as an independent and productive individual. In many instances, where blindness was caused through hereditary factors, the older siblings may fear that they too will become blind, which may greatly influence their attitudes toward the blind family member. This fear may cause them to reject their blind brother, and subsequent guilt that they feel because of this rejection may totally destroy any relationship between the family members. Thus, sibling relationships are a critical factor to take into consideration in the rehabilitation process of the blind.

Fear of Acute Illness

A factor that is often noted as a basis or symptom of anxiety in blindness is the fear of acute illness. Both the client and his family often feel that blindness itself is so great a handicap that the addition of any other illness would be insurmountable. These fears often cause the family to be extremely overprotective of the child to prevent his being hurt by an accident or acquiring some disease that would add further handicapping conditions. Because of the family's fears, the child often grows up afraid of his environment and showing marked symptoms of being a hypochondriac. This condition is also commonly seen in adults who are losing their vision or who have just become totally blind. These fears may be so intense that the client refuses to leave his home and chooses rather to remain under the protective custody of his family. Both psychological and medical consultation may be needed to deal with these kinds of reactions within the client and his family.

Intensified Family Crisis

As in any family situation, there are problems which arise simply as a result of living. However, when a family unit contains a visually handicapped person, the effects of these problems may be greatly compounded. Parents of a blind child may encounter extreme anxiety upon learning that the wife is pregnant. The fear of having another visually-handicapped child may cause intense stress within the family that adds to many of the anxieties the first blind child already feels. Another crisis that often presents problems is the necessity for the family to move to another neighborhood or town. The poorly adjusted family and child may be overly aware of the difficulties they will encounter and more difficulties they anticipate in settling into a new neighborhood. The move may also separate the child from playmates in his neighhood with whom he has been able to establish relations. A move may also take the child out of a school situation that he is comfortable with and place him in a wholly new environment, possibly around children who have never had any experience with a blind person. Families may fear the social pity that sometimes accompanies the recognition that they are the parents of a severely disabled child.

Blinded adults, particularly men, often find themselves left out of family crises. An example of this would be a newly blinded woman whose husband and children leave her out of discussions dealing with family problems. While the family is attempting to keep the wife from worrying about problems, they create a situation where her basic feelings of helplessness and dependency are compounded due to the lack of trust family members have in her. This situation is terribly unfair to the client and complicates her relationship with those she loves. If any of the above-mentioned problems exist within a family unit, it is important for the vocational rehabilitation counselor to help the client and family once again become a close-knit working unit. In some instances, outside family and marriage counseling may be used to alleviate these problems. Where families are forced to move or relocate, they should be made aware of the various rehabilitation services that exist in every state to serve the blind and their families.

Sexual Problems of the Adolescent Blind

A critical stage in any child's development is the counsel and education he receives at the time of puberty. At this time in an adolescent's life, he becomes more aware of his own physical existence and experiences changes within his body that he does not understand. With the blind, this physical awareness may be extremely limited due to the child's inability to compare his own physical being with that of others through the use of vision. Since physical contact is generally socially discouraged except in situations such as athletics, dancing and others, the child may have an inaccurate picture of his own physique and how it differs from that of the opposite sex. Without adequate and appropriate education concerning these differences, the child may grow up without ever understanding this essential part of his own characteristics. Families of blind children often find it extremely difficult to deal with the questions their visually-handicapped children ask about the changes they are experiencing. Also, with these changes come natural sexual urges that seek gratification. The poorly adjusted child and family may encounter embarrassing and anxiety-producing situations during the time of puberty if the child shows inappropriate and socially unacceptable methods of gratifying these urges (Cutsforth, 1951). It is recognized today that sex education can be a major deterrent to such inappropriate behavior with all children, and this certainly applies to the visually-handicapped adolescent.

Sexual difficulties may also arise in the adjustment process of the newly blinded adult. Many times married men and women who have recently lost their sight feel a need to prove to themselves that they are still attractive to the opposite sex. These behaviors do not appear to be as promiscuous as they might seem but rather are often the result of a need to establish or reaffirm self-image and confidence. While this need to reassert self-image often results in overt behavior, it can also affect an adult's sexual activities with his spouse. Due to poor self-concept, many newly blinded men become impotent and generally lose whatever masculine identity they possessed before being handicapped. Psychological or psychiatric counseling is often necessary to alleviate this self-depreciating situation. However, in some instances, the problem is corrected simply as the man accepts and adjusts to his handicap and once again becomes a contributing member to the welfare of the family.

The family of a blind individual can do much to help both the child and adult deal with his sexual needs. If the family is sincerely interested in the welfare of the client and willing to deal with these needs in a mature manner, many of the above-mentioned problems can be avoided.

VOCATIONAL AND MARITAL PROBLEMS OF THE ADULT BLIND

The adult blind individual encounters major adjustments in assuming responsibility for a career and for marriage. Each of these factors will be reviewed.

Vocational Adjustment

At some point in the blind person's life, whether he is congenitally or adventitiously blind, he and his family have to deal with the anxieties that vocational placement may impose. In almost all instances, the thought of employment presents another threat of separation from the family unit. The child who has been protected within the home and the semi-sheltered situation of school faces the possibility and responsibility of work. Usually this means he will be away from the home during the day, away from the family's overseeing guidance and support. This is a threat to the family as well as to the client, and this period of vocational adjustment may be one of the most critical in the visually-handicapped person's life. Psychological and vocational counseling can be of great benefit in reducing the fears of the family and client concerning future vocational endeavors. If these fears are not dealt with, however, the client may remain dependent upon his family and they upon him for the emotional gratification of their own needs.

Decision on Placement

Following the family's and client's acceptance of the idea of vocational placement, they are faced with what type of employment the client should go into. Parents of congenitally blind persons often have extremely high expectations for their child that are above his potential to achieve. Their attitudes are often extended to the client, who, likewise, has an unrealistic concept of his abilities and chooses a vocation that is impracticable or impossible for him to succeed in. On the other hand, some families feel that their child will be fortunate if he can find any employment at all as a visually-handicapped person and reinforce his own feelings of inadequacy about his abilities. Many clients and their families have no concept of what a visually-handicapped person is able to do vocationally and, thus, think in terms of the stereotyped vocations that have long been associated with blindness, such as broom and mop making, chair caning, and sheltered workshop activities.

The architect who loses his sight at age forty also has a difficult vocational decision to make. He suddenly finds himself having to choose a new vocation that will require more training and education, possibly, and one that may greatly reduce the income he has become accustomed to. Many families have difficulty accepting these restrictions and place pressures upon the client to achieve a vocational goal that is beyond his interests and abilities.

Professional vocational guidance and exploration are offered by all state agencies working with the blind, and these services can greatly aid the client in dealing with these difficult decisions. The goal of vocational placement is to help each individual client find remunerative employment within the level of his potential and desire. Vocational counseling is also available for families to help them assist rather than hinder the client in achieving these goals.

Separation Following Placement

After a client has decided upon a vocational goal and has received the training he will need to enter employment, he and his family encounter another threat of separation. From the time the client enters employment, a large part of his life will be devoted to his work. Many families have difficulty accepting this decrease in dependency for them and place a burden upon the client that is often difficult for him to deal with. The less aggressive client who remains dependent upon the poorly adjusted family often finds himself in a situation where they interfere with his productivity by regularly contacting his employer to make sure he is being treated right. The family may also visit the client on the job or telephone him frequently to make sure that all is going well. In such cases, the family can create a situation of difficulty for the client that may result in his dismissal. Hopefully, however, by the time the client has reached the point where he is ready for vocational placement, he should be able to assert himself to his family and control his own vocational activities. The placement and follow-up services of the rehabilitation counselor can often correct unfavorable situations before they become a problem. Further, it is important for the rehabilitation counselor to realize that placement is not the ultimate goal of rehabilitation in itself but, rather, just an integral part of an overall complex process.

Marriage

When vocational adjustment has adequately progressed, there comes the natural desire of the person to find a spouse. Marriage to the family, however, may present the threat of almost total separation, a situation they are unable to accept. In many instances, the blind individual, due to his discomfort around sighted members of the opposite sex, will choose a spouse that is also handicapped. This situation is often disgusting to the family and compounds the basic anxieties that they feel about the limitations blindness imposes. Certainly, it is difficult for two totally blind persons to lead a "normal" life, and often the family's interference in this type of marital situation makes its success impossible. On the other hand, the poorly adjusted family that has made its blind child dependent upon them fears releasing him to the care of someone who may not appreciate the myriad problems the family feels about the situation. This problem is not as common with the adventitiously blind, but it does exist and may be a further deterrent to the fulfillment of an individual's happiness and hopes.

Marital problems often arise between a man and his wife when one of them loses his vision. While it often appears that the sighted spouse wants to leave the blinded person simply because the latter is now disabled, it is frequently noted that this is not the case. What often occurs in essence is the rejection of the sighted spouse by the blind person due to the many feelings of inadequacy and dependency the disabled partner feels about being blind. This rejection is usually not direct in nature but rather the severe and bitter reaction of the blind person toward his own blindness that results in an unbearable situation for his sighted partner. However, it is also not uncommon for the sighted partner to be so threatened by the responsibility of staying with his handicapped spouse that he is unable to deal with this situation and initiates divorce proceedings. Such marital problems need attention and, more often than not, present complicating factors to the rehabilitation counselor in his attempts to help his client, which may take a great deal of time and effort to deal with.

SUMMARY

In this chapter a discussion has been offered to help identify and correct some of the more common problems that are experienced in work for the blind. The section covering common patterns to the adjustment of visual loss dealt with those factors that are generally seen in both the congenitally and adventitiously blind. Some of the more common problems that are indicated by rehabilitation counselors were discussed in the second major section, but it should be understood that "the blind" are human beings and as such react to various situations depending upon their basic psychological makeup. Rehabilitation is not just a process of working strictly with the handicapped person, but may necessitate services that involve families, communities, employers, public attitudes, etc. Understanding the psychological implications of blindness requires an understanding and appreciation of the many factors that affect and influence all of our lives. Blindness has long been recognized as a major disability, but today with the expansion of knowledge about the field and the improvement of services, its prognosis is encouraging.

REFERENCES

Bauman, M. K.: A comparative study of personality factors in blind, other handicapped, and non-handicapped individuals. Article presented to the annual meeting of the American Psychological Association, 1950.

Bauman, M. K.: *A Manual of Norms for Tests Used in Counseling Blind Persons.* New York, American Foundation for the Blind, 1958.

Cholden, L. S.: *A Psychiatrist Works with Blindness.* New York, American Foundation for the Blind, 1958.

Cutsforth, T. D.: *The Blind in School and Society.* New York, American Foundation for the Blind, 1951.

Harriman, P. L.: *Handbook of Psychological Terms.* Totowa, New Jersey, Littlefield, Adams and Co., 1965.

Kurzhals, I. W.: Personality adjustment for the blind child in the classroom. *The New Outlook for the Blind,* 64(5):5, 1970.

Raskin, N. J.: Auditory disability. In Garrett, J. F. and Levine, Edna S. (Eds.), *The Psychological Practices of the Physically Disabled.* New York, Columbia University Press, p. 361, 1962.

Raskin, N. J. and Weller, M.: *Current Research in Work for the Blind.* New York, American Foundation for the Blind, 1953.

Scott, R. A.: *The Making of Blind Men.* New York, Russell Sage Foundation, 1969.

U.S. Department of Health, Education, and Welfare: *Vital and Health Statistics: Selected symptoms of psychological stress.* Rockville, Maryland, 1970.

Warnick, L.: The effect upon a family of a child with a handicap. *The New Outlook for the Blind,* 63(10):299-304, 1969.

(PART SIX)

THE SEVERELY DISABLED

THE SEVERELY DISABLED—
A REHABILITATION CHALLENGE

THE PSYCHOLOGY OF PAIN

MOTIVATION: THE GREATEST CHALLENGE
TO REHABILITATION

Chapter 17

THE SEVERELY DISABLED—
A REHABILITATION CHALLENGE

John A. Fenoglio

I N REALITY, the inabilities of patients to achieve appropriate goals do not represent failure on the part of the client as much as they reflect failure on the part of rehabilitation personnel because the latter have not developed techniques and programs which tap client resources. Client failure, then, cannot be justified on the basis of the rationalization that such severely disabled individuals cannot work (Walker, 1961).

BACKGROUND AND HISTORY
OF VOCATIONAL REHABILITATION SERVICES
TO THE SEVERELY DISABLED

Familiarity with the present rehabilitation program and the disabilities the program serves would cause one to assume that the severely disabled have been adequately served since the inception of the rehabilitation movement. This assumption, however, can be shown to be faulty if one reads authorities in the field. McGowan (1960) stated, "From its beginning in 1920 and continuing for twenty-three years, the scope of the Federal-State rehabilitation program was limited". Massie (1960) also reported, "Services were confined to special assistance in job training, counseling and guidance for the disabled, provision of artificial limbs and other prosthetic appliances, as needed, and placement in a suitable job". Rusk (1971) pointed out that "prior to 1943, a substantial sum of money could be spent on vocational training; however, such training had to be 'training around the disability', for no funds could be spent on eliminating, alleviating, or reducing the disability on the physical capacities of the client."

In addition to program limitations, the types of disabilities represented were significantly different. For example, the history of the paraplegic patients in rehabilitation actually began with World War II. Garrett (RSS No. 210) asserted: "Prior to that war little was heard of these patients, most of whom died, usually within a year, of infection of the bladder". Massie (1960) explained further:

The Barden-LaFollette Act of 1943 broadened the concept of rehabilitation to include the provision of physical restoration services. Initially, the vast majority of physical restoration dollars were expended for the services of physicians and hospitals. This was due, in large measure, to the limited number of rehabilitation facilities. Hill-Burton funds were not available for construction of centers; most states did not have a single comprehensive rehabilitation center; workshops were utilized primarily for continuing employment and few were staffed to provide a variety of rehabilitation services (p. 10).

The Department of Physical Medicine and Rehabilitation was created in New York's Bellevue Hospital in 1946, and was the "first rehabilitation medicine service, with its own personnel and beds, of any civilian hospital in the United States, and probably in the world" (Rusk, 1971).

Such services in hospitals, however, developed slowly in the decade following the creation of the first such programs at Bellevue Hospital. There was a more rapid growth during the period of independent "rehabilitation centers." In many instances these centers were started by local affiliates of the National Easter Seal Society and United Cerebral Palsy, and was limited to the care of orthopedically handicapped children (p. 1).

The 1943 amendments changed "the basic concept of the program" from a scholarship approach to a "need of the client" basis (McGowan 1960). With new additions, such as medical and psychiatric examinations, medical and surgical treatment, hospitalization, training supplies, maintenance, travel, tools, equipment and licenses, the needs of the client were more easily met.

President Dwight D. Eisenhower signed Public Law 565 on August 3, 1954 and stated, "It reemphasizes to all the world the great value which we in America place upon the dignity and worth of each individual human being" (McGowan, 1960). This law was extremely important to the severely disabled in that it encouraged expansion of rehabilitation faculties, workshops and authorization of financing for research studies and demonstration projects to provide new methods and techniques to improve the quality of rehabilitation services. This legislation authorized federal participation in expanding, remodeling or altering existing buildings in order to make them suitable as workshops or rehabilitation facilities for the severely disabled. In addition, special emphasis was given to training personnel through teaching grants, internships and institutes for short-term training courses.

A very important ancillary bill that gave critical support to the rehabilitation effort was the 1954 Medical Facilities Survey and Construction Act which authorized Federal participation in the building of new rehabilitation facilities, chronic disease hospitals, nursing homes and diagnostic and treatment centers. The Randolph-Sheppard Act was broadened to use grant funds for the improvement and expansion of rehabilitation facilities and reduced the financial crisis faced by these support programs. Additionally, the Hill-Burton Act was amended to authorize special appropriations to build medical rehabilitation facilities. These important pieces of legislation established the foundation for massive expansion in the next decade.

The 1965 amendments were the next major change to effect the rehabilitation of the severely disabled. The matching ratio of funding the state-federal program was changed to a 75 percent Federal and 25 percent State basis. This funding allowed new financial resources and provided more services to more people. These amendments established extended evaluation services and allowed vocational rehabilitation involvement in severely disabled cases on a greater scale. This provision coupled with the modern philosophy that rehabilitation services are a "right" rather than a privilege, made it difficult for rehabilitation representatives to deny services by stating "client not feasible."

The extended evaluation amendment allowed up to 18 months for determination of rehabilitation potential of the severely disabled applicant. Services available during this 18-month period included those provided under the regular program. This aided in the utilization of existing facilities and stimulated expansion of others.

Research and demonstration centers and "centers of excellence" assumed leadership roles in technique application of research-based information that materially contributed to the rehabilitation process.

Developmental Ideology

A major question which thus far has eluded an answer is that of a universally accepted definition of disability. For our purposes, the matter of defining who is and who is not disabled is of no concern. Our concern is how does one distinguish who is severely disabled? In the clinical area, precise tables prescribe degree of disability. An example of this rating process is that a mid-thigh amputation or higher produces a 100 percent impairment of the leg and a 40 percent disability of the patient. This logical and physiological process seems to be intelligently and carefully worked out. The logic slips, however, when we look beyond physiology. One amputee rated on the above scale is a professional quarterback, the other an accountant. Each has lost 100 percent of the limb according to the scale but have they both lost 40 percent of their total function? Are these individuals equally disabled or is one more "severely" disabled than the other?

The Congress of Neurologic Surgeons has summarized this dilemma: "The very concept of disability has created a virtual impasse between medicine and the law, which has resulted in hard feelings and unpleasantness on both sides; neither medicine nor law has clearly defined disability and its various aspects" (Burk, 1967, p. 11).

Theories of disability evaluation seem to be divided into three schools: (1) the whole-man theory, (2) loss-of-earning-capacity theory and (3) actual wage loss theory. "The gist of the whole-man theory is that the primary criteria for assessing the loss resulting from injury in work ought to be of a physiological and psychiatric character, and that other, especially economic, factors should play a subordinate role" (Burk, 1967, p. 12). The loss-of-earning-capacity and the actual wage loss theories contend compensable loss as a matter of economic dimension.

Obviously from no more than the above outline of the debate concerning the components of disability, one can perceive that disability definition is purely a matter of perception. Add to this already confused situation the question "Who is responsible for working with disabled people?" and the complexities of the problem enlarge geometrically.

Because disability was seen to be a complex relationship of problems, the concept of the "team approach" began. This concept is closely tied with the beginning of the physical medicine-rehabilitation center that started in the middle forties. Medicine alone could do little more than cure the "illness" and where permanent disability existed there was no "cure". The limits of the physician's capabilities are poignantly stated by Leo Price who noted, "Few doctors have full competence in judging the many different aspects of occupational disability as distinguished from clear-cut biologic disability" (Burk, 1967, p. 11).

The amendments of the forties and fifties resulted in a broadened concept of disability. In order to relate to this broadened concept, the "team" approach to rehabilitation was initiated. One might conclude that this new appreciation of the problems of the disabled demonstrated by team development meant solutions were closer at hand. This conclusion, however, must be tempered with the understanding that "teams" also differ with the conceptualization of disability.

> . . . a common or universal concept of "team" has not prevailed, so that in some instances we find it meaning the skills of many different disciplines, but in others it has taken on a narrower meaning of different skills within the same discipline. If a limited concept of disability as that of a disease and/or impaired physiology is retained, then the concept of "team approach" remains narrow, and we find the team made up of neurologists, urologists, orthopedists, internists, physical therapists, and laboratory technicians. On the other hand, if the broadened concept of disability is accepted, the team is correspondingly broadened to include, in addition to the required medical personnel, psychologist, social worker, vocational counselor, evaluator trainer, minister, employer and the client himself (Burk, 1967, p. 13).

The foregoing discussion has essentially been a look at what a rehabilitation counselor would refer to as development of program and support or resource personnel. Looking introspectively into the rehabilitation program itself, let us view the historical development of the program's relationship with the severely disabled in Texas.

The programs have expanded in Texas, the staff of the rehabilitation commission has grown, supportive resources have developed, counselor training programs have provided specialized training to young potential counselors, and greater numbers of people have received services. In addition to these measures, the research and demonstration projects across the country provided simultaneously, enlightening new insights, techniques and theories to the rehabilitation process. Additional resources became available and with those resources also came increased production expectation. Therefore, more rehabilitation counselors were expected to generate more rehabilitation closures to justify additional monies.

As additional staff increased and more costly services were made available, the increased numbers of cases placed continued pressure on the counselor. Now he must produce more closures and at the same time spread case service funds as far as possible. This dilemma, different from the staggering difficulties faced in the pre-1960 days, is in direct opposition to the needs of the severely disabled client. Counselors under pressure of producing greater numbers of closures on less per capita expenditure find it difficult to spend the time, or the money, on the severely involved cases. This consequence in Texas, led to the development of the program for the catastrophically disabled initiated in March, 1972.

Program Philosophy

For years the overt expression of rehabilitation administration and, in fact, counselors was that the primary aim of rehabilitation was to serve the "severely handicapped." Because of the pressures mentioned above, actions of counselors restricted services to this group. Clients "too severely disabled" were closed as non-feasible, were accepted and provided perfunctory services of a fragmented nature and then closed, or simply were buried under the mass of easier cases on which closure could be more easily foreseen.

At the present stage of the program for the severely disabled, it is not meant to convey that all barriers to the service delivery system have been removed. They have not and will not be removed in the foreseeable future. Critical elements of the problem of restricting services have been removed as will be noted in the next few pages. More importantly, administrative sensitivity to the remaining problems exists, and solutions are being actively sought.

THE PROGRAM FOR CATASTROPHICALLY DISABLED

Counselors report (1) lack of money, and (2) lack of time, as problems most frequently when discussing serving the severely involved case. Reason number one has been removed totally. A special budget was created, aside from the counselor budget, from which any counselor can expend funds without depleting his assigned budget on any case meeting the criteria of the program.

The second reason reported for not working with the severely disabled is a bit more elusive. The amount of counselor time spent with one client is directly correlated to the number of clients dealt with in a given period of time. Therefore, increased time per client equals a decreased number of clients. A decreased number of clients equals a decreased number of closures.

The production expectation of counselors with appreciable numbers of clients qualifying for the catastrophically disabled program has been changed. They are not expected to produce at the rate of those counselors having relatively few cases of this type. This lowered expectation level, however, is something that will require administrative acceptance before the counselor feels comfortable. This type of demonstration takes valuable time.

Criteria for Eligibility

The client must meet basic eligibility requirements of the Commission. Particular care should be taken that clients who do not manifest a reasonable expectation that services will result in gainful employment are not accepted. Gainful employment includes such categories as homemakers and unpaid family workers.

The client's impairment, as determined medically, must fall within one of the following disability groups: (1) Orthopedic deformity or functional impairment, except amputations, where there is absence of a vocationally purposeful function in at least two extremities. For example, an individual with a diagnosis of cerebral palsy affecting both lower extremities would not be eligible for use of these funds if the loss of function in the limbs is minimal and the individual is able to ambulate without significant difficulty. If, however, a similar diagnosis is given but the loss of function in the lower extremities is of much severity as to markedly restrict ambulation, he would be eligible for expenditure of these funds. (2) Absence of amputation of major members, where there is absence of vocationally purposeful function in at least two extremities. (3) Cardiac condition requiring surgical intervention or conditions with a heart classification of III D through IV E.

Historically, the "severely disabled" have been thought of as various disability groups such as cerebral palsy, poliomylitis, quadraplegia, paraplegia, hemiplegia. The criteria outlined above carefully avoids basing eligibility on types or groups of disabilities. Connection with a type of disability leaves out people disabled as a result of innumerable causes. At the same time this disability type system would have automatically included individuals with minimal disability simply because a medical report diagnosed the patient as having a disability stereotyped as a serious malady.

Since the intent of this special programming effort was to assist the counselor with the truly difficult cases, the criteria was written with *function* rather than disability type as the major determinant. Therefore, a client with an above the knee amputation of the right leg and a non-functional left arm resulting from a snake bite, could be eligible. On the other hand, a client diagnosed as having cerebral palsy but having purposeful function of all extremities would likely not be eligible for service under this special program fund.

Frequently, with special criteria as outlined above, the counselor must amass information on a client and submit that information to a central point so that a decision can be rendered before use is made of special funding. In this program this process, too, was carefully avoided. The counselor, who after all is most familiar with the situation, is to make the decision and, following that decision, is to forward supporting medical data for review to the consultant for the severely disabled program. This review seemed essential so that a standard could be maintained.

Placement of Specialist

Special counselors who purposefully enter into a special area of rehabilitation frequently show successes thought impossible by other "not so interested" counselors. In addition, being faced with a designated "row-to-hoe" is significantly different from "picking-the-row-to-hoe". Utilizing the successful experiences of other programs, special counselors are being placed in metropolitan areas, high population concentration areas and special facilities, such as rehabilitation centers and major medical complexes, to work exclusively with the "eligible" catastrophically disabled. These counselors are selected as a result of demonstrated special interest, given special intensive training, provided extra consultative time and are not requested to produce successful closures at the same rate as other staff with less involved cases.

Supportive Programming

Adjunct to this central program for the severely disabled effort are two critically important supportive programs. They are the Hospital Referral Program and the Job Development Program. In essence, these two program endeavors represent the input and output stage of the catastrophically disabled program.

Hospital Referral Program

As has been demonstrated in the Welfare, Social Security, mentally retarded programs and other such areas, early referral is vitally important to the severely disabled client. Dr. Spencer of the Texas Institute for Rehabilitation and Research in Houston has demonstrated that hospitalization periods for traumatic paraplegia and quadraplegia is reduced 30 percent or more if treatment in that center is begun no later than 45 days post injury (Spencer, 1971, p. 5). The rehabilitation hospitalization can be cut more significantly if treatment is started within hours after injury.

Prior to 1960, the rehabilitation program in Texas had fewer than 75 counselors throughout the state. These dedicated former teachers, school administrators, ministers, and so on learned about disabilities through the "school of hard knocks," minimal in-service training, personal associations, and other vicarious methods. They covered vast geographic areas, related to large numbers of people spread over these vast areas and, because of circumstances, had little opportunity to do more than provide a "lick and a promise" type of treatment to their clients.

Fiscal resources were frightfully small and support resources were not available to many counselors. The counselors were expected to be Jacks-of-all-trades, knowing and relating to all disabilities with equal capacity. To understand in depth the various complexities of the amputee, the polio victim, the cerebral palsied, the mentally retarded, the mentally ill and on and on, was virtually impossible.

These counselors were productive and displayed amazing results. These successes were, however, the results of their abilities in becoming very capable catalysts. In most instances, the counselor was able to put together a "team" of people in communities who were able, in individual circumstances, to "rehabilitate" the disabled.

Success with the "severely disabled" was extremely limited because of the many restricting factors mentioned earlier. This was true also of the mentally retarded, mentally ill and other categorically unique groups. This was changed in the early sixties with the advent of "special counselors" for the mentally retarded. This "new breed" was employed to work only with this one disability group. Surprisingly enough, large caseloads evolved where previously few retardates were thought to exist. Even more surprisingly, successes were demonstrated in increasing numbers.

Following this successful endeavor, other specialty areas came into being, such as specialists for the mentally ill, deaf, alcoholic, among others. In addition, special consultative positions were initiated on a statewide basis to provide consultation to the special and general counselors on problem cases. These consultants demonstrated effectiveness in program development, staff training, program evaluation and coordination of activities.

With this in mind, cooperative programming has been initiated to integrate the vocational rehabilitation counselor into the "hospital treatment team" in order to begin the rehabilitation of "patients" even before the treatment phase begins in some cases and at least concurrently with the hospital program in all permanently disabled cases. This program provides joint efforts of the social service staff, physical and occupational therapy programs and rehabilitation. Physical trauma is sufficiently disabling without adding the psychological trauma of an uncertain future. Rehabilitation efforts at this early stage will not preclude the trauma that occurs with regard to the future when a patient's legs are removed, but it can provide help and assurance of positive steps toward a meaningful future. This process allows rehabilitation to get closer to a goal. Dr. Edward Thomas, a leading orthopedic surgeon, was asked the following question: "When should rehabilitation begin?" Dr. Thomas' reply was, "As soon as the patient begins to awake from the anesthesia" (*Verbal report*: Dr. E. Thomas, Orthopedic Surgeon).

Job Development Program

The Job Development Program is proving to be one of the most encouraging efforts of the Texas Rehabilitation Commission. In order for the severely disabled to be employed, there must be a job open in which he can function. The function of the Job Development Program is to provide employment opportunities. This program simply is the inclusion of the employer on the "team." Basically, the efforts at this time are being made by a specialist in job analysis and vocational evaluation. The primary objective is to involve business and industry by educating those sectors about the handicapped, providing an analysis of the jobs in their plants that could possibly be filled by severely disabled individuals, designing job sample screening devices of the selected jobs and finally providing, through the counselor, an applicant to the employer who can effectively fulfill the requirements of the job.

The three-phase approach involves not one "multi-disciplined team" but many "teams" that must carefully overlap and interrelate with one another with such harmony that it appears to be one giant mass moving together with one objective in mind—*the client's need.*

PROGRAM EXPECTATIONS IN WORKING WITH THE SEVERELY DISABLED

With special counselors providing special training, open-ended budgets, lowered production expectations, intensified consultation and other assistance, it is anticipated that greater numbers of the severely disabled population in Texas will be able to achieve a meaningful place in our society. These specialists should be more keenly aware of and alert to the needs of the severely disabled population. With this intensified awareness, problems heretofore unasked will be receiving answers.

It is expected that these specialists involve themselves in a multi-disciplined team if one exists. If one does not exist, which is very likely, one will need to be built. It is expected that these specialists become involved with the family of the clients with whom they work. A California study on rehabilitation of the severely disabled notes the severe disability ". . . usually had a profound impact on the family. At times a complete family became disabled requiring the coordination of many social agencies and special services. Many marriages foundered when the wage earner became unable to earn a wage. These failures in marriage had repercussions in all areas, regarding the beginning of the rehabilitation process" (Garris, 1964, p. 2).

"Unfortunately, not enough attention is paid to the family's role in rehabilitation", states Margolin (1971 p. 100). This inattention possibly cheats rehabilitation personnel out of important guideposts. Margolin continues, "Psychosocial aspects of disability, especially as it involves the family, provides us with clues to what is happening to the patient and what can be done to alter the situation in a positive direction" (p. 100).

The stigma associated with the severely disabled is expected to be reduced. Research indicates that stigmatizing attitudes exist on the part of the nondisabled toward the physically disabled. Stigma plays a vital role in the lives of the severely disabled and in fact studies by English (1971), "clearly indicate that nearly all physically disabled persons are stigmatized to some extent and that for some physically disabled persons stigma is their most

salient or basic fact of life. In many instances stigma appears to be a basis
of further limiting medically impaired persons by turning physical disabilities
into vocational, personal and social handicaps" (p. 19). McGowan (1960)
agrees,

> The rehabilitation counselor and members of related professions may feel that
> they are beyond the pressures of the traditional prejudices of society by virtue of
> their close helping relationship with the handicapped; however, those who have
> made a critical analysis of the total dynamics of the rehabilitation process see
> factors which often mitigate against full acceptance and complete objectivity
> (p. 4).

With the special training provided in the severely disabled program, introspective observation will allow better self-appraisal and will result in the
capability to better assist the client and his family in dealing with the stigmas
of society.

Through a more intensive working relationship with this particular group
of clients, it is expected that a better appreciation of the needs of clients will
be acquired. Basically, the needs of the severely disabled are the same as
those of other human beings attempting to cope with the demands of society.
Spangler (undated) asserts, "However, certain needs may take precedence
over others because of the nature of the disability and the adjustments which
must be made to it and the social environment" (p. 44). The extent to which
these need priorities are understood and applied to the counseling process
will have significant impact on the rehabilitation outcome.

Scientific research and technology is expanding at such rapid rates that
exciting potential exists for dramatic rehabilitation application. Recent
interest in private industries making space research applicable to medical and
rehabilitation needs holds promise of assistive measures unheard of yesterday.
Examples of technological application that have had immediate impact on the
severely disabled are the use of the "eye switch, C.E.G. Helmet, subminiature
biotelementry systems, material preventing decubitus ulcers through reduction of high pressure points and the Ljubljana electronic peroneal brace"
(Culclasure and Eckhardt, 1970). The situation at the present time is that
there are answers if someone will pose the questions. The counselor's task in
working with the severely disabled is formulating the questions.

> The essential quality of the successful counselor in dealing with the rehabilitation
> of the severely disabled is the ability to see things not as they are now, but as they
> could be. If the counselor can define the problem and set up specifications for
> the solution, even a handyman or local mechanic can build the desired item
> (Garris, 1964, p. 14).

PROBLEMS YET TO BE SOLVED

The program for the catastrophically disabled defines disability very
narrowly. Eligibility relates to a functional physical limitation. This narrow
concept was imposed not because of the lack of appreciation of the broader
concept of disability but because of financial limitation. It is desired that this

program evolve a philosophical base that is broad enough to encompass the psychological, social, educational and familial components of disability. If this evolution occurs, the program can relate more effectively to the "severely handicapped".

The acquisition of trained personnel continually presents problems to management of rehabilitation programs. This is particularly true in the program for the severely disabled. Working with this group of people requires tenacity, ingenuity and perceptivity. An appreciation of medical psychological and vocational aspects of the disability is essential. In addition, familiarity with research in many fields is essential. The counselor's personality must fit the job. He should be prepared to probe with the client into areas of concern that are intimate and that frequently will not be brought up by the client at his own initiative. The counselor must be demanding, challenging, supportive and assistive. Most of all, he must *care*. That care incorporates love, affection, acceptance, concern, support and minimizes society's stigma.

The basis of much research in the area of rehabilitation lacks purpose. Objective research, based on scientific methodology, is not only needed but is an absolute must. Research needs to answer simple, basic questions such as "Are the kinds of services offered effective?" and "Would major or minor changes in present services affect the outcome?" The research needed is of the variety that cannot be done by academicians as they lack the ability to define the problem; and it cannot be done by the rehabilitation practitioners as they lack the skill to design scientific models although they can define problems. This simply indicates a need for a closer working relationship between practitioner and researcher.

SUMMARY

O'Connor and Leitner (1971) epitomize the urgent future need for effective rehabilitation of the severely disabled,

> Only when the rehabilitation effort is directed toward the enhancement of the individual in his own eyes in terms of seeing himself as an important and worthwhile person in his important life roles, can the end justify the means or will rehabilitation become a goal as well as a process (p. 19).

The fundamental aim of this program is to add a goal to an existing process.

REFERENCES

Burk, Richard D.: The nature of disability. *Journal of Rehabilitation, 33* (6), 1967.

Culclasure, David F. and Eckhardt, Luida: *Medical Benefits From Space Research.* Report to NASA on SWRI Project, No. 13-2538, 1970.

English, R. William: Combatting stigma toward physically disabled persons. *Rehabilitation Research and Practice Review, 12* (4), 1971.

Garrett, James F.: Psychological aspects of physical disability. Rehabilitation Service Series, No. 210, undated.

Garris, A. G.: *The Rehabilitation of a Selected Group of Severely Disabled Persons.* Final Report of California Department on an Extension and Improvement Grant, VRA-HEW, 1964.

Gracanin, Franjo: *Instruction Manual for Usage of the Ljubljana Electronic Peroneal Brace,* SRA Grant 19-P-58395-F-0, no date.

Margolin, Ruben J.: Motivational problems and resolutions in the rehabilitation of paraplegics and quadraplegics, *American Archives of Rehabilitation Therapy, 20* (4), 1971.

Massie, William A.: *The Role of the State Vocational Rehabilitation Agency in the Development and Utilization of Rehabilitaton Facilities.* Report to Office of Vocational Rehabilitation, HEW, 1960.

McGowan, John F.: An introduction to the vocational rehabilitation process, GTP Bulletin (3). Rehabilitation Service Series, No. 555, 1960.

O'Connor, J. R. and Leitner, L. A.: Traumatic quadraplegia: A comprehensive review. *Journal of Rehabilitation, 37* (3), 1971.

Rusk, Howard A.: *Rehabilitation Medicine* (3rd ed.). St. Louis: C. V. Mosby Co., 1971.

Spangler, Donald P.: *Service Needs of Paraplegics and Quadraplegics.* Report on Research and Demonstration Grant, RD-882, VRA-HEW, undated.

Spencer, William A.: *The Promethean, 9,* (3), 1971.

Walker, R.: Vocational rehabilitation of the quadraplegic. *Archives of Physical Medicine and Rehabilitation,* 1961.

Chapter 18

THE PSYCHOLOGY OF PAIN

Roy C. Grzesiak

INTRODUCTION

Pain is an area that is rarely presented in a purely psychological context. Yet, for the rehabilitation counselor, working with patients or clients with pain is a frequent event. A knowledge of the psychological aspects of pain can prove to be a valuable asset for the counselor. In the ensuing discussion, pain will refer primarily to chronic or intractable pain, for it is the individual suffering from this type of pain with whom the counselor is more likely to come into contact. While acute pain is usually indicative of bodily distress, long-term chronic pain is often symptomatic of a psychoneurotic process. In the latter instance, pain has come to have private meanings for the patient. It is with the psychological mechanisms involved in chronic pain and the variety of meanings pain can acquire, that this chapter will deal.

Chronic Pain and Rehabilitation

It has long been known that physical illness and disability produce emotional changes; these emotional changes can have a marked effect on rehabilitation outcome (Rusk, 1958). Rusk points out that emotional concomitants to physical illness and disability play a role in the rehabilitative prognosis in about 50 percent of all adults and an even greater percentage in child patients (approximately 75 percent).

The rehabilitation patient is unique; he cannot be considered in the same light as other medical and surgical patients. In the first place, whereas diagnosis is often the first step toward a cure for the medical or surgical patient, diagnosis for the rehabilitation patient with a chronic or crippling illness is an admission that complete cure is unattainable (Krupp, 1968). Lindner (1969) points out that the rehabilitation patient is usually a long-term patient. Lindner (1969) also points out that the philosophy of rehabilitation—the notion that the *whole* person is to be rehabilitated—requires that a unique, holistic approach be taken.

The emotional concomitants of chronic physical illness usually set in during the early chronic phase. It is at this point that all major medical inter-

311

ventions have been attempted and the patient must now face the fact that he is at least partially disabled. Krupp (1968) lists some of the common emotional reactions to disabling illness. Depression is a common reaction; and, up to a point, it is adaptive. Denial is also an important adaptive defense; it is important for ego integrity and the overall stability of the personality. Other reactions include conversion symptoms, regression, dependency, hostility, acting out, drug dependence, and narcotic addiction. The latter two can occur when the patient, playing Szasz's (1968) "painful person" game, seduces the physician into the pain game with subsequent iatrogenic addiction.

Pain is a frequent accompaniment of physical disability, and it is not always consistent with the disease process. At this point, *chronic pain* will be defined as *pain that is disproportionate to the physical illness,* or pain that is not related to the underlying somatic pathology, or pain that does not respond to the appropriate medical treatment. Pain can be a mixture of all three definitions. Rusk (1958) notes, and Szasz (1957) elaborates on the fact that pain, conceived as above, has led to the common dichotomization of pain into organic and psychogenic categories. Rusk (1958) points out that while this may be a convenient clinical classification, it often leads to errors in patient management.

Rusk (1953) refers to rehabilitation and convalescence as the third phase of medical care. Rusk (1958) feels that pain may affect rehabilitation in a variety of ways: (1) Pain may prevent the very physical activities that are necessary for rehabilitative progress; (2) pain may lead to sleeplessness and fatigue which slow the process of rehabilitation; (3) pain may necessitate surgical or pharmacological intervention which can either impede or stop altogether the rehabilitation efforts; (4) pain may lead to interpersonal difficulties because of the patient's insistent demands on staff time or because of resentment from fellow patients; (5) pain may lead to bodily preoccupation with subsequent withdrawal from activities; and (6) pain may become a useful tool for secondary gain and staff manipulation. Also, chronic pain has a detrimental effect on motivation, a necessary prerequisite for successful rehabilitation. Cooper, *et al.,* (1950) isolates some psychic factors that serve to perpetuate pain which was originally organically induced. They are the need to hide drug addiction or dependence, compensation neurosis (compensation is used here in the monetary sense), traumatic neurosis, and the exacerbation of pre-existing psychoneurotic tendencies. In the final analysis, Rusk (1958) believes all pain is a psychic phenomenon because of its reliance upon the functioning of the higher nervous centers and its personal or subjective nature. Rusk (1958, p. 238) points out,

> Pain produces emotional changes even in well-adjusted individuals. It increases dependency needs, self-centeredness, and secondary gain. The personality of the patient and his reaction to the disability and to pain will influence his subjective sensation and behavior. Environmental factors also play a role. Pain tends to

appear worse at night because of anxiety, aloneness, and absence of external interests. The patient is more aware of himself at such times. Similarly, pain may be forgotten during recreational activities yet complained of while the patient is in the presence of his physicians.

Therefore, it is obvious that pain is an important consideration in the rehabilitation process. Further, experience has shown that pain cannot be conceptualized as an isolated aspect of the patient; the whole patient, and the meaning of pain for him, must be considered.

The Need for a Psychological Approach to Pain

Pain is no longer regarded as purely a psychophysical phenomenon. Soulairac (1968) points out the functional inadequacy of pain: it is not a useful warning, and it is not adequately related to the biological malfunction underlying it. Also, pain as a signal of the disease process is rarely an early warning signal. More than likely, the disease process has advanced significantly prior to any warning signal, i.e., pain. Soulairac also notes that the idea of a good-doing pain is a fallacy; he views pain as an affective reaction. In other words, pain has emotional components. Sacerdote (1970), a physician, notes that pain can be at times totally psychogenically produced.

Because of the highly subjective nature of pain, Edwards (1950), in a review of pain perception, points out that there is no suitable operational definition of pain. Most research dealing with pain perception has relied on the subject's introspective report. While there has been a wealth of research on pain perception, there are few studies that have relevance for the professional practitioner who must deal with pain patients on a day-to-day basis. Edwards (1950) feels that for experimental findings to have any meaning, it must be possible to differentiate between pain perception and pain reaction. Psychophysical research has demonstrated that the pain threshold varies between individuals and, also, within the individual from one time to another (Barber, 1959).

The use of medical treatments, i.e., treatments that are related to biological functioning, has been notoriously erratic in the ameliorization of chronic pain. Barber (1959) reviewed the use of neurosurgical procedures on the prefrontal lobes in attempts to relieve chronic pain. While he concentrated on leucotomies, he did note other neurosurgical procedures. Barber found that neurosurgical procedures involving the prefrontal lobes relieved pain in some cases but not all. The degree of relief from pain "appears to be a non-specific effect, closely related to the extent of the prefrontal damage" (Barber, 1959, p. 437). It appears that what is altered in the prefrontal procedures is not the patient's pain perception, but rather his attitude toward pain, that is, the emotional concomitants of pain. Barber (1959) also notes research indicating that most patients who have undergone leucotomies can focus on the pain and report pain sensations. Melzack and Wall (1957) refer to some sixteen different surgical procedures that have been designed to alleviate pain; all the procedures have had only moderate success. Cooper and Brace-land (1950, p. 981) suggest that "the conversion of a sensation into a pain-ful experience is largely an emotional reaction." Similarly, Melzack and Wall (1957), in studying the reactions of dogs to painful stimuli, concluded that some components of the pain response require previous experience.

The fact that pain thresholds can be easily influenced by instructions, analgesics, placebos, and hypnosis suggests that there is more to pain perception than a simple, or complex, stimulus-response sequence. The fact that placebos can be potent in pain relief suggests some psychological mediation. Melzack (1961) refers to the ability of attention and anticipation to increase pain perception. He feels the anticipation acts to raise the patient's anxiety which then increases the intensity of perceived pain. Melzack (1961, p. 49) concluded:

> The psychological evidence strongly supports the view of pain as a perceptual experience whose quality and intensity is influenced by the unique past history of the individual, by the meaning he gives to the pain-producing situation, and by his "state of mind" at the moment.

He goes on to say that pain, when conceptualized in this way, becomes a function of the whole individual.

Szasz (1968) takes a more clinical approach to pain in his portrait of *l'homme douloureux*, "the painful person." Szasz believes pain and suffering can become a career, an honorable way to cop-out on life. Much like his concept, the myth of mental illness, he believes pain because it is believed to have a physical basis, allows the individual to abdicate his responsibilities. Essentially, the painful person states: "I am in pain, I am ill, it is not my fault." This is not meant to mean that Szasz sees all persons complaining of pain as having illegitimate symptoms. Rather, he believes that when pain is persistent and "intractable," it can be an experience actively created and fashioned by the self. Chronic pain often indicates that the sufferer wishes to occupy the sick role. Szasz (1968) feels that the social role and identity of *l'homme douloureux* can only be authenticated by his pain and suffering. In his typical loquacious manner, Szasz (1968) speaks of the various levels of professional qualifications the sufferer may hold. The hypo-chondriac is seen as having a B.A. degree in pain. The seriously disabled individual with seemingly delusional beliefs about his body is said to hold a doctorate in pain. Lastly, the patient with "intractable" pain and no dem-onstrable organic disease is said to be worthy of the Nobel Prize in pain. The "painful person" plays a medical game; his goal is to produce undiagnosable and untreatable pain. To the extent that he is successful, the painful person has some control over his environment. Szasz (1968) notes that such indi-viduals seek out medical and surgical intervention to legitimize their role; psychiatric consultation, however, is avoided because it would be a denial of physical illness as such.

That chronic pain is a problem of some significance was noted in the recent NBC News Special, "Pain: Where Does It Hurt Most?" (March 28, 1972). According to the program, chronic pain is a national health problem. Presently, two million Americans are incapacitated by chronic pain and over two and a half billion dollars is paid annually in compensation to pain patients. Also, a new medical specialty was widely introduced to the public, the area of "Painology." In the description of treatment approaches undertaken in this area, considerable attention was given to psychological variables. In fact, many treatment approaches that were observed had a strong behavioral orientation.

This brief introductory review suggests that psychological variables play a role in the perception of pain. The quality and intensity of pain is multideterminied; that is, both physical and psychological factors appear to interact, although there is also evidence that pain can be the result of either factor alone. Because of the highly subjective nature of pain and because pain relief has been variously conceptualized as "freedom from anxiety," "contentment," and "a bemused state" (Barber, 1959, p. 453), a psychological approach to pain seems practical and necessary.

PSYCHOLOGICAL APPROACHES TO PAIN

In this section, the utility of the dichotomy between organic and psychogenic pain will be discussed. Considerable attention will also be given to psychoanalytic and psychodynamic formulations of pain and its meaning within the psychic structure of the individual. While the majority of references to behaviorism will be relegated to the section on treatment, some attention will be given to this area also.

Classical Psychoanalytic Theory

There has been a widespread tendency for classical psychoanalysis to leave "physical" pain in the hands of physiology and medicine. References to pain in the orthodox literature are sparse. Freud made few comments on physical pain, and his interests in pain seemed to center on his pleasure-pain principle. In *Inhibitions, Symptoms, and Anxiety* (1948), Freud comments briefly on "physical pain" and considers the ego's reactions to pain. He offers some tentative formulations regarding the relationships between anxiety, pain, and mourning (Szasz, 1957). Overall, orthodox psychoanalytic theory is structurally inadequate for the integration of pain as a concept.

Bard (1959) speculates on Freud's paucity of references to pain. He notes that Freud's life was a series of illnesses: acute nicotine poisoning, prostatic hypertrophy and bladder dysfunction, a serious heart attack, angina pectoris, and sixteen years living with oral cancer. Bard hypothesizes that Freud's ability to adapt to physical illness may be related to his failure to deal with pain as a theoretical issue.

Extensions of Psychoanalytic Theory

Contemporary psychoanalytic thinking appears to be an admixture of classical Freudianism, ego psychology, and object-relations theory. While it is possible to separate out the various lines of thought, no attempt will be made to do so here. It appears that the mixing of the concepts, within a still reasonably systematic theory, is what allows psychoanalytic psychology to remain viable and useful. While the work of several theorists will be presented, the core of the theoretical exposition will be Szasz's (1957) extension of psychoanalytic theory utilizing object-relations concepts. While not all psychodynamic thinkers agree with Szasz as to the mechanisms involved, his approach is the best defined and most systematic statement on the psychology of pain.

Anna Freud (1952) addresses herself to the role of bodily illness in the mental life of children. She feels that parents tend to alter their attitudes toward the ill child and as a result ". . . the ill child may find himself more loved and fondled than at any other time in his life" (Freud, Anna, 1952, p. 70). The ill child cannot distinguish between the pain that is related to the illness and the pain that is related to the treatment. As a result, the bewildered child must submit passively to both. The effect of this passive submission, the meanings of pain, and the reaction of the child depends on the type and depth of the fantasies aroused. Since discovery of the castration complex, analysts have had ample opportunity to study the impact of surgery on normal and abnormal development. Anna Freud (1952) points out that it is now common knowledge that any surgical procedure (major or minor) can serve as the focal point for "the activation, reactivation, grouping, and rationalization of ideas of being attacked, overwhelmed and/or castrated" (p. 74). Psychoanalytic studies of individual differences to pain indicate that it is not the actual bodily experience that is different but, rather, the degree of psychic embellishment that the pain is given by the individual.

The normal reaction to pain by the individual is to take appropriate measures to avoid it or, when that is not possible, to react appropriately to the pain. Rangell (1953) suggests that deviations from the normal response to pain indicate that the pain may hold morbid or pathological significance for the individual. Seeking pain for its own sake is often an indication that pain has been eroticized as in masochism. Seeking pain can also be an individual's way of expiating himself from real or imagined feelings of guilt. Pain can stand for something else because of its association with a gratifying situation. Rangell (1953) points out that when the reaction to unavoidable pain is inappropriate or disproportionate, it is because of neurotic elements.

Ego psychology has its tacit beginnings in Freud's post-1920 writings, but Heinz Hartmann (1958) was the first to systematically elaborate on ego functions and to make the extension of ego theory into the conflict-free area of functioning. Hartmann believed that not every adaptation to the environment, nor every learning or maturational process, is related to conflict. He divided the ego into the conflict-ridden and the conflict-free spheres; examples of conflict-free functioning are perception, intention, cognition, object comprehension, and so on. Hartmann also mentions the ego's relationship to the body; this is the body ego, a concept that will be of central importance in understanding the psychology of pain. Hoffer (1950, 1952) points out that, according to Freud, the body has to be the first object of the ego. Similarly, the instinct's first object has to be the body.

Szasz's Psychoanalytic Approach to Pain

Szasz (1957) feels that an object relation approach to ego functions allows the freedom to overcome the dualistic mind-body approach. Important for an understanding of Szasz's psychoanalytic approach are several concepts: pain as an affect, ego-orientation, and the symbolic and personal meanings of pain. Formulations related to phantom phenomena will be reserved to a later section of this chapter. Note that this is an attempt to summarize Szasz's theorizing on pain. For an extensive review of his concepts, the reader is referred to his book, *Pain and Pleasure* (1957).

Pain as an Affect

The affective experience of pain is as universal as that of anxiety, but it has received much less attention in the psychoanalytic literature. Szasz (1957) points out that Fenichel (1945) was apparently the first analyst to view pain as an affect. Within psychoanalytic theory there is agreement that the concept of affect is inextricably interrelated with the concept of ego. It is impossible to make a statement about pain relative to the adult ego without using the body as a referent. The experience of pain is fundamentally related to the ego's orientation to the body. Therefore, Szasz sees pain as a warning signal (an ego warning) about a bodily state. Within this framework, the body is an ego object. At this point, a formal definition of object relationship is needed.

> In the concept of "object relationships" attention is focused on a process of mutual interaction between the ego and another system. Whatever the nature of this system, it may be called an "object" (Szasz, 1957, p. 56).

While Schilder (1953) used a similar concept, Szasz points out that Schilder's definition of ego is not consistent with psychoanalytic theory but refers to something more analogous to the self construct. The ego is defined as a "cohesive organization of mental processes" (Freud, 1949).

When pain is defined as an affect, it can be considered much the same as anxiety. Anxiety is the danger of losing a needed object (originally the mother), and pain can be interpreted analogously "as a warning of the danger of the loss of a part (or the whole) of the body" (Szasz, 1957, p. 59).

Ego Orientation

The concept of ego orientation is of central importance to Szasz's psychoanalytic approach to pain. Schilder (1953) maintained that the body is ego-close while the world is ego-distant. Szasz's (1957) concept is similar. Pain is the affect referring to ego-body orientation while anxiety is the affect referring to ego-object orientation. The ego, as an experiencing system, evaluates the danger in its relationship to the body and experiences some shade of pain. In this respect, pain indicates the danger of the disruption of the continuity of the body and the potential loss of a body part. Pain can also be a reaction to and a warning against the danger of excessive stimulation. This latter function, of course, is more in keeping with the traditional psychophysical definitions of pain. The former function, on the other hand, allows pain to take on more personal or individual connotations and, therefore, is more important when pain is considered within a clinical context.

Any discussion of ego functions needs to take into account developmental considerations. Within the area of psychoanalytic theory, there is still disagreement as to how the primitive ego develops. The position taken here is that the earliest ego states involve bodily feelings, and further, that the ego's first object is the body. Szasz (1957) feels that, for the early ego, the body as an object is more important than people as objects. Szasz (1957) briefly summarizes the ego's relationship with objects at three levels of development. The first level, the neonatal period and part of early infancy, is the familiar stage involving the differentiation of ego and non-ego. At this time, there is no object differentiation and affect is best described as undifferentiated pain-anxiety (unlust). The second level, the period of roughly four months to nine months, is that point in the developmental sequence at which the infant knows the difference between his own body and that of the person who is caring for him. At this time, the beginning of ego orientation toward either the body or objects is possible. Similarly, the early affective experience, primitive pain-anxiety, becomes differentiated into pain (relative to the body) and anxiety (relative to objects). At the third level we are considering the adult ego. At this level, there should be generally complete differentiation between body and objects. Also, as the result of experience and growth, both pain and anxiety are overdetermined. In addition, both anxiety and pain can serve as defenses, each one against the other. While psychoanalytic theory has given little emphasis to the ego's defenses against pain, clinical experience demonstrates a relationship between pain and anxiety. Anxiety can serve as a defense against illness and pain as in the stoical patient. Similarly, in the hypochondriac or hysteric demonstrating pain, that pain is often a defense against the experiencing of anxiety. This relationship has been noted in patients undergoing analytic treatment; the stoic begins to experience pain and the hysteric or hypochondriac begins to experience anxiety concomitant with a lessening in somatic symptomatology as the defensive structure of the personality is altered. Szasz (1957) points out that there are times in everyone's life when body security and continuity are threatened. He gives examples: childhood, puberty, pregnancy, menopause, old age, and times of illness or injury.

There are three general categories of ego orientation according to Szasz's (1957) theory. The first is the silent feeling of bodily well-being. This refers to a preconscious awareness of the body and its functions when no conscious attention is focused on the body. The second category is that of increased interest in the body. Szasz (1957) makes it clear that here he is not referring to the observer's interest but rather to the ego's interest in body function. All manner of feelings such as pain, itching, burning, etc., that indicates that there is increased cathexis of the body by the ego, is included in this category. The third category refers to decreased interest in the body. Here we are referring to a lack of interest on the part of the ego in the body as an object. Examples of decreased ego-cathexis in the body are again the stoic who feels no pain in the presence of severe illness or injury, hysterical anesthesia, and the schizophrenic patient who inflicts serious injury on himself without demonstrating pain. It is, of course, the second category that is relevant in considering the pain patient. This is the patient who, for psychodynamic reasons, cannot give up his pain. He has so much investment in his body and so little of importance in the world around him, that pain takes on chronic or unexplainable qualities. This brings us to the next consideration in the psychology of pain.

The Symbolic and Personal Nature of Pain

Pain cannot be viewed merely as an isolated phenomenon involving only the experiencing ego; it is also a social phenomenon. Szasz (1957) again uses a tripartite categorization.

The first category of pain is what Szasz (1957) refers to as the primary model of pain. This is pain as a signal of biological malfunction. This pain is not learned but acquired spontaneously in early childhood. This is the simple stimulus-response (S-R) concept that is fundamental to the concept of sensation. This type of pain is "objective"; the experiencing system does not elaborate or embellish it, so inherent in this model is the notion that any similar intact organism would experience pain similarly. In addition to pain's signal function, it is also a message to the ego to take evasive action to protect the integrity of the body. The primary model of pain is a single organism model—a one-body frame of reference.

The second category of pain can be distinguished when another person is brought into the field. This is of course inevitable, for, as Anna Freud (1952) was noted as saying earlier, the parent can hardly help but alter his responses to the ill child. In the course of childhood, the expression of pain leads other persons to minister to the child in an attempt to alleviate his discomfort and suffering. So while the original expression of pain is spontaneous and not in essence goal-directed, the consequences establish pain as a fundamental method of asking for help or attention. Pain, therefore, is more complex than the primary model would have us assume; it now refers to one or both of the above categories. Szasz (1957) refers to the first category as the *medical* meaning, and the second category as the *communicative* meaning of pain. It is important for the individual experiencing pain to be able to communicate the dangerous state adequately. To the degree that there is discrepancy between sufferer and observer, the likelihood increases that the observer will label it *mental* or *psychogenic* pain. This discrepancy or failure to reach agreement on the nature of pain between sufferer and observer, or patient and professional, can be considered as a failure to reach consensual validation. In other words, the communication is not having its proper intent communicated to someone outside of the subject's experiential field. The point under elaboration is that pain is a symbolic communication that may or may not be a "significant symbol," as Mead (1962) would call it, depending upon the intent of the individual communicating the pain message and the interpretation of the person receiving the communication.

In Szasz's (1957) third category of pain, the communicative meaning of pain is the central issue. As such, one person addressing himself to another with a pain communication is the focus. Crucial to understanding the meaning of this third category is knowing to whom the pain communication is being addressed. Pain may be a command to a particular person from whom assistance may be expected. Pain may be addressed to a particular person because the sufferer feels that person owes him. Pain may also signify rejection, aggression, or a myriad of other interpersonal communications.

The meaning of a particular bodily feeling depends on several factors: (1) Most important is the life history of the individual; (2) whether or not the body-as-an-object is being used to work out or re-enact a conflict, also deserves attention; and (3) if it is a conflict, the meanings should become apparent by considering the illness, the nature of the pain, and the interpersonal nature of the pain communications. In summary, Szasz (1957, p. 90) re-iterates:

> We can state the differences between the three categories, or levels of symbolization, of *pain* most clearly and succinctly in terms of the things to which *pain* points as a referent. In the first category it points to the body; in the second it points ambiguously to both body and other people; and in the third category its referent is some particular person.

This then is an overview of Szasz's psychoanalytic extension involving object relationships toward a theory of pain that should have relevance for the practicing clinician as well as the theorist. The theory will perhaps become clearer, and the ego mechanisms better understood when it is applied to the psychology of phantom sensations and phantom pain in a later section of this chapter.

Behaviorism and Pain

Behaviorism in this context will refer to the approaches that have their roots in learning theory and reinforcement paradigms. While it is possible to make distinctions between behavior therapy, behavior modification, and other operant or instrumental approaches, such a distinction is not of value here.

Because pain is a highly personal "internal state" that has a data base primarily in introspective report, behavioral theory does not deal with pain *per se*. Pain, as an internal process, is not amendable to the rigorous, operational definition that is required within the behavioral approach. However, it was apparent in the communicative meanings which Szasz (1957) connotes to pain, that pain does have an instrumental function for the individual. As such, behavior modifiers have dealt with "pain behavior." "Pain behavior" refers to those aspects of the patient's behavior that, by virtue of the response by the environment, have maintaining effects on the behavioral concomitants of pain (Fordyce, Fowler, Lehmann, and DeLateur, 1968).

While there is no systematic theory of pain within the behavioral framework, there is considerable evidence that some aspects of the pain response are learned. Melzack and Scott (1957) demonstrated with laboratory dogs that some aspects of the pain response require experience. According to Neal Miller (1951), when human subjects acquire a learned drive on the basis of pain, the cues do not elicit a hallucination of pain but rather a part of the original pain-fear response. Specifically, that part of the response called fear. Miller feels that fear is much more learnable than pain, although he does note clinical evidence suggesting that, in some cases, pain may be learnable. Michael (1970) suggests that pain has both operant and non-operant components. He notes that the wide individual differences in reaction to pain are a function of the operant component and it is this component that may be strengthened by reinforcement such as staff attention, drugs on demand, and the like.

THE PSYCHOLOGY OF THE PHANTOM

Phantom sensation and phantom pain, particularly the former, is encountered so often that Serafetinides (1968) suggests that it is unavoidable following amputation. While phantom sensation is an almost universal phenomenon following amputation, phantom pain is much less frequent. Kolb (1954) found the incidence of painful phantom to be very small. Ewalt, Randall, and Morris (1947), with a sample of 2,284 amputee patients (404 with extensive psychiatric work-ups), found only eight cases of phantom pain. Clinical experience and empirical studies (Szasz, 1957; Ewalt, *et al.,* 1947; Simmel, 1959) indicate that the individual with phantom pain has serious personality problems. Relative to phantom pain, Szasz (1957, p. 150) makes the point,

> Such everyday clinical problems as the differentiation between so-called organic and psychogenic pain . . . call attention to the blind alley into which we are led by the question "Where is the pain?"

Any attempt to explain phantom phenomena psychologically must lead to a discussion of the body image or body scheme. Flescher (1948, p. 157) states:

> In neuropathology the concept of "body scheme" is based on the fact that besides

sensations conveyed by sight, touch, and the receptors of muscles and tendons, as well as the entero-receptive receptors (of the viscera), we possess a global and direct impression of the wholeness of our body as a tri-dimensional image."

He goes on to say,

> The pathology of the body scheme shows a very remarkable phenomenon: the phantom limb. Patients who have suddenly been deprived of a limb by amputation, retain for a certain length of time the image or the sensation of possessing it.

There have been neurological, psychiatric, and psychoanalytic attempts to explain the phantom. This section will deal primarily with the psychological approaches, and particularly with the psychoanalytic attempts at understanding the nature of the phantom. Again, the theoretical approach of Szasz (1957) will serve as the core for the psychoanalytic explanation. This will be followed by an overview of other theoretical approaches and an application of the psychological theory to a "scientific" critique.

Psychoanalytic Approach to Phantom Phenomena

Szasz (1957, p. 150) asks the interesting question about the nature of ego adaptation: "What happens if the dangers about which the affects of anxiety and pain warn the ego do in fact materialize?" In the case of the loss of an object, the dynamic process of mourning is well known; in fact, it is considered a necessary adaptive process on the part of the ego in reaction to a disequilibrium in its relations with objects. Important in this process according to Fenichel (1954) is the *time factor*: the ego, to maintain its integrity, converts a sudden loss into a gradual loss thus allowing time for an adaptation in its object environment. Szasz (1957) uses the same process to explain phantom sensations. He calls the gradual process the "psychic metabolism."

TABLE 18-I*

MOURNING AND PHANTOMIZATION

Loss of:	Object	Part of the Body
Adaptive response:	Introjection of object	Phantomization
	Internal object replaces what is lost in external reality.	Phantom organ, or body part, replaces lost organ or part.
	Mourning	Phantom "sensation"
Resolution:	Detachment of cathexes from introjected object. Formation of new object relationships.	Shrinking of phantom and its ultimate disappearance. Formulation of a new "body image."
	A new ego-object integration becomes established.	A new ego-body integration becomes established.

*Reprinted with permission of Dr. Thomas S. Szasz.

Thus, mourning and phantomization use of the same ego mechanisms (see Table I) for adaptation and resolution of the sudden loss. The process works as follows: the ego cannot tolerate the sudden disruption of the body image so the object (the body part) is introjected and the internal object (the phantom body part) replaces the lost external object (the amputated or lost body part). This results in the phantom sensation which is the ego's body image analog to mourning. This process of "psychic metabolism" allows the ego time for a reintegration of the body image. As time passes, the ego decathects from the introjected object (the phantom) and a new ego-body integration is formed. It is during this reintegrative phase that the phantom sensation becomes distorted and gradually shrinks away. Szasz (1957) points out that this process only applies to the loss of those body parts that are part of the body image; for the ego, no other parts of the body are said to exist. This does not mean, however, that phantom sensations are restricted to the limbs and other external anatomy; any part of the body of which one has ever had any awareness can, upon its loss or injury, be experienced as a phantom. In this respect, Szasz speaks of "visceral phantoms"; he warns, however, that he uses the term "visceral" in a purely historical sense and not an anatomical or physiological one. "A phantom limb similarly represents the use of an anatomical designation for an essentially historically conditioned event" (Szasz, 1957, p. 168). The psychological approach calls attention to the need to differentiate between the body image and the observer's view of the body. The patient must be the primary source of data.

As noted above, while phantom sensations are common following amputation or spinal cord injury, the incidence of phantom pain is rare. Also, although phantom sensations tend to disappear with time, phantom pain, once established, tends to persist either continually or intermittently for years. Ewalt, *et. al.,* (1947) noted that patients experiencing phantom pain were patients who had considerable psychopathology. They concluded that "phantom pain is merely the interpretation of a phantom sensation by certain individuals who show psychopathology" (p. 123).

There are differences in the reported quality of pain from individuals with direct injury and those with phantom pain. In the case of a bodily injury, pain is often reported to be sharp, acute, stabbing and agonizing. The patient suffering from phantom pain, on the other hand, complains of chronic, twisting, tearing, pulling, and annoying pain. Just as he made the analogy between mourning and phantom sensations, he draws a similar analogy between the mechanisms involved in paranoia and phantom pain. Szasz notes that many of the behaviors involved in the two processes are similar. The paranoid makes noisy claims about the persecutory delusion; similarly, the patient with phantom pain makes noisy claims about his "persecuting object", the painful limb or missing body part. Both types of patients tend to engage the staff's attention with annoying, pestering behavior.

Szasz's (1957) formulations involve a comparison of a delusion of persecution with phantom pain (see Table II), and the mechanisms are essentially as follows. Like with mourning and phantomization, the precipitating event is a loss—the former of an object and the latter of a body part. The loss activates the ego defenses, leading to denial of the loss and the appearance of a phantom body part in the form of a sensation. However, in the paradigm leading to phantom pain, there is also a denial of the affect associated with the loss—i.e., pain. Szasz (1957, p. 159) notes,

> As in the case of a delusion of persecution, countercathexis may or may not be applied to keep the defense effective. This takes the form of projection and leads, for example, to the erroneous perception of amputations (or of suffering, pain) in other people with intact bodies.

The final step in this process is the return of the denied, both in terms of the body part and the associated affect. The convergence of denied material, the loss of a body part and the pain associated with it, lead to the final symptom, phantom pain. In phantom pain, as in the persecutory delusion, "the once familiar and loved object, the body part, returns in the form of something strange and threatening" (Szasz, 1957, p. 159). The symptom of phantom pain serves two purposes: (1) it allows for partial discharge of the previously denied affect; and (2) it is a renewed and ultimate denial of the original loss.

TABLE 18-II*

PARANOIA (DELUSION OF PERSECUTION) AND PHANTOM PAIN

Mechanism	*Delusion of Persecution*	*Phantom Pain*
Precipitating event:	Loss of object (e.g., loss of heterosexual love object)	Loss of body part (e.g., amputation)
Defense mechanism (1) denial (A "claim"):	1. Denial of loss of object: introjection of object	1. Denial of loss of body part: Phantom
(2) Projection (Countercathexis—a "counterclaim"):	2. Denial of regressively reactivated conflict-producing drive (homosexuality) "No, I am not a homosexual. He is a homosexual."	2. Denial of affect (pain) "No, I am not amputated. He is amputated."
Return of the denied (as something alien and threatening):	Reappearance of: 1. Lost love object (persecutor) 2. Denied drive or need (homosexuality)	Reappearance of: 1. Lost body part (phantom) 2. Denied affect (pain)
Symptom:	Delusion of persecution	Phantom pain
Economic function of symptoms:	1. Partial discharge of otherwise ego-alien drive (homosexuality), and 2. "Ultimate denial" of loss of object: "He persecutes me—it cannot be, therefore, that he does not love me, that I have lost him."	1. Partial discharge of previously denied affect (pain), and 2. "Ultimate denial" of loss of body part: "It hurts—it cannot be, therefore, that it is not present, that I have lost it."

*Reprinted with permission of Dr. Thomas S. Szasz.

For Szasz (1957), the symptom of phantom pain appears to be the result of an adaptive mechanism that goes awry. Fischer (1968, p. 325) takes a similar view; he states,

> In phantom pain, the symptoms arrest the readaptive effort at an unacceptable pathological level to protect against other disruptive ego manifestations associated with inner instinctual conflicts.

Simmel (1959) does not agree with Szasz on the importance of denial of affect as a central aspect of the formation of phantom pain. She feels that patients who have severe phantom pain soon after surgery present a very different clinical picture. These patients are usually acutely anxious and depressed and, rather than denying their affect, they are being overwhelmed by it. She does, however, agree with Szasz that many patients with chronic, severe phantom pain present a clinical picture similar to the paranoid.

A psychological approach to phantom limb and phantom pain offers the professional who works with these patients a more personal framework for viewing the symptomatology of the patient. As seen above, it is possible to put these symptoms into a frame of reference that is consistent with contemporary psychodynamic thought. It was noted that the relative rarity of phantom pain suggests that its origin is strongly influenced by psychological factors and perpetuated by neurotic concomitants.

Phantom Pain: A Theoretical Overview and Attempt at Integration

Three general, and broad, categories of theory have been used to attempt explanations of phantom phenomena. Two, the peripheral theory and the central theory, have their base in neurophysiology and neurology. The third, the need or fantasy approach, is primarily a psychodynamic approach to the phantom.

Peripheral theory assumes that phantom sensations are the result of various sources of irritation in the stump. Examples of irritants are scar tissue, neurotoma, lack of oxygen, and nerve destruction. Weinstein (1969) points out that, although there is a rational basis for the peripheral theory, it is generally not acceptable. Phantom sensations often appear immediately after amputation or in cases with deafferentation or spinal anesthesia where there is no neural input from the periphery. The peripheral theory is also inadequate for explaining so-called visceral phantoms.

Central theory, according to McDaniel (1969), has been proposed by Simmel and Weinstein. This approach attributes phantom sensations to activity within the cortical projection areas that had previously served the missing body part. There is ample evidence to support this approach. It has been observed that phantom sensations can be elicited by stimulation of the somatosensory cortex. Also, phantom sensations can be apparently permanently eliminated by ablating or inducing a lesion in the appropriate cortical area. McDaniel further notes that "the central theory assumes that the somatosensory cortical representation of the body is the genetic neural framework of the body-image and also the source of phantom perceptions (McDaniel, 1969, p. 101). Generally, central theory seems to be consistent with the empirical findings on brain function related to phantom phenomena.

The theory, however, tends to consider phantom limb and phantom pain together. It has already been pointed out that phantom limb or phantom sensations are, for all practical purposes, universal, while phantom pain is quite rare. The question is also raised whether neurosurgery should be the treatment of choice for the patient complaining of phantom pain.

Fantasy theory is generally held to be the theoretical explanation of the patient's phantom as a function of his imagination; he has the phantom because he needs it emotionally. The theoretical presentation outlined in this chapter would have to be placed under the rubric of "need or fantasy" theory. This approach will, of course, be defended here. McDaniels (1969) refers to this approach as *fanciful,* and Weinstein (1969) rejects this view by citing "abundant evidence." His evidence, however, does not contradict a psychodynamic formulation. Because "need or fantasy" is ill-defined in this context and generally unacceptable because of its simplistic connotations, this approach will be referred to as the psychodynamic approach—"psychodynamic" referring to the forces of the mind which include such factors as ideas, attitudes, affects, and adaptational maneuvers.

The defense will consist of two approaches. First, a discussion of the interrelationship between psychodynamic and neurological approaches, and second, a point-by-point demonstration that psychodynamic theory can explain the phantom even in the light of Weinstein's (1969) "abundant evidence."

A Psychodynamic Explanation

While psychodynamic approaches are acceptable to this author, the fact remains that most psychodynamic approaches do not drop out the underlying concomitant neurophysiological processes. Henry Murray speaks of this with his principle of regnancy (Hall and Lindzey, 1970). This is the idea that the personality has a physiological substratum and all behavior is related to concurrent functional activities within the central nervous system. Hartmann (1952, p. 19) makes this point also:

> In the ego's relationship with the body, we can now describe three aspects: the postulated physiological processes underlying activities of the ego, the apparatuses that gradually come under the control of the ego and which in turn influence the timing, intensity, and direction of ego development; and third, but not necessarily independent of the two others, those special structures that underlie what we call the body ego.

The receptotopic organization of the cerebral cortex or the somatosensory homunculus may very well be one of these special structures that underlie the body ego. The point is, however, that psychodynamic explanations are not necessarily inclined toward an arbitrary dismissal of physiology.

The "abundant evidence" cited by Weinstein (1969) suggests that he allows no variance for the psychological approaches that have their basis in psychology rather than physiology. The evidence cited by Weinstein will be examined and explained to be consistent with a psychodynamic approach. Note, refutation of central theory is not the objective here; rather, the point is to illustrate the complementary nature of psychodynamic and central theories.

Weinstein (1969, p. 80), in his first criticism of fantasy theory, states: "Sensations are a most drastic manifestation of a need. There are no other psychological 'needs' that result in hallucinations. Thus, orphans do not hallucinate their absent parent." Apparently Weinstein is not using the term "hallucination" in its clinical context. Regarding hallucinations, Fenichel (1945, p. 425) notes: "Hallucinations are substitutes for perceptions . . . Inner factors are projected and experienced as if they were external perceptions." Therefore, with the exception of some toxic and metabolic dysfunctions, one could draw the conclusion that hallucinatory phenomena are a function of psychological factors, be they "needs," wish-fulfillments, or otherwise. While sensations are considered by Weinstein to be "a most drastic manifestation of a need," false perceptions would also seem to have a dramatic element. Yet both are frequently encountered in the clinical setting. Perhaps it is the notion of the clinical context, the implicit reference to psychopathology, that is upsetting when considering the physically disabled patient. Yet what could be more taxing, more demanding of the patient's adaptive resources, than a traumatic amputation. From the frame of reference of the patient, the loss of limb, whether forewarned or sudden, is certainly a trauma requiring marked utilization of adaptive or adjustive maneuvers. That these adaptive functions should be ineffective in a small number of cases is not surprising since clinical experience indicates that there are people that just do not possess the adaptive resiliency to bounce back, so to speak, from a major trauma. One last point, while psychological "needs" can induce hallucinations, physical needs can do likewise. Hallucinations are often concomitants of alcoholic, diabetic, and uremic conditions. Hallucinations also occur with vestibular irritation.

Weinstein's (1969, p. 80) second criticism is that, "Phantoms are universal in some populations of patients; fantasies are never so consistent." The weakness of this point lies in the specification of certain undefined populations of patients. Were the populations defined, the evidence would indicate that phantoms occur principally where the loss of a body part is sudden. One of the most notable findings concerning a group of patients that do not have phantom phenomena is Simmel's (1956) study of patients with leprosy. These patients lost digits but did not experience phantoms. This finding is consistent with an ego framework because of the unique disease process involved in leprosy whereby the loss of function and tissue destruction is a gradual process. This gradual process does not pose a sudden and over-whelming threat to the ego-body integration. According to Szasz (1957), the adaptive nature of the phantom is to allow for a gradual acceptance of the experience; in leprosy the loss itself is a gradual process. The interesting finding that phantoms do occur, although with much lower frequency, in individuals with nonfunctional limbs such as found in congenital aplasia is difficult to fit into a strictly psychological framework. The psychological theory presented here relies heavily on the ego as an experiencing system; in the case of congenital aplasia, the phantom sensation would have to be regarded as wish fulfillment. However, the small incidence of phantoms in congenital aplasia is more consistent with the central theory which would allow for sensations without previous experience.

Weinstein's (1969, p. 80) third point is that "If phantoms are fantasies, it is difficult to understand why they are so often: (1) painful, (2) telescoped, (3) shrunken, and (4) misshapen. Fantasies typically involve wish-fulfillment rather than such undesirable distortion." First, fantasies of the phantom, as indicated earlier, are not so often painful. In fact, the painful phantom is relatively rare. The distortion, shrinking, and telescoping of a phantom limb is an aspect of the readjustment process, what Szasz (1957) refers to as the psychic metabolism. As the ego moves toward a new integration and develops a revamped body-image, the phantom goes through a fading-out process often with considerable distortion of the sensation. Even if fantasies typically do involve wish-fulfillment, that does not mean that the fantasy is going to be pleasurable or benevolent. While phantoms no doubt are to a large extent the result of wish-fulfillment, the persistent, chronic phantom takes on many of the qualities of a delusion. As such, Fenichel's (1945, p. 426) comments regarding hallucinations seem appropriate: "However, most schizophrenic hallucinations are not pleasurable and do not seem to represent simple wish-fulfillments. Often they are extremely painful or frightening." While implying that patients with phantom pain are schizophrenic would be a foolhardy application of a much misused label, it should be remembered that numerous investigators have remarked on the psychopathology found in patients with chronic phantom pain (Kolb, 1954; Ewalt, *et. al.*, 1947; Szasz, 1957; Simmel, 1959; and Fischer, 1968).

> It seems evident that the "need" for a missing limb does not differ among young children. However, the proportion of phantoms of appendages in children of the same age is a monotonic function of the age at which the amputation occurred or whether it was congenital (Weinstein, 1969, p. 80).

He goes on to say that if "need" were to dictate the existence of a phantom, then age would be *irrelevant*. This, of course, is inconsistent with the theory of ego development. What this seems to indicate is that the stability of the body image or ego-body integration is a monotonic function of age. The younger the child, the less stable the body image. Therefore, it is expected that phantoms would increase in frequency as a function of age.

"It has been frequently reported that phantoms of amputated limbs frequently tend to shrink, fade, or telescope in time; such phenomena are difficult to understand in the framework of a fantasy theory" (Weinstein, 1969, p. 80). On the contrary, such phenomena are easy to understand within the psychodynamic theory presented in this chapter. As already noted, the tendency to shrink, fade, or telescope in time is a function of the psychic metabolism; the process of adaptation to the loss.

The observation that a patient under spinal anesthesia often perceives his anesthetized legs as phantoms also points to the stability and continuity of ego-body integration. Since the body image is a total gestalt, from an experiential framework, it is not unexpected that the patient would continue to experience the totality of his body (as a whole) even though sensory input from specific areas has been temporarily blocked.

Other Explanations of Phantom Phenomena

A review of this nature suggests that our theoretical approaches are necessarily incomplete at this time. It is apparent that psychodynamic explanations do have difficulty with certain aspects of phantom phenomena. Likewise, there are gaps in physiological and neuroanatomical explanations of the phantoms. What is impressive is the fact that virtually all vicissitudes of phantom phenomena can be explained by combining psychodynamic and central formulations. Man is not either a psyche or a soma but rather a psychosomatic or, if you prefer, a somatopsychic unity. Yet, theoretical explanations tend to dichotomize the two, no doubt because of the inherent difficulties with a monistic approach. Also, the failure of the psychosomatic approach to find emotional components to physical diseases and particularly the failure in the area of psychosomatic specificity, a specific psychological conflict for a specific physical illness (Stein, 1972), has led many researchers away from monistic approaches. According to Stein, much of psychosomatic research was too heavily weighted on the hypothesized psychogenic components. Redlich and Freedman (1966) note that the trend toward discrete studies designed to evaluate a sequence of processes with the analysis of multiple factors, rather than overinclusive projects designed to explain everything at once, will probably be of benefit to the area of psychosomatics.

It would seem that a holistic approach to the individual with phantom pain is in order. An approach that encompasses both the physiological and the psychodynamic would be particularly valuable to the practicing professional. That an integration of physical and psychological concepts can be accomplished, at least in theory, is demonstrated by Freeman (1969) who related the neurological theorizing of Hughlings Jackson to the psychodynamic formulations of Sigmund Freud. Just as there are striking similarities between the concept of body image as a psychodynamic phenomenon and body image as a function of the somatosensory cortical homunculus, there are marked similarities between Jackson's notions of cortical evolution-dissolution and Freud's concept of regression. There are, of course, inconsistencies in any complementation of this nature. For the purpose of exploratory research, however, concentration on the similarities might prove to be more empirically heuristic since the inconsistencies are based on theoretical formulations presently extant. Following a course of research based on the similarities could conceivably shed new light on an area and, hopefully, alter what had previously been considered inconsistent. A psychological framework can be useful in explaining the various aspects of phantom phenomena and it offers the practicing professional a referent for conceptualizing the psychological processes involved in patients with such symptomatology.

THE MANAGEMENT OF PAIN

The patient suffering from chronic or intractable pain is, for all practical purposes, a medical problem. Acute pain, often indicative of a medical emergency, is necessarily restricted to treatment and management by the physician. For the chronic patient, however, whose pain is suspected to have emotional parameters, the psychologist working within a medical setting can be useful. The well-trained professional psychologist has knowledge of a number of therapeutic approaches that may aid the pain patient. These approaches range from traditional counseling and psychotherapy to the new, esoteric, primarily exploratory techniques such as biofeedback and alpha training. This section is an overview of treatment procedures that are often within the purview of the psychologist. Some techniques, such as hypnosis, have an extensive literature regarding their use in the control of pain. Others, such as counseling and various forms of psychotherapy, have little specific reference to pain control and usually refer to that tenuous, overused concept of adjustment in relation to physical disability. Behavioral techniques have only recently began to make inroads toward the pain patient. Biofeedback techniques such as various forms of autonomic conditioning have yet to be extensively applied to pain control but their promise is exciting to consider.

Hypnosis

While hypnosis is most often associated with psychiatry and psychology, it has had, and will continue to have, relevant application in virtually every medical specialty (Schneck, 1953). Pattie (1967) places the beginning of hypnotism with Mesmer (1734-1815); he feels references to hypnotism prior to Mesmer are primarily accounts of magic, witchcraft, miracles, demon possession and so on. As hypnosis becomes free from the mystical connotations for so long associated with it, it is finding more acceptance for use in controlling pain and in other health problems (Hightower, 1966).

Meares (1968) believes that patients are culturally conditioned against psychological approaches to pain control. This is notable in the widespread belief that, when one is in pain, he should take a pill or get an injection. Yet, hypnosis has been found to be a useful tool in pain control. Stokvis (1956, p. 81) states: "Hypnotherapy, applied as a symptomatic treatment, is especially indicated in those cases of organic diseases in which the patient has neurotically elaborated his physical suffering."

An excellent review of the psychological mechanisms involved in hypnosis is provided by Meares (1968). In addition, he notes the advantages and disadvantages of each mechanism relative to pain control.

Suggestion: This term is probably one of the more common associations one would make to the word *hypnosis*. The reggressive process involved in hypnosis dulls the logical critical faculties and allows the mechanism of suggestion to function more freely (Meares, 1968). The patient is given the suggestion that he is comfortable and that the painful area is "easy and natural." Meares (1968) points out that this procedure is usually effective as long as the patient remains in the regressed hypnotic state. However, even with strong posthypnotic suggestion, the control of pain usually breaks down when the patient is out of the hypnotic state.

Denial: Meares (1968) notes that denial can be an effective defense against minor psychological conflicts. Denial as a hypnotic mechanism is used by reducing the patient's anxiety and by suggesting relaxation and a state of calm both in mind and body. Denial, even hypnotically induced, is not effective for the patient with severe pain; it is difficult for the patient to maintain the state of denial.

Masochistic Elaboration: The experience of pain can be eroticized, or invested with sexual qualities, that make the pain experience sensually pleasant. While this approach can be very effective, Meares (1968) points out that it involves a distortion of basic psychological values. He goes on to state: "However effective this might be, it is obviously wrong to use such a mechanism, lest we initiate a perversion in the patient's personality" (p. 55).

Dissociation: This is the hypnotic mechanism that is usually associated with the control of pain. While dissociation is a natural mechanism, its elaboration within the hypnotic state often allows the patient to stand aside, so to speak, from his pain. The patient is not emotionally involved with his pain and, according to Meares (1968), the affected area is described as numb or "dead." Meares (1968) feels this is an effective technique for operative procedures but, for the control of pain, the patient must be taught autohypnosis so that he can produce the dissociated state himself. The danger here is that the patient could become too reliant on the dissociation and run the risk of impairing the overall integration of his personality.

Pure Pain: Meares (1968) feels there is a technique that does not suffer from the disadvantages of the mechanisms described above. This approach allows the patient to experience pain in its pure form. Meares (1968, p. 56) states: "The pure sensation of pain, in the complete absence of any alert preoccupation with the part, loses its hurt." The process involves several psychological mechanisms. Through the atavistic regression of passive hypnosis the patient's level of anxiety is reduced along with a lessening of the psychological factors that exacerbate pain perception. The patient is aided to identify with the therapist who demonstrates that painful stimuli are not disturbing to him. By identifying with the therapist and introjecting his attitudes toward pain, the psychological embellishment of pain is reduced to a minimum. Meares (1968) then uses hypnosis combined with a simple conditioning paradigm in which the patient is subjected to increasingly severe stimuli which would ordinarily produce pain. Care is taken during this procedure to never actually hurt the patient. The patient is then taught autohypnosis and required to practice the procedure several times daily until he is proficient. The end result of this approach is a decreased level of anxiety and an increased threshold for pain perception.

Just as the variables involved in therapeutic process are today under careful scrutiny, the same questions are being asked relative to hypnosis. Gordon (1967) cites numerous studies indicating that it is not so much the hypnotic trance that has an ameliorating affect on pain, but rather the degree of involvement the hypnotist invests in the individual patient. He goes on to point out that uncontrolled interpersonal variables may have been at work in other studies referring to hypnosis and pain. Meares (1968) places emphasis on the central importance of the hypnotist as a model for identification in the treatment of the pain patient. A similar approach to the hypnotic control of pain is taken by Szasz (1957, p. 124) who states:

> The latter (hypnotist) deliberately sets himself up and imposes himself upon the subject as his sole object of legitimate interest. The ego is, in effect, commanded to abandon its investment at least for the time being, in all other objects and to focus exclusively on the hypnotist. As the ego relinquishes its interest in the body, affects pertaining to this orientation do not arise."

Hypnosis has proven to be a useful tool in the management of the pain patient. It has also proven useful with other types of rehabilitation patients where pain may or may not be a factor. Crasilneck and Hall (1970) have found hypnosis useful in working with patients who have suffered traumatic or vascular injury to the central nervous system. They feel that it is not generally known that hypnosis is useful in this type of case; but, in several instances, they report that the introduction of hypnosis into the treatment plan proved to be a turning point in the rehabilitation program. Lehew (1970) has found hypnosis a useful approach to pain control in patients with musculo-skeletal disorders. Not only does hypnosis aid in controlling pain in these patients, it also aids in muscle relaxation and allows for a higher level of activity with earlier recovery and rehabilitation. Hypnosis provided relief from pain in a variety of cases ranging from simple tension headaches to terminal cases of cancer (Hightower, 1966).

Hypnosis has been found particularly useful with the following types of patients according to Crasilneck and Hall (1970): (1) patients with poor motivation for rehabilitation; (2) patients displaying extreme anxiety, negativism, and depression in the face of rehabilitative efforts; (3) patients who had apparently given up their will to live or desire for recovery; and (4) patients who could not communicate effectively for either neurological or motivational reasons. This listing by Crasilneck and Hall (1970) reinforces the belief that hypnosis has a useful place in rehabilitation psychology.

Counseling and Psychotherapy

References to the use of counseling and psychotherapy in the treatment of the pain patient are scarce. There are, however, numerous references on the use of psychotherapeutic techniques with the physically disabled or rehabilitation patient. When the rehabilitation patient is not able to adapt to his disability after an appropriate period of "mourning," it is generally held that the disability has come to have private meaning for him. That the patient's efforts at adaptation have failed or proved to be maladaptive suggests a neurotic or infantile approach to resolving the conflicts precipitated or exacerbated by the disability, and it is in these cases that a psychotherapeutic relationship is indicated. Pain can interfere with readjustment, and chronic pain is often the result of an unsuccessful attempt at adjustment. As such, chronic pain is believed to have neurotic underpinnings. Chronic pain was defined earlier as pain disproportionate to the physical illness, or pain not related to the somatic pathology, or pain that does not respond to appropriate medical treatment. In referring to psychological treatment of the pain patient, it should be kept in mind that these are references to patients whose pain meets one or more of the above criteria. As such, pain can be considered as symptomatic of psychological conflict and psychotherapy can be appropriately indicated.

Speaking on psychotherapy for patients with physical symptoms and particularly pain, Rangell (1953) notes that the treatment may be brief or extensive depending on the nature of the underlying conflict situation. A few interviews may be sufficient if the conflict situation is relatively simple and easy to localize. On the other hand, if the conflict is deeply rooted in the character structure of the patient, a long-term depth approach to treatment may be necessary. Alexander (1950) points out that it is feasible for medical management and psychotherapy to be carried out concurrently. He does, however, note exceptions. When the organic illness is serious, even though believed to have strong psychosomatic components, psychotherapy must be limited to support. Also important is the fact that any purely medical "cure" of a psychosomatic illness is usually short-lived. In view of this, it is important that there be a good line of communication between the physician in charge of the medical aspects of the case and the psychotherapist.

Psychotherapy with the physically ill is unusually difficult and complex. Physical illness can have different meanings at different levels for the patient (Bard, 1959). Because of the nature of physical illness, there is a greater likelihood of countertransference manifestations on the part of the therapist. Redlich and Freedman (1966) point out the importance of trans-ference-countertransference factors in working with the medical patient. They also note that the medical practitioner seldom has sufficient psychological sophistication to be cognizant of these primarily unconscious factors that impinge on the doctor-patient relationship. Moreover, Redlich and Freedman feel that the medical non-psychiatric specialist is often reluctant to admit the presence of such factors in his relationships with patients. In essence, they question what the psychiatrist has to offer regarding bedside manners.

This is perhaps a good point to take a brief excursion into the realm of the psychologist's more traditional function—diagnostic testing—and its impli-cations for psychotherapy and management of the patient with physical problems. The important and illuminating role projective techniques play in understanding the psychological nature of physical illness is emphasized by Shorr (1955). The psychologist doing diagnostic testing with the physi-cally disabled patient is usually not concerned with differential diagnosis according to Bardach (1968). More important are questions regarding mo-tivation, the patient's view of his disability, and suggestions for aiding in the management and rehabilitation of this particular patient. Rusk (1953), in advocating an interdisciplinary approach to the rehabilitation patient, states:

> The main point is that after the patient's personality is thoroughly known by psychiatric examination, psychologic study, and social service investigation, then each problem, as it comes up, can be handled with the full knowledge of the limitations of the patient, psychologically and physically (p. 452).

Bardach (1968) illustrates how Maslow's hierarchical system of needs can be used to help determine the level of management and treatment approaches necessary for the rehabilitation patient. The depressed patient, for example, is temporarily functioning at a lower need level, probably safety and security needs, and needs supportive help while the patient whose prepotent needs appear to be for self-esteem and self-actualization is ready for long-term planning including vocational counseling or psychotherapy as indicated.

The increasing demand for relevant psychological treatment has led to increasing emphasis on short-term psychotherapy (Bellak and Small, 1965; Wolberg, 1965; Barten, 1971; Small, 1971). Short-term psychotherapy is characterized by goal-setting (usually symptom removal and restoration of an adequate level of psychological functioning), time limits, and differences in therapeutic techniques, the most important of which relate to transference phenomena. Stein, Murdaugh, and MacLeod (1971) have found that pa-tients who develop psychiatric difficulties in the aftermath of physical illness often respond quite well to short-term psychotherapy. These authors feel that brief psychotherapy is the treatment of choice for this type of patient. Stein, *et al.* (1971) suggest some principles that can prove useful in the psycho-therapeutic treatment of patients with physical illness. First, they note that treatment goals should be limited. The goals are usually limited to restoration

of psychological functioning to a previous, more adaptive level, social adaptation, and the relief of symptoms. Second, treatment should be initiated as soon after symptom manifestation as possible. Third, treatment should focus on the precipitating stress, and fourth, there should be a good deal of flexibility in the treatment program. Stein, *et al.,* also point out the importance of formulating the clinical material early when attempting brief therapy. Here again guidelines are offered; useful themes to focus on are denial, narcissistic injury, and the patient's cognitive understanding of the illness. Cobb (1962) also emphasizes the importance of clearing up any misconceptions the patient may have about his illness as one of the initial aspects of counseling with medical patients.

Sector psychotherapy, a procedure delineated by Deutsch and Murphy (1955), has its theoretical origins in psychoanalysis. Unlike psychoanalysis, sector psychotherapy is goal-limited and the therapist takes a more active role. This approach seems particularly useful with psychosomatic complaints and with physical problems that have a neurotic component.

> We speak of sector psychotherapy as being goal-limited and planned because, as a rule, due to exigencies of time, one symptom or set of symptoms is taken and its relationship to figures in the past explored and linked up to figures in the present (Deutsch and Murphy, 1955b, p. 13).

In sector psychotherapy the positive transference is used to facilitate therapeutic understanding and associative anemnesis is substituted for free association. The idea is to come to a psychodynamic understanding of the symptoms by exploring relevant and recurrent themes in the patient's communications. The patient's communications have several meanings; some are conscious and others are unconscious. In addition, the patient usually communicates in a double language; one aspect is verbal and the other is somatic. It is important to keep the patient's communications focused on the set of symptoms or sector that is the problem area. The skilled therapist, by using associative exploration, can determine the psychodynamic picture underlying the set of symptoms by linking past conflicts with present conflicts and then communicates this insight to the patient. Especially relevant to this chapter are two case illustrations that demonstrate the psychodynamic picture underlying phantom pain (Deutsch and Murphy, 1955a). While it is impossible to present a cogent summary of these two detailed accounts, they do both demonstrate the importance of conflicts stemming from the early loss of an object (parent) and a preference in the patient for using denial as a means of getting around difficulties.

An Adlerian conception of pain has been given by Waldman (1968). He sees pain as a "friction." While he does not address himself to the rehabilitation patient (he refers to the hysteric and the malingerer), the motives for pain are consistent with some of the previous theoretical explanations. Pain is seen by Waldman as "a tactic in the evasion of life's obligations and responsibilities" (p. 490). This bears similarity to the motives of *l'homme douloureux,* Szasz's (1968) painful person. The psychotherapeutic approach to pain as a fiction involves interpreting the significance and meaning of the pain to the patient.

Actually, the majority of rehabilitation patients present no serious psychopathology, and intensive psychotherapy is usually not indicated. Fishman (1962) sees psychotherapeutic assistance sought most often because a patient's motivation is insufficient for progress through the rehabilitation program. The psychotherapist can often facilitate the patient's progress. Neff and Weiss (1965) suggest a tandem approach when the patient is resisting efforts at vocational rehabilitation. While adjustment to a disability within the rehabilitation setting may be a major achievement for some patients, another crisis can arise when the patient is faced with aspects of the rehabilitation program that indicate he is coming ever-closer to re-entering the outside world. The prospect of returning to a world of relatively nondisabled people poses a new threat to the rehabilitation patient. It is at this point that the psychotherapist can provide warmth and support, essentially become a mother-figure while the vocational counselor maintains a more realistic, fatherly orientation urging the patient to test his resources against reality. Neff and Weiss (1965, p. 818) state: "This mother-father tandem, in relation to the patient-client tandem, sometimes facilitates more rapid progress because the role division minimizes the intensification of resistance."

A somewhat existential approach to working with the physically disabled is offered by Kir-Stimon (1970). He feels that it is not the specific nature of the disease that is important but the way it has changed the patient's relationship to himself and his world. Physical disability can have a devastating effect on one's self-concept, and the task of the patient is to truly be his "self" in relation to both himself and the world about him. Often the first real interpersonal test the patient can make of his own worth as a person is with his therapist or counselor. On this point Kir-Stimon (1970, p. 74) writes:

> . . . communication must be on a one-to-one level, not as able-bodied to disabled, or doctor to patient. The encounter is one in an existential sense between one human being and another with commitment on both sides.

This is essentially a core factor in psychotherapy with all individuals— i.e., the variables of therapist congruence and genuineness that have been found of therapeutic value across virtually all psychotherapeutic modalities. Kir-Stimon goes on to state, "How free the patient becomes to release and handle his suffering will depend in great deal on how free we feel to work with him" (1970, p. 74). A somewhat similar approach is suggested by Cobb (1962) in working with the terminal cancer patient, a patient that often has a great deal of pain. While many counselors and therapists are uncomfortable with the terminal patient, all that is required is often a real, warm relationship. The psychologist can be effective in that, as an empathetic and, when appropriate, sympathetic individual, he can be with the patient and share the patient's fears, dreads, and so on. Possibly the correct role in this context is not so much that of therapist or counselor as it is that of "person." The degree of variance between being a "therapist" and being a "person" is certainly food for thought.

The schools of thought briefly represented in this section on counseling and psychotherapy have ranged from a psychoanalytic orientation to a humanistic, somewhat Rogerian, framework. Such therapeutic diversity may be unexpected in a chapter that offers primarily a psychoanalytic approach to the theory of pain. Such is the nature of theory. Many authors have commented on the fact that our theoretical systems of personality and psychopathology have advanced far beyond our capability to apply them therapeutically. As such, a broad range of approaches needs to be considered. This is especially true in rehabilitation psychology where there is no good overall integration of theory extant. Consequently, in the applied setting, the pragmatist has probably fared better than the purist. To those who would object to this tacit advocation of an eclectic, or maybe practical is a better word, stance because of its "unscientific" quality, Guntrip's (1971) remark that to be orthodox is unscientific would seem appropriate. It seems that to be effective with the pain patient is much more important at this time than the degree to which a therapist confines himself to the tenets of a particular theoretical system.

Behaviorism and Similar Approaches

Behaviorism had its beginnings with the work of Watson (1913). While Watson's classic case, little Albert, was a paradigm for neurotic symptom formation, there was little interest in the therapeutic application of behavioral principles prior to the late 1940's. The field received its first real impetus when Lindsley (1960) published a paper on the application of operant principles to chronic schizophrenia, and Wolpe (1954) published his reciprocal inhibition technique. In 1958 Eysenck applied the name "behavior therapy" to the new learning theory approaches to personality and psychopathology. Since the 1950's, the field of behavior therapy and behavior modification has been making rapid progress in a variety of psychological areas including rehabilitation psychology. Behavioral approaches have made advances in two interrelated areas. The first is the treatment of the individual patient. The second area is more of a training function in which a variety of health and allied medical personnel are taught principles of behavior that are related to the total care of the patient.

Reviewing the use of behavior modification techniques in rehabilitation, Michael (1970) notes that the disabled patient finds many of his previous reinforcement opportunities are no longer available. In addition, there are likely to be new punishment contingencies, the most notable being the pain that often accompanies a physical disability. Because of the wide individual differences that occur in reaction to pain, it is believed that pain can have a significant operant component. Pain that has an organic basis or pain that is appropriate for a specific physical disability can also take on instrumental value because of its potency in aiding the patient to manipulate his environment. Fordyce, Fowler, and DeLateur (1968) point out that, because of the responses others make to a patient's complaints of pain, the environment can be shaped in such a way that pain behavior is actually reinforced. Fordyce, Fowler, Lehmann, and DeLateur (1968) define "pain behavior" as the operant behavior by which we become aware of another person's pain. The above authors believe that the practice of providing pain relieving drugs on demand may also serve to maintain pain behavior. The alteration of ward practices so that drugs were administered only on a regular time basis instead of on demand was found to considerably reduce pain behavior. It should be noted that when the patient can function without his "pain behavior," he is much more open to the rehabilitation efforts of the staff.

Behavior therapy has also proved to be a useful adjunct in treating the patient with neurological disease. Di Scipio and Feldman (1971), while recognizing that a suspected or known brain lesion is usually a counterindication to behavior therapy, report a successful case study where behavior therapy combined with physical therapy proved effective after the latter alone failed. The behavior therapy consisted of muscle relaxation training and systematic dessensitization. In this case, severe anxiety resulting in a fear of walking complicated the attempts at physical rehabilitation. Relaxation techniques have proved valuable in a variety of problems. Bobey and Davidson (1970) found that relaxation techniques are the most effective psychological technique for altering pain tolerance.

An experimental area that is presently making inroads in applied areas is bio-feedback. Over the past decade or so, there has been a proliferation of research that indicates that a variety of autonomic responses, previously believed to be beyond any voluntary control, can be manipulated by operant procedures. Gannon and Sternbach (1971), using operant alpha conditioning techniques, had moderate success in treating a patient who had suffered for years with severe headaches. The patient was trained to induce a high alpha state and when he was able to do so, he reported symptomatic improvement. It was noted in this study that, if the patient already had a headache, he was unable to concentrate enough to induce high alpha. While this study is far from definitive, the authors do feel this area could prove valuable in pain control. The implications of biofeedback for rehabilitation and, particularly psychosomatic medicine, are monumental. Operant techniques, particularly those involving bio-feedback, may eventually be a major treatment mode in a variety of medical fields.

Operant procedures have proved useful in pain control (Fordyce *et al.*, 1968; Gannon *et al.*, 1971), incontinence (Wagner and Paul, 1970; Tomlinson, 1970) and a variety of fears related to somatic functions (Furst and Cooper, 1970; Gentry, 1970; Di Scipio *et al.*, 1971). The earlier reference to

Miller (1951) and his belief that it is usually the fear component of the pain-fear reaction that is conditioned is important in considering the value of behavior therapy for somatic phobias. The patient with a physical disability, especially if it is painful, is more likely to have increased somatic concerns that can reach phobic proportions. Desensitization procedures provide a heuristic technique for dealing with problems of this nature.

Again, an eclectic position is going to be advocated. Behavior therapy has been shown to be particularly useful when the problems and symptoms involved can be well-defined and well-localized. For the rehabilitation counselor who is attempting work with a client exhibiting pain behavior, a first question should refer to the nature of the gain that the client can receive from his behavior. While the counselor should not appear overly suspicious of the patient's complaints, it is important to remember that all behavior is motivated and that this adage holds true for much of pain behavior. By exploring the nature of the client's pain complaints, his beliefs regarding his pain, and his present and future goals relative to his perception of his disability, the counselor can usually gain insight into the specific reinforcement contingencies that serve to maintain pain behavior. By doing so, the counselor can gain some understanding of the depth of the problem and feel more confident in making a disposition of the case, whether it be a decision to try to help this client through the problem, a decision to refer him for more intensive professional help, or whatever.

When the counselor attempts to work with the client, an interesting approach is offered by Woody (1971). This approach, called psychobehavioral counseling, allows the counselor, on the basis of his own philosophy of man, to adopt either a psychodynamic or a behavioral frame of reference but yet remain cognizant of the important therapeutic variables delineated by both schools of thought. In working with the client, the types of behavior demonstrated by the client, be they in action or in words, often are the best indicators of the severity of the pain problem. A Rogerian approach suggests that the counselor let the client lead the way. A behavioral approach suggests that the behavior should lead the way. A combination of these two approaches in the counseling situation—i.e., letting the client lead the way and observing his behavior—will usually stand the counselor on good ground and often lead to successful short-term counseling.

The mental hospital as a therapeutic community is a well-known concept. The same concept has value for the general and rehabilitation hospital. Shontz (1962) notes the value of using the hospital as a therapeutic community for the chronically ill. Neff and Weiss (1965, p. 815) state: "While individual therapy or counseling may be required, the treatment process is at least as much involved with the provision of an appropriate psychological environment which will assist the patient to overcome his feelings of deprivation, loss, and self-derogation." The concept of a psychologically healthy environment for the rehabilitation patient is implicit in many of the cited behavioral studies—i.e., much of the overall program is carried out by the nursing staff and their aides. This is inevitable because (1) most hospital services are overloaded, and (2) it is the nursing staff that has the most day-to-day involvement with the patient. In the psychiatric area, there has been considerable attention given to the role of nursing and ancillary services in the overall management of the patient within the hospital setting (Ayllon and Michael, 1959; Daniels, 1970). It would seem that more and more attention will be given to the role of nurses, attendants, and aides in the total treatment plan of the rehabilitation patient. This is an area where the psychologist is ideally suited for providing staff training. This seems to be a trend in that the psychologist is finding more and more demands for his services in the training of other professionals and sub-professionals in the psychological aspects of hospitalization and the efficacious management of patient communities.

SUMMARY

There is considerable need for a psychologically based theory of pain. The fact that pain is so susceptible to a variety of psychological manipulations suggests that pain often has a significant psychological component. Chronic or intractable pain is a deterrent to rehabilitation. It affects motivation, leads to withdrawal, results in somatic preoccupation, and generally prevents the patient from engaging in activities of a rehabilitative nature.

Considerable attention has been given in this chapter to the psychoanalytic aspects of pain, particularly the psychic meanings of pain and the ego mechanisms involved. This approach appears to offer the broadest and most comprehensive psychological explanation of pain. While it is acknowledged that pain can have a legitimate organic basis, it is pointed out that chronic or intractable pain often has psychoneurotic components. Pain has traditionally been dichotomized into the two categories of organic and psychogenic pain. The value of this dichotomy has been questioned; it can lead to errors in patient management. From the patient's standpoint, pain hurts; and its etiological base is not important. Phenomenologically, all pain can be regarded as legitimate. The patient or client is trying to communicate something. Pain can have a signal function relative to the workings of the body. On this function, numerous instances can be found where pain, as a signal, is too late. Pain can also serve as a warning to the ego that the overall integrity of the personality is in danger. A variety of interpersonal meanings can also be found for pain; these range from a cry for help to a demand for attention and retribution. The personal and private meanings pain can have for the individual are related to his past history. Many of the neurotic embellishments given to pain have their origins in childhood; surgery of any kind can have a marked affect on the child's attitudes toward illness and pain.

A psychoanalytic theory, utilizing the concept of object relationships, for pain was discussed and applied to phantom phenomena. Phantom limb appears to be an almost universal reaction to loss of limb. From a psychological standpoint, phantom limb is the result of the ego's attempt at adaptation to the loss. Essentially, a sudden loss is converted into a gradual loss allowing time for a new ego-body integration or body image. Phantom pain, however, is a relative rarity and, once established, often becomes chronic. Phantom pain appears to be the result of the ego's attempts at resolution going awry with subsequent maladjustment. In addition to the psychological explanation of phantom phenomena, two primarily neurological approaches, peripheral theory and central theory, were briefly noted. Central theory with its emphasis on the somatosensory organization of the cortex appears to be the more promising of the two approaches. The complementary nature of central theory and psychodynamic theory was also discussed.

In reviewing psychological approaches to the management of pain, an attempt was made to survey all primarily psychological treatments that could conceivably be within the purview of the psychologist or counselor. Relative to pain control, hypnosis has the most extensive literature. The advantages and disadvantages of various hypnotic mechanisms were discussed. The combination of hypnosis and simple conditioning to reduce anxiety and raise the level of pain tolerance appears to be the most efficacious. A variety of psychotherapeutic and counseling techniques were presented; and, for the individual counselor, the appropriate technique is primarily a matter of personal preference, psychological sophistication, and training. Behavioral approaches have been making headway in the treatment of the pain patient. Muscle relaxation training and, when indicated, systematic desensitization have proven effective with a variety of physical problems including pain. Newer techniques that have an essentially operant base such as the various forms of bio-feedback show much promise in rehabilitation work.

In counseling the pain patient, the counselor should always remember that the client is also a person and that the relationship is of therapeutic value. Genuineness and congruence on the part of the counselor or therapist have been found again and again to be potent factors in the therapeutic process. The counselor who is open to the client's experiences and feelings, open to his own feelings and reactions, and feels free to share the phenomenology of the relationship, will find that he can be helpful to the pain patient and other clients with physical and psychological difficulties.

REFERENCES

Alexander, F.: *Psychosomatic Medicine.* New York, Norton, 1950.

Ayllon, T. and Michael, J.: The psychiatric nurse as a behavioral engineer. *Journal of the Experimental Analysis of Behavior, 2:*323-334, 1959.

Barber, T. X.: Toward a theory of pain: Relief of chronic pain by prefrontal leucotomy, opiates, placebos, and hypnosis. *Psychological Bulletin, 56:*430-460, 1959.

Bard, M.: Implications of analytic psychotherapy with the physically ill. *American Journal of Psychotherapy, 13:*860-971, 1959.

Bardach, J. L.: Psychological assessment procedures as indicators of patients' abilities to meet tasks in rehabilitation. *Journal of Counseling Psychology, 15:*471-475, 1968.

Barten, H. H. (Ed.): *Brief Therapies*. New York, Behavioral Publications, 1971.

Bellak, L. and Small, L.: *Emergency Psychotherapy and Brief Psychotherapy*. New York, Grune and Stratton, 1965.

Bobey, M. J., and Davidson, P. O.: Psychological factors affecting pain tolerance. *Journal of Psychosomatic Research, 14:*371-376, 1970.

Cobb, B.: Cancer. In Garrett, J. F. and Levine, E. S. (Eds.), *Psychological Practices with the Physically Disabled*. New York, Columbia University Press, 1962.

Cooper, I. S., and Braceland, F.J.: Psychosomatic aspects of pain. *Medical Clinics of North America*, pp. 981-993, July 1950.

Crasilneck, H. B., and Hall, J. A.: The use of hypnosis in the rehabilitation of complicated vascular and post-traumatic neurological patients. *The International Journal of Clinical and Experimental Hypnosis, 17*(3):145-159, 1970.

Daniels, D. N.: Milieu Therapy. In Rosenbaum, C. P., *The Meaning of Madness*. New York, Science House, 1970.

Deutsch, F. and Murphy, W. F.: *The Clinical Interview*. Vol. I.: *Diagnosis*. New York, International Universities Press, 1955a.

Deutsch, F. and Murphy, W. F.: *The Clinical Interview*. Vol. II.: *Therapy*. New York, International Universities Press, 1955b.

Di Scipio, W. J. and Feldman, M. C.: Combined behavior therapy and physical therapy in the treatment of a fear of walking. *Journal of Behavior Therapy and Experimental Psychiatry, 2:*151-152, 1971.

Edwards, W.: Recent research on pain perception. *Psychological Bulletin, 47:*449-474, 1950.

Ewalt, J. R., Randall, G. C. and Morris, H.: The phantom limb. *Psychosomatic Medicine, 9:*118-123, 1947.

Eysenck, H. J.: *The Scientific Study of Personality*. New York, Wiley, 1958.

Fenichel, O.: The ego and the affects (From *Collected Papers of*). New York, Norton, Vol. 2, pp. 215-227, 1954.

Fenichel, O.: *The Psychoanalytic Theory of Neurosis*. New York, Norton, 1945.

Fischer, H. K.: The problem of pain from the psychiatrist's viewpoint. *Psychosomatics, 9:*319-325, 1968.

Fishman, S.: Amputation. In Garrett, J. F. and Levine, Edna S. (Eds.), *Psychological Practices with the Physically Disabled*. New York, Columbia University Press, 1962.

Flescher, J.: On neurotic disorders of sensibility and body scheme: A bioanalytic approach to pain, fear and repression. *International Journal of Psycho-Analysis, 29:*156-162, 1948.

Fordyce, W. E., Fowler, R. S. and DeLateur, B.: An application of behavior modification technique to a problem of chronic pain. *Behaviour Research and Therapy, 6:*105-107, 1968.

Fordyce, W. E., Fowler, R. S., Lehmann, J. F. and DeLateur, B.: Some implications of learning in problems of chronic pain. *Journal of Chronic Diseases, 21:*179-190, 1968.

Freeman, T.: *Psychopathology of the Psychoses*. New York, International Universities Press, 1969.

Freud, A.: The role of bodily illness in the mental life of children. *The Psychoanalytic Study of the Child* (Vol. VII). New York, International Universities Press, 1952.

Freud, S.: *Inhibitions, Symptoms, and Anxiety.* London, Hogarth, 1948.

Freud, S.: *An Outline of Psychoanalysis.* New York, Norton, 1949.

Furst, J. B. and Cooper, A.: Combined use of imaginal and interoceptive stimuli in desensitizing fear of heart attacks. *Journal of Behavior Therapy and Experimental Psychiatry, 1*:87-89, 1970.

Gannon, L. and Sternbach, R. A.: Alpha enhancement as a treatment for pain: A case study. *Journal of Behavior Therapy and Experimental Psychiatry, 2*:209-213, 1971.

Gentry, W. D.: In vivo desensitization of an obsessive cancer fear. *Journal of Behavior Therapy and Experimental Psychiatry, 1*:315-318, 1970.

Gordon, J. E. (Ed.): *Handbook of Clinical and Experimental Hypnosis.* New York, Macmillan, 1967.

Guntrip, H.: *Psychoanalytic Theory, Therapy, and the Self.* New York, Basic Books, 1971.

Hall, C. S. and Lindzey, G.: *Theories of Personality* (2nd ed.). New York, Wiley, 1970.

Hartmann, H.: The mutual influences in the development of ego and id. *The Psychoanalytic Study of the Child* (Vol. VII). New York, International Universities Press, 1952.

Hartmann, H.: *Ego Psychology and the Problem of Adaptation* (trans. by David Rapaport). New York, International Universities Press, 1958.

Hightower, P. R.: The control of pain. *American Journal of Clinical Hypnosis, 9*:67-70, 1966.

Hoffer, W.: Development of the body ego. *The Psychoanalytic Study of the Child* (Vol. V). New York, International Universities Press, 1950.

Hoffer, W.: The mutual influences in the development of ego and id: Earliest stages. *The Psychoanalytic Study of the Child* (Vol. VII). New York, International Universities Press, 1952.

Kir-Stimon, W.: Counseling with the severely handicapped: Encounter and commitment. *Psychotherapy: Theory, Research, and Practice, 7*:70-74, 1970.

Kolb, L. C.: *The Painful Phantom: Psychology, Physiology, Treatment.* Springfield, Thomas, 1954.

Krupp, N. E.: Psychiatric implications of chronic and crippling illness. *Psychosomatics, 9*:109-113, 1968.

Lehew, J. L., III: The use of hypnosis in the treatment of musculo-skeletal disorders. *American Journal of Clinical Hypnosis, 13*:131-134, 1970.

Lindner, R.: A seminar in doctor-patient relationships in a rehabilitation medicine setting. *Psychosomatics, 10*:354-359, 1969.

Lindsley, O. R.: Characteristics of the behavior of chronic psychotics as revealed by free-operant conditioning methods. *Diseases of the Nervous System,* Monograph Supplement, *21*:66-78, 1960.

McDaniel, J. W.: *Physical Disability and Human Behavior.* New York, Pergamon, 1969.

Mead, G. H.: *Mind, Self, and Society.* Chicago, University of Chicago Press, 1962.

Meares, A.: Psychological mechanisms in the relief of pain by hypnosis. *American Journal of Clinical Hypnosis, 11*:55-57, 1968.

Melzack, R.: The perception of pain. *Scientific American, 204*(2):41-49, 1961.

Melzack, R. and Scott, T. H.: The effects of early experience on the response to pain. *Journal of Comparative and Physiological Psychology, 50*:155-161, 1957.

Melzack, R. and Wall, P. D.: Pain mechanisms: A new theory. *Science, 150*:971-979, 1957.

Michael, J.: Rehabilitation. In Neuringer, C. and Michael, J. (Eds.), *Behavior Modification in Clinical Psychology*. New York, Appleton-Century-Crofts, 1970.

Miller, N. E.: Learnable drives and rewards. In Stevens, S. S. (Ed.), *Handbook of Experimental Psychology*. New York, Wiley, 1951.

Neff, W. S. and Weiss, S. A.: Psychological aspects of disability. In Wolman, B. B. (Ed.), *Handbook of Clinical Psychology*. New York, McGraw-Hill, 1965.

Pattie, F. A.: A brief history of hypnotism. In Gordon, J. E. (Ed.), *Handbook of Clinical and Experimental Hypnosis*. New York, Macmillan, 1967.

Rangell, L.: Psychiatric aspects of pain. *Psychosomatic Medicine, 15*:22-37, 1953.

Redlich, F. C. and Fredman, D. X.: *The Theory and Practice of Psychiatry*. New York, Basic Books, 1966.

Rusk, H. A.: Rehabilitation and convalescence: The third phase of medical care. In Weider, A. (Ed.), *Contributions toward Medical Psychology*, Vol. I. New York, Ronald Press, 1953.

Rusk, H. A.: *Rehabilitation Medicine*. St. Louis, Mosby, 1958.

Sacerdote, P.: Theory and practice of pain control in malignancy and other protracted or recurring painful illnesses. *International Journal of Clinical and Experimental Hypnosis, 18*:160-180, 1970.

Schilder, P.: *Medical Psychology*. New York, International Universities Press, 1953.

Schneck, J. D. (Ed.): *Hypnosis in Modern Medicine*. Springfield, Thomas, 1953.

Serafetinides, E. A.: Neuropsychiatric aspects of pain. In Soulairac, A., Cahn, J. and Charpentier, J. (Eds.), *Pain*. New York, Academic Press, 1968.

Shontz, F. C.: Severe chronic illness. In Garrett, J. F. and Levine, E. S. (Eds.), *Psychological Practices with the Physically Disabled*. New York, Columbia University Press, 1962.

Shorr, E.: The emergence of psychological problems in patients requiring prolonged hospitalization. In Harrower, M. (Ed), *Medical and Psychological Teamwork in the Care of the Cronically Ill*. Springfield, Thomas, 1955.

Simmel, M.: Phantoms in patients with leprosy and in elderly digital amputees. *American Journal of Psychology, 69*:529-545, 1956.

Simmel, M.: Phantoms, phantom pain and "denial." *American Journal of Psychotherapy, 13*:603-613, 1959.

Small, L.: *The Briefer Psychotherapies*. New York, Brunner-Mazel, 1971.

Soulairac, A.: On an experimental approach to pain. In Soulairac, A., Cahn, J. and Charpentier, J. (Eds.), *Pain*. New York, Academic Press, 1968.

Stein, M.: The what, how and why of psychosomatic medicine. In Offer, D. and Freedman, D. X. (Eds.), *Modern Psychiatry and Clinical Research*. New York, Basic Books, 1972.

Stein, E. H., Murdaugh, J. and MacLeod, J. A.: Brief psychotherapy of psychiatric reactions to physical illness. In Barten, H. H. (Ed.), *Brief Therapies*. New York, Behavioral Publications, 1971.

Stokvis, B.: The application of hypnosis in organic diseases. *Journal of Clinical and Experimental Hypnosis, 2*:79-82, 1956.

Szasz, T. S.: *Pain and Pleasure*. New York, Basic Books, 1957.

Szasz, T. S.: The painful person. *The Journal-Lancet, 88*:18-22, 1968.

Tomlinson, J. R.: The treatment of bowel retention by operant procedures: A case study. *Journal of Behavior Therapy and Experimental Psychiatry, 1*:83-85, 1970.

Wagner, B. R. and Paul, G. L.: Reduction of incontinence in chronic mental patients: A pilot project. *Journal of Behavior Therapy and Experimental Psychiatry. 1*:29-38, 1970.

Waldman, R. D.: Pain as fiction: A perspective on psychotherapy and responsibility.

American Journal of Psychotherapy, 22:481-490, 1968.

Watson, J. B.: Psychology as the behaviorist views it. *Psychological Review, 20*:158-177, 1913.

Weinstein, S.: Neuropsychological studies of the phantom. In Benton, A. L. (Ed.), *Contributions to Clinical Neuropsychology*. Chicago, Aldine, 1969.

Wolberg, L. R. (Ed.): *Short-Term Psychotherapy*. New York, Grune and Stratton, 1965.

Wolpe, J.: Reciprocal inhibition as the main basis of psychotherapeutic effects. *AMA Archives of Neurological Psychiatry, 72*:205-226, 1954.

Woody, R. H.: *Psychobehavioral Counseling and Therapy*. New York, Appleton-Century-Crofts, 1971.

Chapter 19

MOTIVATION: THE GREATEST CHALLENGE TO REHABILITATION

G. Frank Lawlis

REHABILITATION is a process of psychological growth, and as such a certain amount of an imbalance of homeostasis occurs. The client has to want to help himself; otherwise, regardless of how much a rehabilitation counselor, nurse, doctor, or therapist of any kind wants to help him, he will not reach success. A cut finger or broken bone may mend without a client's concern, but rehabilitation demands a certain amount of desire on the client's part to overcome his limitations and re-educate himself to his world.

The problem of motivating people is a universal one, and it is not limited to rehabilitation. The term is applicable to any situation where one person desires to influence the behavior or actions of others, including child training, education, politics, advertising, courtship, and psychotherapy.

The concept of motivation has been a central aspect of the dynamics systems of psychology from Freudian psychoanalysis to neo-behaviorism. Littman (1958) pointed out that it developed out of a recognition of the inadequacy of the sensory psychology of the last century, and he referred to the concept of motivation as constituting a revolution in psychology. While there are various conceptions of motivation in psychology, there is agreement upon the necessity for such a concept. There has been as little agreement, however, upon identifying the motives underlying behavior as there was upon listing the instincts of which motives seem to be the successors.

THEORETICAL BACKGROUND

The concept of motivation underlies all approaches to the analysis, understanding, and control of behavior. To the man on the street, psychology has both the answers to why he behaves as he does and the ability to control his behavior; and it is true that behavior can be directed and controlled to some extent in some situations. We can condition or influence both animals and children by reward and punishment. In fact, Skinner (1971) has made a plea in his book, *Beyond Freedom and Dignity,* for a society in which everyone can be happily engaged in constructive activity as a result of operant conditioning. His reasoning indicates that once a rational system of reward

346

and punishment can be established for society, then the individuals will not be frustrated by irrational goals. Consequently, there would be no need for the individual to seek freedom from the system because he would be happy there.

While the danger of complete control of behavior by psychological manipulation is presently very distant, the implications of such control are significant (Patterson, 1959). We are interested not in controlling or manipulating people without their knowledge or awareness and consent but with helping them to become aware of and to accept voluntarily different goals or changed behavior. Operant conditioning appears to be capable of inducing some interesting, if limited, changes without the knowledge and cooperation of the individual; but most of us are more interested in voluntary changes in behavior.

So there is left the problem of influencing people to do what they should do, what is obviously good for them, what society wants them to do, and what would benefit society, without negating their freedom of choice. On the physiological level this may appear to be simple—the organism is hungry, so it reacts to food or searches for food (Littman, 1958); but experiments too numerous to be reviewed here indicate that even at basic level, it is not so simple. What if the organism is experiencing two or more different needs? Which determines its behavior?

Is there a hierarchy of psychological needs as Maslow depicts (1954)? Or is there a single, dominant need, which subsumes all other needs? Freud was attracted by the latter idea and thought that he had found this need in the sex instinct or libido. Freud was not actually a monist, in spite of this, since he also recognized an ego instinct; and his theory of instincts went through many changes (Bibring, 1958).

Adler (1965) depicts a feeling of inferiority as the prime motivational construct by which organisms direct their energies; however, the more existential theorists, such as Viktor Frankl (1959), consider the desire to find meaning in life as the energy force. Maslow (1954), as we noted above, finds a hierarchy of motivational needs, such as physiological factors, safety, love, belongingness, and self-actualization. Cattell, *et al.* (1964), considers motivational drives to be factors which he has found in his psychological analysis researches, such as fear, mating, narcism, pugnacity, and assertiveness.

Perhaps the most pervasive influence in today's society is the phenomenologist's solution to the primary motivation of man. Simply stated, quoting Combs and Snygg (1959, p. 45), it is this: "From birth to death the maintenance of the phenomenal self is the most pressing, the most crucial, if not the only task of existence . . . Man seeks both to maintain and enhance his perceived self." All other needs, drives, and motives can be subsumed under this basic, universal need. It includes, but it is more than, the preservation of the organism. Thus the preservation of the phenomenal self may at times supersede the preservation of the biological organism. This concept of motivation not only has simplicity and even the virtue of parsimony; it clarifies or eliminates the confusion which we face when we try to understand the multiplicity of drives and motives, often contradictory or opposed to each other, which are attributed to human beings.

REVIEW OF THE LITERATURE

The concept of motivation is an ambiguous one to be sure; however, we can learn what conditions appear to be related to motivation in rehabilitation. Three areas of research are presented in the literature here reviewed: correlates of motivational indices in rehabilitation settings, correlates of motivational indices in counseling, and considerations of the term *remotivation,* or behavior modification techniques.

Correlates of Motivational Indices in Rehabilitation Settings

Numerous studies dealing with predictability as it relates to successful or unsuccessful outcomes in rehabilitation, have been conducted in recent years (Ayer, Thoreson, and Butler, 1966; Danielson, 1965; DeMonn, 1963; Drasgon and Dreher, 1965; Ehrle, 1962; Heilbrun and Jordan, 1968; Lesh, 1968; Lesser and Darling, 1953; McPhee and Maglry, 1960; Rabinowitz, Johnson, and Reilly, 1964; Sankovsky, 1968). One of the earliest studies dealing with the rehabilitation center dropout was undertaken by Wardlow (1964) at the Hot Springs Rehabilitation Center in Arkansas. Wardlow reported that approximately 30 percent of the clients enrolled dropped out of training before scheduled completion. Utilizing a questionnaire and selective intedviewing, he attempted to classify the reasons for self-termination for a nine-month period. For the sixty-four persons dropping out during this period, sixteen categories were established to "set forth what is believed to be the real reason why each of the . . . dropouts left the Center." *Homesickness* was reported to be the most frequent reason for self-termination, followed by *to enter employment, family problems,* and *inability to adjust to Center routine.* Less frequent reasons given were *financial difficulties, inability to learn,* and *lacking in motivation.*

While Wardlow's study was limited to a descriptive survey, it did succeed in focusing emphasis on the need for more sophisticated research and served as a prototype for a study later conducted by Sankovsky (1969) at the Pennsylvania Rehabilitation Center.

Sankovsky's study concentrated, as did Wardlow's, on the reason the individual gave for terminating his rehabilitation program. Sankovsky postulated that certain key constructs could be identified from the reasons given for leaving and that these would reveal the basic problem and needs of the individual precipitating the self-termination. He developed a matrix of categories based on reasons for leaving given by 238 self-terminators and classified them as follows:

1. *Dependency:* a strong attachment for home; homesickness.
2. *Dissatisfaction:* either client or parent dissatisfaction with services, policies, procedures, or progress at the Center.
3. *Emotional and adjustment reasons:* an inability to adjust to Center routine, a feeling of stress, an inability to identify with the handicapped population.
4. *Personality and family problems.*
5. *Lack of motivation.*
6. *Other.*

Four judges independently sorted the reasons given for leaving into the categories established, and achieved 91 percent agreement with the author. Of the total of 238 dropouts, 23 percent were classified as leaving because of homesickness or dependency; 21 percent, dissatisfaction; 22 percent, emotional and adjustment problems; 14 percent, personal and family problems; 4 percent, lack of motivation; and 16 percent, no reason given.

Sankovsky (1969) recommended that if the dropout rate is to be reduced, a method must be devised

> (1) to identify the potential dropouts within the first few days after admission or before, and (2) to provide intensive therapeutic programs to neutralize the tendency of these dropouts to self-terminate their programs of rehabilitation services (p. 28).

An attempt to satisfy the first of these recommendations was reported by Perlman (1968) in a recently completed study. Perlman extracted eighteen demographic variables and scores on the Minnesota Multiphasic Personality Inventory (MMPI) and Army General Classification Tests (AGCT) from the case records of 285 dropouts and 285 graduates from vocational training at the Pennsylvania Rehabilitation Center. Utilizing this data, he examined the feasibility of combining test data with selected demographic variables, with the objective of increasing predictive efficiency in the identification of potential dropouts. In addition, the problem of the development of a predictive model for the identification of potential dropouts was explored, using multivariate statistical methods.

Perlman reported that the psychometric data (MMPI and AGCT) failed to differentiate significantly between dropout and graduate, and it was excluded in the predictive phase of the study. He did report significant differentiation between the graduates and dropouts on the basis of five variables when they were subjected to discriminant analysis. The following five variables were retained in the final model as the most efficient for predictive purposes: (1) pre-selected training goal at entry; (2) sex; (3) age at entry to the PRC; (4) age at onset of disability; and (5) years of work experience. Predicted group membership for 570 clients resulted in 63.50 percent correct classification and 36.50 percent misclassification.

Perlman concluded that the prediction of dropouts, based on selected demographic variables, was a feasible approach and recommended cross-validation in other rehabilitation settings. He also suggested that additional demographic variables   not available for his study be investigated—e.g., socioeconomic factors, prior scholastic achievement.

Several related studies have directed themselves to attempting to define and describe the personality and motivational variables contributing to the behavior of rehabilitation clients, but the lack of consistency in findings and the inconclusiveness of results have added little knowledge of value to the rehabilitation practitioner. For example, several authors have attempted to establish some relationship between intelligence and rehabilitation outcome, but uniform agreement is still lacking. Lesser and Darling (1953) reported that, based on follow-up, proportionately more clients of average and above-average intelligence were found to be employed. A number of investigators —Ayer, Thoreson, and Butler (1966); Rabinowitz, Johnson, and Reilly (1964); Sankovsky (1968); and Perlman (1968)—concluded that there was no relationship between intelligence level and the ultimate rehabilitation outcome.

Other studies have been reported in which client interests were used to attempt to predict rehabilitation outcome. McMahon (1964), in a sample of eighty-eight clients who completed training and eighty-four clients who self-terminated their program, reported no significant differences on the Kuder Preference Record that would discriminate between completers and non-completers. Samuelson (1958), in a study of vocational school trainees, concluded that although some relationship existed between certain interests and subsequent achievement, the relationship was not significant and of limited usefulness for ultimate prediction.

The MMPI has been a favored instrument of a number of investigators in attempting to predict rehabilitation success or failure, but again the results have been contradictory or inconclusive. Ayer, Thoreson, and Butler (1966) reported that the Masculinity-Femininity Scale (MF), the Correction Scale (K), and the Psychopathic Deviate (Pd) Scales, in conjunction with intelligence and age at time of application, had significant beta weights in a regression equation for predicting rehabilitation success. None of the MMPI scale scores were found to be significantly predictive independently.

Sandness (1968) reported the MMPI pattern of Depression (D), Hysteria (Hy), and Psychopathic Deviate (Pd) Scales as approaching but not reaching significance in distinguishing the successful from the unsuccessful group. Perlman (1968) reported only one significant finding—the Schizophrenic (Sc) Scale for males as distinguishing between program completers and dropouts.

Despite the recognition of the critical importance and determinative influence of client motivation, only limited study has been devoted to attempting to define and describe specific motivational variables contributing to the behavior of rehabilitation clients. Many of the studies reported (Barry and Malinovsky, 1965; Danielson, 1965; Phillips, 1957; Suinn and Paulhe,

1966; Wispe, 1965) carry theoretical or conceptual significance, but relatively few have attempted to apply or assess predictive measures of client motivation.

Barry and Malinovsky (1965) have provided a singularly outstanding reference in their monograph, *Client Motivation for Rehabilitation: A Review,* which describes and discusses the concept of client motivation as used by various rehabilitation specialists. In summarizing this work, they state:

> It can be seen that the concept is used very broadly in most instances, sometimes to the extent of being **almost meaningless**. Research dealing with client motivation for rehabilitation in most cases has profited more from the more specific definition of client's behaviors and characteristics subsumed by the term motivation . . . There are few indications from the research that certain approaches or descriptive systems are less useful than others (p. 58).

In summary, a review and analysis of the literature concerning the problem of the rehabilitation center dropout, leads to several conclusions: (1) the state of research and investigation in this area exists at a rather elementary level and is largely exploratory—i.e., the comparative newness of comprehensive rehabilitation facilities and the subsequent development of the dropout problem have dictated that present research be basic, preliminary, and, in part, oriented toward eliminating certain areas of study while offering direction toward more feasible or productive areas; (2) that research on the handicapped, in relation to success or failure of rehabilitation efforts, has been primarily limited by the nature of the experimental design—that is, the unsuccessful client or the dropout is studied after he has terminated his program or comes to a standstill in progress, and the research approach has been to analyze whatever information was readily available; (3) there exists a need to supplement actuarial notions of success or failure with concepts "more explicitly related to social psychological models of the rehabilitation process itself" (Rabinowitz, Johnson, and Reilly, 1964, p. 7).

Correlates of Motivation in Counseling

The counselor is often asked to perform many tasks, and one of the most essential is to determine what personality dynamics are operating in an individual. On the basis of his judgments and through his counseling, the counselor can help the client readjust or integrate his life so that rehabilitation can be achieved. The questions arise: When is a person motivated? What dynamics underlie his performance?

Hughes (1960) has indicated that acceptance of one's disability is essential for happiness and mental health. Therefore, motivation could be defined as a drive for self-acceptance and a positive correlation to success in rehabilitation. Litman (1962) used this model and hypothesized strong positive relationships between the client's positive self-regard and self-acceptance with orthopedic rehabilitation procedures. In support of this theory, a negative self-concept was associated with performance below expectation for one-hundred disabled clients, whereas positive self-concept predicted good response to rehabilitation procedures.

Super (1957) and Small (1958) have pointed out that motivational problems often result when one's chosen occupation is not consistent with his aspirations, self-concept, or role expectations. In other words, the more incongruent an individual's goals are with his self-concept, the less able he is to move toward those goals. Reimonis (1964) supported this disparity model with his findings to the effect that achievement motivation varied directly with the disparity between life goals and present status. His study sample consisted of forty Veterans Administration domiciliary adults.

In this regard, Herzberg and Hamlin (1961) have presented a type of motivational theory that involved a motivational drive for personal growth. They considered a critical factor in psychotherapy to be an orientation for growth rather than an inverted pattern of seeking satisfaction toward environmental influences (hygiene factor).

Frantz (1962) designed a study to investigate the relevance of this theory to rehabilitation. Thirty clients (nineteen men and eleven women) undergoing physical medicine rehabilitation, were asked to describe in some detail four critical incidents—two of which helped and two of which interfered with their progress in rehabilitation. All of the critical incidents and related materials were classified as to whether they were growth oriented or environmentally oriented. Predictions made about the success or failure in rehabilitation of the group were compared against the Katz Index of Independence (Katz, 1959, 1963). The results confirmed the hypothesis that those clients with predominantly growth motivations were much more often successfully rehabilitated than clients with hygiene motivation.

Hamlin and Nemo (1962) also confirmed the theoretical position of growth orientation as predictive of rehabilitation with twenty-three improved patients, two who continued to work and live in a VA hospital, and twenty-three unimproved chronic schizophrenic patients. The improved schizophrenics obtained higher growth scores reflecting their tendency to seek satisfaction in self-actualizing experiences.

There have been several researchers who have found healthy attitudes and independency to be favorable to motivation in rehabilitation. Kelman (1962) observed that *improvers* in a nursing home were found to be generally more independent, to manifest less intellectual deterioration and less emotional instability, and to show more interest in the rehabilitation treatment as compared to the *worseners*.

Vernier, *et al.* (1961) reviewed a series of projects dealing with the psychological and social aspects of tuberculosis. One of their studies dealt with the quality of adaptation to hospitalization that showed that clients making the *best* adjustment to the hospital setting were older, more passive, and less intelligent than those clients judged by the staff as making poorer adaptations.

Paradoxical results with regard to rehabilitation outcome and passivity or dependency have been shown in two studies using the identical instrument, the Motivational Analysis Test (Cattell, 1964). In a discriminant analysis between seventy-five chronically unemployed and seventy-five stably employed males, Lawlis (1971) found that the chronically unemployed group was more fearful of personal relationships, generally more anxious, and characterized by less integrated or unrealistic motivation in attempts to deal with their aspirations as individuals. Even more noteworthy, the most predictive variable of employment was high self-sentiment in job stability.

Contrary to these findings, Little (1970) found that the most predictive variable in determining rehabilitation *failure* in the Hot Springs Rehabilitation Center was high self-sentiment. Other studies, such as described and demonstrated by Tiffany, Cowan, and Tiffany (1970) in their excellent book, *The Unemployed,* have consistently shown that when non-institutionalized criteria are utilized as motivational indices (employment, study work habits, achievement of important life goals, etc.), independence and high self-concept predict motivation toward these goals. On the other hand, when institutional indices (adaptation to rules, following a training plan, etc.) are utilized as criteria for motivational indices, dependency and passivity are strong predictors of success. We wonder what goals are considered to be indicative of *good* motivation.

Pfonts, Wallace, and Jenkins (1963) examined the nature of the relationship between the referral source of 218 clients in an adult psychiatric outpatient clinic, the client's motivation for treatment, and the extent of contact with the clinic. Clients were rated as minimally, moderately, or strongly motivated on the basis of a verbalized desire for help, appropriateness of their expectations regarding help, and their efforts to obtain help. The higher the level of motivation, the greater was the probability that the client would make progress in treatment. The study further suggested a causal relationship between the positive and negative feelings of a client toward his actual referral source, and his subsequent use of the clinic. Lief, Lief, Warren, and Heath's (1961) results replicated the implication that minimally motivated clients with negative attitudes toward their referral sources tended to refuse services, while minimally motivated clients with positive attitudes toward their referral sources accepted services.

Smith and Fink (1963) attempted to examine the degree to which measures of orientation, intelligence, personal adjustment, social adjustment, and motivation were related to improvement in physical mobility and independent living. Utilizing a multiple regression coefficient, they found motivation and personal adjustment to be the best indicators of rehabilitation potential.

The conclusions of the previous research review appear to be the following: (1) that self-concept theory and its implications to the various constructs of dependency, growth needs, etc., are relevant to the nature of the goals to which we ascribe for rehabilitation clients; (2) that mental health correlates (ego strength, lack of depression, etc.) are predictors of continued good outlook and performance; and (3) that *motivation* is a vague term even though we use the term in a multitude of models.

Remotivation Tactics

There have been some attempts to remotivate clients for rehabilitation through the means of behavior modification techniques. The broad category of behavior modification involves a specific behavior to be either rewarded or punished consistently, thereby increasing or decreasing the frequency of that act.

When we consider motivated behavior, psychologists usually make a distinction between goal attainment and goal-directed behavior. For example, if a man is hungry and consumes food, he is manifesting goal attainment. However, what mannerisms he manifests in order to get the food is goal-directed behavior. We have considered goal attainment as correlates to motivation thus far in this review, with terms such as *rehabilitated, employed,* etc.; however, goals are difficult to change or measure and consequently uncontrollable by the counselor. On the other hand, if the individual goal is known, goal-directed behavior can be influenced by successive steps toward that goal. Thus an individual can be remotivated or modified to behave in specific ways in order to achieve his goals.

Four terms have been used by Birch and Veroff (1968) to identify sources of effect on goal-directed action: *availability, expectancy, incentive,* and *motive. Availability* means simply that the individual must perceive that his goal can be met within his capability. The past history of the individual is important to availability in at least two ways. First, we have the concept of habit in which a course of action is most likely to occur. This is extremely relevant to that person's past history of successful goal attainment in that a person tends to attain a goal in very similar ways to those he has learned in the past. Interestingly, an individual habitually reacts to the goals he recognizes, whether or not they are efficient. Second, the likelihood that a goal is suggested to a person should be a function of the overall frequency with which the goal has been found relevant in the past. For example, the goal of vocational placement for a welfare client may not have been too relevant or important to him in the past. This history would prove to be a factor in his future motivation.

Expectancy is the perceived probability by the individual in that his activity will lead to his particular goal. The client must fully understand and believe that his goal is fully contingent upon his own behavior, and his reward will be forthcoming. Otherwise, his goal-directed behavior has no purpose and will eventually cease. Trust also plays a big part in this factor. Past associations create a perceived credibility that pay-off will ultimately come.

Incentive is basically the attraction or repulsion of the goal, whereas motive is the overriding strength toward the incentives. For example, a steak sandwich may be an incentive object, but that incentive is significantly more valuable if the individual's *motive* for food in general is obsessive.

Researchers have taken the four factors and planned experiments with both animals and humans in modifying their goal-directed behavior. Although the approach is presented in an over-simplistic manner, the principle of behavior modification is considered to be a priority for general use. The general approach has been to specify the goal, either induced or derived by some source. For example, hunger is easily induced in rats by sheer deprivation. The qualification that the goals are deemed to be relevant to this motive of the subject is a critical factor.

The subject is then confronted with the behavior upon which the goal or reward is contingent, i.e., the desirable behavior. This process may be as simple as saying, "In order that A is attained, B must be done." Animals and young humans have the problem of understanding the association and have to be shown the process in a step-at-a-time manner by successive efforts. As the subject approximates the goal-directed behavior, he is given an association to the goal. These approximations continue until he finally *learns* the desired behavior. At that point he is only rewarded for that desired behavior. For example, Skinner used this method to *shape* pigeons to peck at a ring to obtain food. As the pigeon would step closer to the ring, he was fed a pellet of food. When the pigeon accidentally hit the ring, he was immediately fed. Afterwards he was fed or rewarded only for hitting the ring. Further specifications can be made until the goal is reached (the pigeon or other subject gets full), or the goal is found to be unattainable (unavailability), or the subject loses faith that he will be rewarded (expectancy loss).

What are the basic goals relevant to man? There are no global answers to this question since individuality plays such a major part. Maslow describes the basic needs of physical requirements, safety, love, belongingness, self-esteem and self-actualization as prime goals of man. For example, by deprivation of food or water, hunger or thirst can be motivators for goal-directed behavior. Thus, a rat can be *taught* to push a lever to get a drink or food pellet. Sleep and sexual goals have also been used for goal attainment in animal studies, but research ethics have prohibited human treatment. Storrow (1962) used money as a motivating force in order to improve work performance criteria for mental retardates. Zelhart (1970) used several different kinds of rewards in reading behavior for his juvenile delinquent samples. He found that he could effect behavior change in classroom reading with trading stamps, coins, points to get off probation, and privileges.

Madison and Herring (1960) used the client's own achievement as a reward by providing clients with a graphic, easily visualized record of their progress. They investigated the performance on five motor-skill tasks of an experiment group of seventeen clients with an equal number in the control group. All the clients had suffered some injury to their hands. Although the performances of the two groups were not statistically different on any one test, the experiment group did show uniformly greater improvement on all five tests.

Mason (1961) used hypnosis as a method of inducing asphasic clients toward recovery. His nine clients developed new behavior patterns consistent with positive attitude change.

Filer and O'Connell (1964), in a carefully designed study of disabled VA patients, found that patient-specific goals and rewards had very favorable results. That is, the researchers made no attempt to reinforce all patients equally, but each individual had his own set of reinforcers.

Global roles can be reinforced as well as specific behavior, according to A. B. Sweney (1972). He has found that people relate in general styles according to the ways they are treated by their superiors or perhaps the ways they *perceive* their superiors. Sweney's instruments ascribe three subordinate roles of submissiveness, cooperativeness, and rebelliousness in relationship to three superior roles of authoritarianness, democratic leadership, or permissiveness. In other words, one role encourages the role playing of another. His results indicate that authoritarian roles invoke subordinates to be submissive; whereas permissive superiors encourage rebellious roles in their subordinates. Perhaps another way of describing the latter relationship is that the superior *allows* his workers to be rebellious.

In Sweney's model, these two relationships are described as *maintenance* relationships because people play roles merely to maintain their organization. The democratic-cooperator relationship is described as a *goal-directed* relationship. Good examples are the relationships that exist in the Army in the conditions of war and peace. In war conditions, men relate in cooperative relationships because the goals are obvious, and they have to relate or else all is lost. The term *democratic* may not label such men as Patton in the most popular definition. Sweney, however, would define such a man as democratic in that he was willing to consider the ideas of others if the goals could be attained regardless of the engendered motivation. On the other hand, a peace-time Army encourages back-stroking roles just to maintain the existing structure.

The relevant point to the field of motivation is that maintenance role playing is nonconclusive to goal attainment. The more the client is encouraged to be rebellious or submissive, the more likely little if any movement is being made toward solutions.

There is some evidence to show that these maintenance roles are evident in chronically unemployed people. In clinical observations by Tiffany *et al.* (1970) and statistical analysis by Lawlis (1971), the chronically unemployed were divided into two groups, a highly dependent or submissive group and a rebellious group.

The conclusions of these studies are that roles can be reinforced and that some of these roles are more productive than others. The more a counselor can relate democratically and in a goal-directed manner to his client, the more that client will be encouraged to also be goal-directed and cooperative. Consequently, the counselor must look within his own orientation of counseling for maximum production.

Although a summary of behavior modification techniques would only reiterate the overall successes of changing one specific behavior, there is little evidence that such behavior change will continue once the reward conditions are relaxed or even if the behavior change is reflected in the self-concept of the client. The conclusion seems to confirm that clients can be sensitive to conditions about them, either negatively or positively. The perceptive counselor can capitalize on the properties of the environment as seling for maximum production.

A CONCEPTUAL MODEL

The above review of research literature leads to the conclusion that there is no one approach to motivation. Therefore, in order to make application to rehabilitation practice, a model of motivation could be developed. The *model of experienced control* by Tiffany, Cowan, and Tiffany (1970) was theorized to be an explanation for the phenomena of the feeling of powerlessness and, consequently, lack of motivation of disadvantaged groups. The expansion of this model has tremendous value for the data presented thus far.

The model outlines not one, but two sources of motivation: internal (A) and external (B) forces.

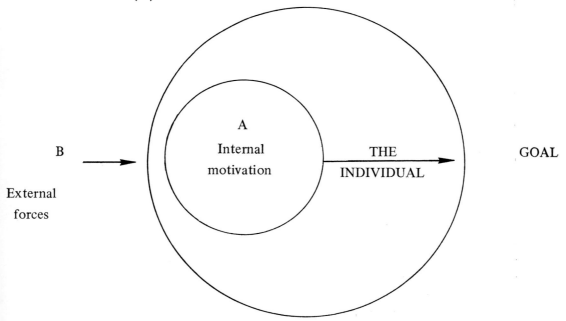

Figure 19-1. Motivation Model

The internal forces are those within each individual to which he directs his energies. These constructs can be sexual, career, power, etc., whatever forces tend to drive a person to achieve a goal that is not directly perceived in his environment. It is always interesting to note how the internal goals are developed, because they seem to develop in childhood in quite mysterious ways. For example, there was the client who had the desire for powers as a burning internal force in his life because his father lost his job when the client was young. The trauma and resultant anxiety left him with a tremendous motivation toward that goal. Another example is the client who wanted to be a beggar because his brother had always been more successful than he. Therefore, he chose another style of life that was less threatened by success.

Research appears to support the theory that the label *unmotivated* denotes, at least, a correlation to unrealistic or unintegrated internal goals. The principle implied at this point is that if the goals of clients are to be realized, the latter must have the ego strength, the energy, and realistic aspirations to carry them out.

The second part of the model shows the environmental forces that impinge upon the individual. Most of us are not so insensitive or self-actualized that we do not attend to the external rewards of the world. As indicated in the section on behavior modification, goals have value only as self-determiners. However, in order to obtain such goals, the individual has to attend to those external conditions that regulate the probability of goal achievement. The research by the behavior modification scientists dramatizes the importance of positive *and* negative attributes of the environment. This principle implies that, regardless of internal forces within the individual, he *can* achieve satisfaction with more immediate goals. Thus, there are appropriate goals that are enforced upon all of us, such as eating, money making, and sleeping; and contingencies for achieving these things constitute the bulk of our economy. So, why not make similar systems for those persons who have *less* tolerance for delayed gratification, and thereby achieve society goals as well?

Everyone has his pet theory of motivation; yet the primary point of this paper is to say that there are "different strokes for different folks." That is, all people are not necessarily motivated by the same constructs or environment. Paul Zelhart (1970) and G. Frank Lawlis (1968, 1971) found that there were several Arkansas juvenile delinquents that would not respond to counseling of any sort, yet were excellent clients in behavior modification approaches. They reasoned that the internal forces of these juveniles were either directed toward asocial goals or became dysfunctional to interpersonal intervention, and that therefore environmental controls would be most effective in *re*motivating these clients. On the other hand, they also found a category of juvenile delinquents that did not respond to behavior modification because they considered the system as irrelevant to their personal motivation constructs. These particular clients were amenable to counseling and personal re-education. The two researchers reasoned that intelligence might be a factor between these two groups.

In support of the model of at least two different motivational systems, Lawlis (1971) found two distinct groups of personality types within a chronically unemployed group in rehabilitation training. The descriptions of the types implied a motivational structure to their environment. One type was a self-inhibiter, while the other was more aggressive in expressing goals. Although the implications have yet to be demonstrated, the former group might be more amenable to counseling and self-exploration, whereas the latter group might need a more rational environment wherein to achieve.

Another thought-provoking study was performed by Lawlis and Rubin (1970), in which at least three different personality types were depicted in a twice-replicated study with alcoholics. Again, individualized treatment could be theorized along that line of self-styled motivation and is explored in their published work (Rubin and Lawlis, 1970). Although an attempt was made to research this personalized approach, a change in state laws and municipal policies made it impossible to analyze the data with objective outcome measures, such as return to hospital, unlawful behavior, etc. The data was extremely promising.

At this point a critical variable appears to be the emotional affect associated with either goal or reinforcement. Ellis (1962) has developed the theory that people have emotional wrappers attached to their goals in such a way as to inhibit, or possibly facilitate, their motivation. In his terminology, an individual (A) perceives object (C). For example, the perception (A) of the individual may be of a vocational choice of garbage collector (C). He may have an emotional effect (B) associated with C such as "degrading," "second class," "dirty," etc., that repulses him from considering that vocational choice. Lawlis (1968) found that chronically unemployed people did have differing values attributable to money. Although there was no constant interval for the increase in actual monetary value, he found indications that his chronically unemployed group did value one-dollar bills more highly than his stably employed group; however, the reverse was true for five-dollar bills.

The conclusion so important to the model and to the implications for rehabilitation, is that the person defines the object in terms of his own affect. Nothing is neither good or bad; for each one of us it has to be one or the other. We define things as positive or negative, although we do so in ways of which we are often unaware. If we are ever to conceive of motivating people, this emotional wrapper must be modified.

In concluding the section on a theoretical model, it should be pointed out that no attempt can be made to systematize all research results into one person. People are different from all vantage points, and *this statement includes counselors*. Therefore, motivational dynamics not only apply to what is going on in the counselor's mind or environment, but also what is going on *between* the counselor and client. That relationship has its own dynamics, forces that facilitate or hinder both parties. As indicated earlier, sometimes *in absentia* counseling can be more valuable than talking. On the other hand, there has been too much lack of communication between counselor and client.

Suffice it to say, the unmotivated client will not rehabilitate himself. That statement is definitional. The challenge to this situation rests in the counselor's hands. As pointed out by Tiffany *et al.* (1970), there are many physically disabled persons with the need of medical services who will rehabilitate themselves because of their healthy past histories. What lies ahead for the rehabilitation counselor is the clientele that needs the counselor as the primary service, persons who will not rehabilitate themselves as a result of their own energy source. The skills of the counselor become paramount to this challenge.

APPLICATIONS TO REHABILITATION

The theoretical background, research evidence, and model just described generate suggestions and implications for effective counseling procedure with clients. This section is devoted to speculation for counseling approaches that would maximize the likelihood of success with clients who appear *unwilling* to rehabilitate themselves. The implications are divided into the following areas: misconceptions about motivation and counseling, research utilization, and innovative approaches to counseling with the unmotivated.

Basic Misconceptions

There are three basic misconceptions that counselors have about motivation. First of all, there is no such thing as an *unmotivated* client! He may not be motivated to achieve the same goals as the counselor, or his drive to achieve might reach for unrealistic goals, but at least he is motivated to do *something*. The only time he is not motivated is when he is dead. A second misconception implies that all people reach for the same goals. We have heard it said many times that middle-class Americans constantly strive to project their needs on other classes, and then call these other sub-cultures *unmotivated* when similar rewards do not arouse behavior. The frustrating element comes in when counselors attempt to overcome this class or culture barrier *without at least an appreciation* of other beliefs and socialization. Thirdly, motivation is often confused with *method* of achievement, instead of being referred to achievement itself. For example, Thomas Edison was often described as *unmotivated* because he lived in his world in non-conformity. Many people perceive, think, synthesize and consequently act in bizarre methods *to achieve their ends*. Yet counselors often confuse these methods, inefficient as they may be, with defective motivational structures.

What misconception can be projected to the relationship in counseling, and how may it be overcome? The most obvious suggestion is to direct the counselor to analyze his own needs, personality, and motivational dynamics. As described in an earlier part of the chapter, Sweney (1972) has shown that the superior roles have different effects with the subordinate roles. That is, an authoritative counselor would have a more positive influence upon the motivation of a submissive client than a rebel client. A permissive counselor would have the most beneficial effect on a rebel client, and a democratic counselor could deal more effectively with a cooperative type of client than the other types. The counselor should analyze his own power mechanisms in relation to the type of client with whom he is dealing.

A further application to the before-mentioned suggestion is the use of evaluation for goal-seeking behaviors. Sometimes counselors choose goals or encourage the client to choose goals that are unrealistic. The process of rehabilitation is made of many small steps, rather than two or three king-sized steps. However, we often counsel with clients about too many king-sized steps at once. For example, we often start talking immediately to a client about his vocational choice; certainly this is a giant step when we consider how many choice points and learning we went through before we came to our own vocational choice. Yet, we expect our client to come to a sudden decision. When gradual, one-at-a-time, smaller steps are overlooked, motivation and drive are lost due to the lack of evaluative counseling so necessary for an integrated effort.

Motivation is a complex construct that has a variety of meanings. In rehabilitation, we conceive of this construct as the degree to which the client improves. However, improvement does not come out of a mass effort, but only through individuals. The crucial point is that there are factors in the client's world which build him up as well as tear him down. It is a major challenge to the counselor to learn to use his knowledge, his intuition, his interpersonal skills, and whatever sources are available, in developing the client's own unique manner of reaching rehabilitation goals.

Research Utilization

What extensive knowledge the counselor has at his disposal is usually referred to as *research utilization*. Programs in all areas of rehabilitation have invested in very expansive systems for the counselor to retrieve information in a very short duration of time and extension of effort. With the volumes of research available, why has the field not been more successful in solving the problems of the *unmotivated* client? Several answers explain this issue well: (1) The information can only be used as a part of the counselor himself. Information itself does not provide a significant impact until the counselor integrates it into his overall functioning. Therefore, the counselor must have the time and training to learn. (2) Much of the information is redundant or in direct opposition to existing outcome studies rather than building toward more comprehensive researches. Perhaps this is more of a blast toward journal editors than researchers, but it appears that there is some device in the screening of papers or projects that prohibits new concepts or results from being published; yet thousands of rather mundane results are formulated each year. (3) The applications of research findings are often not presented clearly for rehabilitation counselors. Rather than expressing findings as being applicable to rehabilitation practice, research results are only assumed to be applicable.

Some New Approaches

The innovative approaches that can be considered by the counselors are derived only partly from the research and theory presented in this chapter. First of all, the counselor is encouraged to formulate his counseling practice on a social as well as psychological basis. Much counseling has been based entirely upon white, middle-class constructs that have nothing to do with the client's constructs. I am sure this criticism of counselors is not new in these days of civil rights; however, it is equally true that it is possible that the counselor can be helpful to people of all races if consideration for their backgrounds can be made.

The counselor is encouraged to understand not only the psychological dynamics going on inside an individual, but also whatever cultural influences may affect behavior. Feelings are universal in their presence in human beings. We all feel anger, love, frustrations, etc., to some extent. As Eric Hoffer wrote in his book, *The True Believer* (1958), we are all Hitlers or Mussolinis inside; but we control our potentialities in one respect or another.

The presence of feelings does not predict similar behaviors, however. These manifestations are often governed by our past, our culture, our personal life styles. For example, the Mexican-American or Indian client would probably react quite differently to his feeling of frustration than his Anglo counterpart possibly because of a traditionally more authoritarian family structure. In short, the counselor not only has to be a psychologist, but a sociologist, historian, and educator as well.

In this context, the counselor can effect motivation by helping the client direct himself toward responsibility for his own behavior. In other words, by the understanding and acceptance of what makes a person behave in the way he does, the counselor and client together can shape the latter's environment into a more rational place in which to live, as well as provide impetus for the client's personality integration.

The question is often asked: How can a counselor set up an effective behavior modification program for an individual? He does not have to do this. The client will set up for himself if he is allowed. People want to achieve goals that are realistic, and experience has shown that most people, including children, are quite capable and willing to set up their own reinforcement systems. Therefore, it is highly recommended that the client take the major responsibility in deciding his own program, thereby creating in the context of the person's own psychological and social background, a program for goals and responsibilities that are intrinsically his.

Relative to this approach on the part of the counselor, the client will be receiving invaluable training in decision making. This is probably the most significant impact of the counselor in the whole program. Within this context, the counselor is first of all a person with real needs and limitations of his own. With the therapeutic ingredients of empathy, warmth, and genuineness, the counselor can relate not only the structure of his agency but his own way of dealing with decision making. In this way, the counselor can serve as a social model, perhaps, to the client, but more importantly as a relater of important factors for decisions. For example, test results and job market requirements can be considered as significant factors.

These conclusions are not intended to be new objectives for rehabilitation. The counselor, especially the vocational counselor, is still faced with his job of vocational placement. What is emphasized in this chapter, however, is a desire to consider motivation toward that objective in the client's field. The old theoretical formula of abilities plus job requirements equal satisfaction without the considerations of the system in which that person operates, his psychological and social structure, and the client's own planning, simply does not apply to today's clientele. What is needed from the counselor is a *sensitivity* to these factors, a willingness to share the responsibility of the program if need be, and an honest attempt to engage in meaningful discussion. Ability to instigate integrated motivation in a client toward a goal becomes a personal matter instead of a mechanized construct. After all, motivation is only a term used to explain behavior. It does not explain how to modify that behavior. In the end, all *re*motivation is a personal matter.

REFERENCES

Adler, A.: *Understanding Human Nature.* Greenwich, Connecticut, Farcett Publications, Inc., 1965.

Ayer, M., Thoreson, S. and Butler, A.: Predicting rehabilitation success with the MMPI and demographic data. *Personnel and Guidance Journal,* 44(6):631-637, 1966.

Ballis, R. C.: The usefulness of the drive concept. In M. R. Jones (Ed.), *Nebraska Symposium on Motivation.* Lincoln, University of Nebraska Press, 1958.

Barry, J. R. and Malinovsky, M. R.: Client motivation for rehabilitation: A review. *Rehabilitation Research Monograph,* No. 1, University of Florida, 1965.

Bibring, E.: The development and problems of the theory of instincts. In. C. L. Stacy and M. F. DeMartino (Eds.), *Understanding Human Motivation.* Cleveland, Howard Allen, 1958.

Birch, D. and Veroff, J.: *Motivation: A Study of Action.* Belmont, California, Brooks-Cole, 1968.

Cattell, R. B., Horn, J. L., Sweney, A. B. and Radcliffe, J. A.: *The Motivational Analysis Test.* Champaign, Illinois, Institute for Personality and Ability Testing, 1964.

Combs, A. W. and Snygg, D.: *Individual Behavior.* New York, Harper, 1959.

Danielson, R.: Relationships among ego-strength, motivation, and degree of success in rehabilitation activity. *Rehabilitation Counseling Bulletin,* pp. 82-88, March 1965.

DeMonn, M. M.: A predictive study of rehabilitation counseling outcomes. *Journal of Counseling Psychology, 10*:340-343, 1963.

Drasgon, J. and Dreher, R. G.: Predicting client readiness for training and placement in vocational rehabilitation. *Rehabilitation Counseling Bulletin, 8*:94-98, 1965.

Ehrle, R. A.: The predictive value of biographical data in vocational rehabilitation. Unpublished doctoral dissertation, University of Missouri, University Microfilms, 1962. No. 61-6033.

Ellis, A.: *Reason and Emotion in Psychotherapy.* New York, Lyle Stuart, Inc., 1962.

Filer, R. N. and O'Connell, D. P.: Motivation of aging persons. *Journal of Gerontology, 19*:15-22, 1964.

Frankl, V. E.: *Man's Search for Meaning.* New York, Washington Square Press, 1959.

Frantz, R.: Motivational factors in rehabilitation. Unpublished doctoral thesis, Western Reserve University, 1962.

Hamlin, R. M. and Nemo, R. S.: Self-actualization in choice score of improved schizophrenics. *Journal of Clinical Psychology, 18*:51-54, 1962.

Heilbrun, A. B. and Jordon, B. T.: Vocational rehabilitation of the socially disadvantaged: Demographic and intellectual correlates of outcome. *Personnel and Guidance Journal,* pp. 213-217, November 1968.

Herzberg, F. and Hamlin, R.: The motivation-hygiene concept of psychotherapy. *Mental Hygiene, 45*:394-401, 1961.

Hoffer, E.: *The True Believer,* New York, Harper and Row, 1958.

Hughes, G. R.: Self-resignation: A mighty foe. *Journal of Rehabilitation, 26*:18-19, 1960.

Katz, S.: Definition of terms for index of independence in activities of daily living. *Journal of Chronic Disability, 9*:55-63, 1959.

Katz, S., Ford, A. B., Maskowitz, R. W., Jackson, B. A., and Jaffe, M. W.: Studies of illness in the aged: The Index of ADL, a standardized measure of biological and psychosocial function. *Journal of the American Medical Association, 185*:914-919, 1963.

Kelman, H. R.: An experiment in the rehabilitation of nursing home patients. *Public Health Reports, 77*:356-366, 1962.

Lawlis, F.: Perception of money as related to employment stability. *Discussion Papers,* Vol. 1, no. 21, Arkansas Rehabilitation Research and Training Center, 1968.

Lawlis, F.: The hard-core unemployed: Unidimensional or multidimensional personality. *Rehabilitation Counseling Bulletin,* pp. 13-18, March 1971.

Lawlis, F.: Motivational factors reflecting employment stability. *Journal of Social Psychology, 84*:215-223, 1971.

Lawlis, F. and Rubin, S.: 16 PF study of personality patterns in alcoholics. *Quarterly Journal of Studies on Alcohol,* pp. 318-327, June 1970.

Lesh, T. U.: Prediction of vocational rehabilitation success. *Rehabilitation Counseling Bulletin,* pp. 9-13, September 1968.

Lesser, M. and Darling, R.: Factors prognostic for vocational rehabilitation among the physically handicapped. *Archives of Physical Medicine and Rehabilitation, 34*:73-81, 1953.

Lief, H. I., Lief, V. F., Warren, C. O. and Heath, R. G.: Low dropout rate in a psychiatric clinic. *Archives of General Psychiatry, 5*:200-211, 1961.

Litman, T. J.: The influence of self-conception and life orientation factors in the rehabilitation of the orthopedically disabled. *Journal of Health and Human Behavior, 3*:249-257, 1962.

Little, N.: The rehabilitation center dropout: A demographic and motivational assessment. Unpublished Ed.D. thesis, University of Arkansas, 1970.

Littman, R. A.: Motives, history, and causes. In M. R. Jones (Ed.), *Nebraska Symposium on Motivation*. Lincoln, University of Nebraska Press, 1958.

McMahon, T. J.: A comparative study of the Kuder Preference Record of interest patterns of select groups. Unpublished Master's paper, Pennsylvania State University, 1964.

McPhee, W. and Maglry, F.: Success and failure in vocational rehabilitation. *Personnel and Guidance Journal, 38*:497-499, 1960.

Madison, H. L. and Herring, M.: An experimental study of motivation. *American Journal of Occupational Therapy, 14*:253-255, 1960.

Maslow, A.: *Motivation and Personality*. New York, Harper and Row, 1954.

Mason, C. F.: Hypnotic motivation of aphasics. *Journal of Clinical Experimental Hypnosis, 9*:297-301, 1961.

Patterson, C. H.: *Counseling and Psychotherapy: Theory and Practice*. New York, Harper, 1959.

Perlman, L.: The development of a predictive model for the detection of potential dropouts from vocational tarining in a comprehensive rehabilitation center. Unpublished doctoral dissertation, Pennsylvania State University, University Microfilms, 1968. No. 69-5581.

Pfonts, J., Wallace, M. S. and Jenkins, J.: An outcome study of referrals to a psychiatric clinic. *Social Work, 8*:79-86, 1963.

Phillips, E. L.: The problem of motivation: Some neglected aspects. *Journal of Rehabilitation*, pp. 10-12, March-April 1957.

Postman, L.: Is the concept of motivation necessary? Review of M. R. Jones (Ed.), *Nebraska Symposium on Motivation in Contemporary Psychology, 1*:229-230, 1956.

Rabinowitz, H. S., Johnson, D. E. and Reilly, A. J.: A preliminary study of program dropouts from vocational services. *Rehabilitation Counseling Bulletin, 8*:2-7, 1964.

Reimonis, G.: Disparity theory and achievement motivation. *Journal of Abnormal and Social Psychology, 69*:206-210, 1964.

Rubin, S. and Lawlis, F.: A model for differential treatment for alcoholics. *Rehabilitation Research and Practice Review, 1*:53-58, 1970.

Samuelson, C.: Interest scores in predicting success of trade school students. *Personnel and Guidance Journal, 36*:538-541, 1958.

Sandness, D. G.: The MMPI as a predictor in vocational rehabilitation. *Rehabilitation Counseling Bulletin*, pp. 111-113, December 1968.

Sankovsky, R.: An analysis of factors associated with self-discharge at the Pennsylvania Rehabilitation Center. Unpublished Master's paper, Pennsylvania State University, 1965.

Sankovsky, R.: *Identifying the Program Dropout at a Comprehensive Rehabilitation Facility*. Research and Training Center in Vocational Rehabilitation, University of Pittsburgh, 1969.

Sankovsky, R.: *The Prediction of Successful and Unsuccessful Rehabilitation Outcomes: A Review of the Literature*. Research and Training Center in Vocational Rehabilitation, University of Pittsburgh, 1968.

Skinner, B. F.: *Science and Human Behavior*. New York, Macmillan, 1953.

Small, L.: Some psychological aspects of job placement. Paper presented at Workshop on Motivation and Rehabilitation Counseling, Springfield College, Springfield, Massachusetts, 1958.

Smith, J. and Fink, S. L.: The relationship between physical improvement and psychological factors in chronically ill patients. *Journal of Clinical Psychology, 19*:289-292, 1963.

Storrow, H. A.: Money as a motivator. *Journal of the American Public Welfare Association, 20*:199-204, 1962.

Suinn, R. M. and Paulhe, G. P.: A note on types of work motivation. *Rehabilitation Counseling Bulletin,* pp. 102-105, March 1966.

Super, D.: *The Psychology of Careers.* New York, Harper, 1957.

Sweney, A.: Management styles and subordinate roles. Speech delivered to the Psychology Department, Texas Tech University, Lubbock, Texas, May 1972.

Tiffany, D. W., Cowan, J. R., and Tiffany, P. M.: *The Unemployed: A Social-Psychological Portrait.* New Jersey, Prentice-Hall, 1970.

Vernier, C., Barrell, R. P., Cummings, J. W., Dickerson, J. H. and Hooper, H. E.: Psychological study of the patient with pulmonary tuberculosis: A cooperative research approach. *Psychological Monographs, 75*:510, 1961.

Wardlow, D.: *A Nine-Month Dropout Study.* Hot Springs Rehabilitation Service, 1964.

Wispe, L. G.: A psychologist looks at motivational problems in training. *Occupational Outlook Quarterly,* pp. 13-15, December 1965.

Zelhart, P.: *Personal Communication.* University of Arkansas, 1970.

(PART SEVEN)

THE EMOTIONALLY DISABLED

The Mentally and Emotionally
Handicapped

Chapter 20

THE MENTALLY AND EMOTIONALLY HANDICAPPED

Clifford S. Knape

THE NEUROPSYCHIATRIC CLIENT presents a rehabilitation challenge of great complexity. A large number of conditions are included, ranging from precisely demonstrable organic lesions to loosely described functional behavior variables. In the latter categories, diagnosis is frequently uncertain and subjective for many of the neuropsychiatric categories. While much progress has been made in the treatment of the mentally and emotionally handicapped in the last decade, treatment still is comparatively protracted and runs an uncertain course. Finally, despite great improvement in the attitudes of society toward neuropsychiatric clients, the community still offers substantial resistance to the assimilation and rehabilitation of such individuals.

MAJOR CATEGORIES OF MENTAL AND EMOTIONAL ILLNESS

The rehabilitation specialist will encounter several types of mental and emotional illness. A brief description of the most prevalent categories follows.

Psychotic Reactions

In the active phases of this condition, the individual demonstrates behavioral distortions, falsifications of reality, and other symptoms in gross or subtle degrees. In remission, or improved phases, these symptoms may disappear, only to have a subtle effect which allows the individual to interact realistically and effectively with his environment. The term *insane* is the legal and colloquial equivalent of the medical term *psychotic*.

Neurotic Reactions
(psychoneurotic reactions)

In the crisis phases of this condition, the individual over-reacts or over-inhibits emotionally, worries without specific fears, and otherwise behaves in non-adaptive fashions. The degree and duration of these behaviors, including the inability to meet the ordinary demands of life, distinguish the neurotic person from the normal. When the condition improves, the neurotic person resumes effectiveness to the degree of improvement.

Personality Disorders

This group encompasses a wide spectrum of pattern and trait disorders, many involving moral and character deviations. Many alcoholics, sex deviates, vagrants, swindlers, and other such socially maladjusted persons belong to this category. It is important, however, not to confuse behaviors such as excessive drinking, sex deviation, and others, as arising *only* from personality disorders, as some such behaviors arise from psychoses, neuroses, sub-cultural models and expectancy, etc.

Mental Retardation

This group includes the functionally and statistically definable persons of low mental ability. Medical and psychological terminology today favors the descriptions of *mild, moderate, severe,* and *profound* to indicate the degree of retardation, avoiding the less specific and emotionally-charged nouns *moron, imbecile,* and *idiot* which were formerly used. Schools classify retardates as *Educable* and *Trainable,* based generally upon scores of *50 to 69* and *below 50,* respectively, on a standard individual test of intelligence such as the Revised Stanford-Binet or the appropriate Wechsler.

ILLNESS OR PROBLEMS-IN-LIVING

A psychiatrist, T.S. Szasz (1960) voiced the long-festering dissatisfactions with psychiatric terminology in an article with the provocative title "The Myth of Mental Illness", published in the *American Psychologist,* the official journal of the American Psychological Association. Szasz, long concerned with moral conflicts and ethics in psychiatric conditions, originally addressed himself specifically "to sociopathological problems of living . . . not the whole field of psychiatry" (Szasz, 1960, p. 118). Szasz supported his characterization of mental illness as a myth by denying that "all problems in living . . . (can be) attributed to physiochemical processes which in due time will be discovered by medical research" (Szasz, 1960, p. 113).

A psychologist, O.H. Mowrer (1960), contributed to the discussion with an article entitled " 'Sin,' The Lesser of Two Evils". Mowrer contended, with Freud, that neurosis reflects a conscience-hold on the individual and, when the individual "confesses . . . and makes what poor attempts he can at restitution, then the superego (like the parents of an earlier day—and society in general) forgives and relaxes its stern hold; the individual is once again free, 'well' " (Mowrer, 1960, p. 304).

A prompt rebuttal to both Szasz and Mowrer appeared in the *American Psychologist* (Ausubel, 1961), and the lines for discussion were rather cleanly drawn. These lines have tended to become vague in the last decade, as voices and opinions have proliferated and emotions have heightened. Opinion is by no means fixed by professional affiliation, although generally psychologists lean to the illness-is-a-myth approach and the psychiatrists lean to the illness-is-a-physiochemical-imbalance approach. It is subjectively felt that psychologists who were working in mental hospitals prior to 1954—when the "breakthrough" in tranquilizers and other psychopharmaceuticals occurred—generally support the physiochemical imbalance approach. As the popular press has picked up glimmerings of the professional disagreement and has linked it with attacks upon overuse of medications, an unfortunate resistance to proper continuation of a medicine regimen (properly prescribed by qualified psychiatrists and other physicians) has developed among neuropsychiatric patients and their families.

Rehabilitation specialists can increase the effectiveness of their efforts by encouraging the continuation of the prescription established by the client's physician. Rehabilitation specialists who wish to investigate further will find it profitable to review the articles cited in this matter so the limited application of the contentions presented will be clear. An appreciation of the biochemical aspects (causes *or* results) is also valuable, and can be obtained by reading the research summary prepared by the staff of the National Institute of Mental Health (Staff, NIMH, 1964), Woolley's article in the popular press (Woolley, 1965), and Woolley's earlier classical summary (Woolley, 1952). A fine overview of this matter is found in *Biological Treatment of Mental Illness*, edited by Rinkel (1966).

PSYCHOTIC SYMPTOMS AND BEHAVIOR

While full descriptions of symptoms and nosological pigeon-holes are the province of texts on abnormal psychology common to the educational background of rehabilitation specialists, an overview of these symptoms, perhaps organized somewhat differently than the standard approach, is appropriate. In reviewing these symptoms, readers should bear in mind that the *duration, intensity,* and *resultant personal ineffectiveness* distinguish the abnormal from the normal experience. All readers will be able to see many correlates in their own experience with the symptoms to be described as the symptoms are common experiences of mankind, abnormal only when intense and prolonged enough to remove or substantially reduce the ability of the individual to function in his everyday world.

Psychotic symptoms may be summarized under four types of disorders: disorders of thought; disorders of perception; disorders of emotional response, mood; disorders of motor functions.

Disorders of Thought

Disorders of thought may be related to the *progression* of thought or the *content* of thought. Progression disorders may be flights of thought, demonstrated as a very high verbal production, jumping from one chain of thought to another without discernible connectives. Another common progression disorder is found in blocks, or retarded thought. Here the thoughts are markedly slowed or blocked. Content disorders are delusions or obsessions. Delusions may be exactly defined as firm, fixed, and false beliefs not rooted in the culture. For example, The Nazi belief in the superiority of the German was firm, fixed, and false, but since it was culturally inculcated, the individual holding such belief was not abnormal.

Common types of delusions are those of grandeur (expansive misconceptions of self-worth), delusions of persecution (misconceptions of the acts and statements of others as being antagonistic, imagined antagonisms of individuals and groups toward the person harboring the delusion, and other feelings of being under attack or severe criticism), delusions of self-accusation (feeling that one has committed "unpardonable" sins, of worthlessness, and other self-depreciatory attitudes), delusions of identity (belief that one is "really" someone else, usually a famous or infamous person), and other false beliefs. Obsessions, also related to the psychoneurotic symptomatology, consist of the morbid domination of the affected individual's thoughts by a single idea.

Disorders of Perception

Disorders of perception are quite common in the psychoses. The psychotic is prone to misinterpret sensory impulses and stimuli, and is unable to spontaneously correct his misinterpretation. A misinterpreted sensory stimulus is known as an *illusion,* and of course is commonly experienced by everyone. The normal person, however, is able to correct his misinterpretation by logic or by investigation, whereas the psychotic individual persists in his misinterpretations without reference to logic. Illusions are especially common in toxic disorders.

Another disorder of perception is found in *hallucinations,* which are reactions to imagined sensory stimuli. Illusions and hallucinations may be referrable to any of the senses—auditory, optical, olfactory, tactile, or gustatory. This falsification of reality is not analogous to any normal reaction, but hallucinations may occur in otherwise normal persons during periods of toxicity or fevers. Auditory hallucinations are very commonly combined with delusions of persecution in the paranoid states, whereby the affected individual "hears" voices of known or unknown persons disparaging him unmercifully.

Disorders of Emotional Response

Disorders of emotional response and mood are quite characteristic of the psychoses. The response may be over-reactive, under-reactive (flattened), or inappropriate. Inappropriate response is sometimes incorrectly perceived by workers who project their own value system into the situation and expect a certain emotional response from the client. The client's values and experiences, however, may be such that the indicated emotional response *is* appropriate. For example, an individual may be describing the breaking up of a marriage, and the rehabilitation worker may be "empathizing" with feelings of sadness—for the client, however, the situation may be one causing relief, relaxation of tensions, lowering of uncomfortable levels of responsibility, etc.; therefore, his reflected emotion may be one of pleasure and relief. It is most important that counselors and others seek to ascertain the client's background before emotional reactions to certain life-changes are predicted, or rather, expected.

Disorders of Motor Functions

Disorders of the motor functions may reflect themselves in hyperactivity, hypoactivity, grimacing, postural oddities, and muscle tensions. The typical catatonic immobility and "staring into space" is an example of a motor disorder. Occasionally the catatonic will retain a position until it is physically altered by someone else, adopting then a new position and retaining it in a fixed manner. This condition, existing in the acute phases, is cited as *waxy flexibility*.

SYMPTOMS OF THE NEUROSES

The symptoms of the neuroses are anxieties, obsessions, compulsions, phobias, and conversion-hysteria. Technically, loss of memory as in amnesia is considered a psychoneurotic manifestation, but for the most part such intellectual impairments are connected with organic psychoses.

Neurotic Anxiety

Neurotic anxiety differs from the usual anxiety in that the neurotic person is anxious about generalities and unknowns whereas normal anxiety attaches itself as a rule to a specific situation. The neurotic feels that "something bad is going to happen," but he does not have any specific cause or expected development to identify. Of course, the non-neurotic occasionally has this "free-floating" anxiety also, but in the neurotic, it is persistent, very intense, and prevents adjustment to the normal activities of living.

Conversion Reactions and Hysterias

Conversion reactions and hysterias are neurotic symptoms of fairly definite confidence, as these symptoms generally have no normal, non-organic correlates. The individual develops organic impairment of the various senses or motor functions, as in hysterical blindness, hysterical deafness, hysterical paralysis, some forms of aphasia, digestive disorders, back disorders and other organ signs not physically or neurally based.

Obsessions

Obsessions are found in both psychosis and neurosis. In these symptoms, the affected individual's thoughts are dominated by a single or very restricted number of thoughts. This overconcentration upon single topics has normal correlates, of course, but the degree and duration is slight compared to the neurotic type of obsession.

Compulsions

Compulsions are reflected by repetitive, non-logic-directed actions, postures, and behaviors. The morbid adherence to a fixed pattern or sequence of movements, actions, and postures may be found in either psychosis or psychoneurosis.

Phobias

Phobias are unreasoning, strong, and persistent fears. These fears are not amenable to logic, and are frequently seen by the affected person as "foolish," yet the fears are dominating and disabling when found in the neurotic pattern. Everyone is familiar with a number of Greek-compounded words describing the specific object or situation to which the phobia is attached.

SECONDARY SYMPTOMS OF THE NEUROSES

The neurotic patterns may be so painful that the secondary symptoms of disassociative reactions, somatization reactions, asthenic reactions, hypochondriacal reactions, depressive reactions, and others emerge.

Dissociative Reactions

Dissociative reactions are the amnesias, multiple personalities, and fugues (amnesia coupled with escape-travel). The multiple-personality syndrome, so common in fiction, is extremely rare clinically. The dissociative reactions must be distinguished from prepsychotic and psychotic disorders of the intellect and memory.

Somatization Reactions

Somatization reactions are the psychosomatic illnesses, and are myriad. Special types of somatization reactions may be seen in the asthenic (chronic fatigue) reaction and in the hypochondriacal (over-concern with bodily function) reaction. In the somatization reaction proper, the merging symptom is specific and referrable to a system or function of the body, whereas non-specificity characterizes asthenia and hypochondria.

Depressive Reactions

The depressive reactions represent strong self-depreciatory feelings, resulting in a self-evaluation of worthlessness coupled with an outlook of hopelessness. Frequently depressive reactions are precipitated by an actual loss in the affected individual's life, but they are dynamically based, as a rule, on long-felt self-concepts of inadequacy, worthlessness, and other self-depreciatory viewpoints. The neurotic form of depression differs from the psychotic form in subtle ways involving the evaluation of the psychotic disorders enumerated in preceding paragraphs.

SYMPTOMS OF PERSONALITY DISORDERS

Symptoms of the personality disorders are found in the atypical, antisocial, maladaptive, and "selfish" behaviors themselves, and once again depend upon persistency and intensity for separation from the normal problems of maturing and becoming a conforming and moral member of the society in which the individual lives. Emotional instability, passivities, and aggressions mark the behavior patterns of some of the personality disorders.

In the *instability reactions,* the individual reacts with excitability in everyday stress situations, being unpredictable in his response to others and to the problems of life. In the *passivities,* the response may be either one of helpless, indecisive dependence or disguised aggressiveness such as procrastination, stubborness, or childlike pouting. In the aggressions, the typical response is one of irritability, tantrums, and impulsive destructive actions.

Other personality disorders are self-defining. In view of difficulty of diagnosis, the rehabilitation specialist must be very complete in his reports of contact with these persons, as the medical consultant depends upon extremely tenuous threads to distinguish among the personality disorders and between them and either psychosis or psychoneurosis.

SYMPTOMS OF NEUROPSYCHIATRIC CONDITIONS

Discussion of the symptoms of the neuropsychiatric conditions is difficult because of the overlapping nature of the phenomenological observations basic to diagnosis. A simplified statement of the symptoms can be found in a popularly distributed pamphlet (Milt, 1959), which is recommended to rehabilitation workers in general, as well as those specializing in neuropsychiatric caseloads.

TREATMENT METHODS

Treatment of the neuropsychiatric patient has vastly improved in effectiveness in the last decade, and there is promise of even greater improvement in the future. In general, treatment involves three aspects: physical-chemical alteration of the patient, changes in environment of the patient, and changes by communication with the patient.

Medical Treatment

In the physical-chemical procedures, drugs, shock, and surgery may be employed. These are medical approaches entirely, but the rehabilitation specialist must know about possible side-effects and residuals of such treatments. Any of the drugs used in treatment may have hypersensitivity effects as well as less dramatic side-effects. The hypersensitivity effects are generally quickly and dramatically apparent and may be noticed during the medical observation and supervision phases of the treatment. Some of these effects, found in patients taking major or minor tranquilizers, psychic energizers or antidepressants, are as follows: skin rashes, convulsions, liver malfunction, blood effects, and rarely, addictions. Rehabilitation specialists should report such effects to the medical consultant immediately, as hypersensitivity effects a direct change in treatment modality.

Less dramatic and more frequent side-effects of the major tranquilizers are weight gains, insomnia, sensitivity to sun, drowsiness, dried-out mouth and nose sensations, blurry vision, heartbeat disturbances, urinary difficulties, constipation, and sex-potency-expectancies and performance. This latter side-effect, related so intimately with psychological expectancy, is a major cause for interruption of prescribed courses of drug treatments. This side effect is probably found much less frequently among patients who have not heard the matter discussed at length or those who have experienced satisfactory potency after taking the drugs and prior to hearing of the matter. In any event, the rehabilitation specialist should not initiate inquiry into the manifestation of this possible side-effect, and should respond reassuringly to those clients who initiate the discussion of this matter. Such clients should be referred to physicians for evaluation and treatment as medically indicated. Some rehabilitation specialists may feel that discreet inquiry, perhaps restricted to the wife, is appropriate, but this feeling overlooks the real possibility of causing the symptom by expressing the direct or indirect concern in this subtle area of effectiveness. Accordingly, rehabilitation specialists should not bring up the subject with the client or with the client's wife.

Similar side-effects are found in patients taking minor tranquilizers and the antidepressants or psychic energizers. Blood pressure disturbances are frequently found in clients using chemotherapies, with consequent dizziness or easy fatiguability. Rehabilitation specialists must work closely with the medical consultant and other physicians, as appropriate, in recognizing and reporting such side effects and their impact on the physical and mental capacities of the client.

In addition to the more transitory nature of side-effects, there are residuals of some forms of the physical-chemical treatment modalities. Psychosurgery leaves neurological and intellectual residuals, widely variant from individual to individual. The various forms of shock treatment have effects upon memory and may possibly have subtle effects upon intellectual functioning similar to those found in "minimal" brain damage, especially if such shock treatments are numerous. In a recent psychological study of one of the author's clients, minimal brain damage signs, including expressive aphasia, were demonstrated quite clearly, although no causative factor could be identified whatsoever unless one accepted ninety-two electric shock treatments as that factor. Close observation and reporting are essential in contacts with patients who have had extensive shock treatment or psychosurgery of any sort, as medical follow-up in such cases is tremendously aided by proper and complete reports from the rehabilitation specialist.

Environmental Manipulation as Treatment

In addition to the physical-chemical alteration of the patient, treatment also includes changes in the environment of the patient and changes in the conceptualizations of the patient by communication. The environmental changes generally are designed to reduce the tensions and stresses of his former environment, and may involve the use of sheltered employment, changed employment, foster homes, and other such environmental manipulations. This treatment is generally associated with the physical-chemical alteration efforts and also with the treatments based on communication.

Treatment by Conceptional Change

The efforts to change the concepts of the patient by communication with him fall into such categories as psychotherapy, psychodrama, play-therapy, group therapy, and other techniques. The preferred terminology in counseling psychology and in rehabilitation professions differs from that in clinical psychology, social work, and medicine. Generally, the latter three professions prefer the term *psychotherapy* to refer to the communicative approaches to alteration of concepts, while counselors and rehabilitation workers prefer the term *counseling*. While it is patently not scientific for any one profession to preempt a term such as *psychotherapy* or *counseling* as pertaining only to its own techniques, there are advantages in using the term *counseling* to describe the relationship involved in the rehabilitation professions rather than the less specific term *psychotherapy,* which runs the gamut from psychoanalysis to supportive therapy offered during brief contacts with the patient. *Counseling,* particularly if the adjectival specification *rehabilitation* is prefixed, more clearly establishes the focus and the aims of the relationship involved. Additionally, in a teamwork approach to treatment which typifies the methods in neuropsychiatry, the professionals involved can better be perceived as cooperating team members, rather than members of a competing team, if technique-terminology is as specific and non-overlapping as possible.

It should be clear, of course, that *counseling* as used in this discussion, is a specialized form of treatment seeking alteration of concepts and behaviors of the client through insight-development and motivation-strengthening. That this definition also suffices for the term *psychotherapy* in no wise vitiates the argument advanced for specific terminology, as differences in methodology and protocol constitute the professional differentiations.

Psychotherapy to the psychoanalyst, for example, may involve directive forms of interpretation to the patient, whereas counselors and rehabilitation specialists lean to the non-directive efforts at insight on the part of the patient. Psychotherapy to the psychiatrist may include any number of methods in the treatment sphere, aided or unaided by drugs, whereas counseling is undertaken without the assistance of drugs or other medical approaches. These differences in methodology, naturally, do not force distinctions in the depth of the technique nor in the effectiveness of the technique, as these variables will depend upon the skill of the professional and upon the readiness, susceptibility, and accessibility of the patient.

DIMENSIONS OF THE PROBLEM

Statistics as to the number of persons with neuro-psychiatric conditions are not easily interpreted. Crawford (1965, p. 2) points out that "the task of determining who in a population is mentally ill defies exact solution at this time . . . Even if only diagnosed cases are identified and studied, comparability may be lacking." The problem of epidemiology in this area of medicine centers on the lack of adequate reporting, the elimination of duplications caused by different treatment courses and readmissions of the same treatment sources, and finally the lack of any confident and comparable diagnostic categories.

In common with most estimates, the staff of the National Committee Against Mental Illness reports that "about one in every ten persons is now suffering from some form of mental illness" (Staff, NCAMI, 1961, p. 1). This estimate is based upon a survey of an urban area, but it is in agreement with every other estimate available on the incidence of mental illness.

Schlaifer (1962, p. 7) describes the origin of the "one in ten" figure as being the uncertain guess he made before a Congressional committee, noting that he was "very concerned that some Congressman would ask, 'Where did you get those figures?' . . . Fortunately, no one asked . . . During that year, however, many doctors and organizations quoted those figures because they were in the *Congressional Record*." Despite this uncertain origin, all studies seem to support the one-in-ten incidence, and Schlaifer (1962, p. 7) also reports on a recent "study which came up with almost exactly the same figures."

This one-in-ten figure is applicable to the number of emotionally disturbed children in our classrooms. The staff of the National Congress of Parents and Teachers reported, on the basis of a California survey, that "at least three children in each average classroom can be regarded as having problems of sufficient strength to warrant the appellation of 'emotionally disturbed child' " (Staff, NCPT, 1964, p. 12).

CAUSES OF EMOTIONAL DISTURBANCES

By statistical definition, the retarded constitute about three percent of the population, but the exact epidemiological data are very hard to obtain. One cannot merely count non-institutionalized special education (retarded groups) students and add thereto the institutionalized population in schools for the mentally retarded, for additive and subtractive errors occur by such procedure. For example, many persons classified as mentally retarded may be so emotionally disturbed that adequate measurement of the basic mental ability is not possible. Such errors may account for the fact that 372, or almost five percent, of the resident population in Texas schools for the mentally retarded have intelligence quotients higher than 70, and the fact that almost one-in-five of these non-retarded residents have intelligence quotients higher than 85. (Staff, The Board for Texas State Hospitals and Special Schools, 1964, p. D-17). This type of net-additive error may be compensated wholly or partly by the subtractive errors inherent in incomplete reporting of retarded persons past school age or privately maintained. At any rate, one does not need epidemiological counts to assign the three percent incidence to retardation, as this is a statistical reflection of mental ability testing and classification.

Within the neuropsychiatric category, the most common cause (26 percent) for first admissions to mental hospitals is cerebral arteriosclerosis, including senile psychoses resulting from circulatory disturbances in the brain (Staff, MCAMI, 1961, p. 5). Schizophrenia is next, with a reported 23 percent incidence among first admissions, and alcoholism is third, with a 14.3 percent incidence (Staff, NCAMI, 1961, p. 5). Personality disorders, with 6.2 percent, and psychoneurotic reactions, with 5.8 percent (Staff, NCAMI, 1961, p. 5), are certainly underestimated because of the relatively small percentage of persons with these disorders seeking admission to mental hospitals. Until reports of private treatment are adequate, and until duplications in available reports are eliminated, one must agree with Crawford (1965, p. 2) that the problem of incidence of neuropsychiatric conditions defies solution. In the meantime, one may accept the one-in-ten figure for overall estimate, and reserve judgment on the exact distribution of such persons within the neuropsychiatric totals. More than half of all hospital beds in the country are filled by neuropsychiatric patients and this fact alone would justify the American Medical Association's citation of mental illness as "the major health problem facing the nation today" (Staff, Council on Mental Health, AMA, 1962, pp. 3, 11).

DISORDERS OF PERSONALITY AND DEVELOPMENT

One is led into imponderable problems, almost moot but so pertinent to the rehabilitation function that argument, moot or not, is required. These imponderables are as follows: First, what proportion of criminals are mentally ill? Second, what proportion of alcoholics are mentally ill? Third, what proportion of sex offenders are mentally ill? Fourth, what rehabilitation prospects do the foregoing classes of persons manifest?

Criminality and Mental Illness

First, consider the relationship between criminality and mental illness. Unquestionably, this is a complex matter, but it is easily seen that this has significance for the rehabilitation specialist. Some criminal actions arise out of purely psychotic perceptions; for example, the assault of a paranoid patient upon the imagined source of his "persecution". Other criminal actions arise out of less obvious psychotic perceptions; for example, a patricide or matricide based on dynamics in the parent-child relationship. Many criminal actions result from sociopathic personality disorders. The report of the 1962 National Congress on Mental Illness and Health (Staff, Council on Mental Health, AMA, 1962, p. 68) contains these remarks by Dr. P. Q. Roche:

The concept of the sociopathic personality has gained great interest in the study of illegal conduct. Sociopathic conduct has come to be equated with incorrigibility and there is a growing conviction that the sociopathic pattern is properly regarded as a mental disorder. By some, it is considered a kind of mental disturbance warranting the diagnosis of psychosis. In the sociopath there is a conspicuous absence of connections with the deeper social emotional accompaniments of experience and a lack of identification of such persons with their fellow human beings—an incapacity to feel the hurt in others . . . Early care is highly desired not only for a child, but also, since pathogenic factors are almost invariably uncovered, in other persons around the child. Once established, sociopathic patterns are difficult to change . . . The family physician's participation in and active support of community endeavors to detect and treat early manifestations of psychological stress in children and young persons cannot be over-emphasized (p. 68).

Criminality based on sub-cultural models can be corrected by the successful substitution of legal-conforming models; hard-core sociopathic behavior, however, is not so simply attacked. Here the motivation to conform must be so clearly related to the sociopathic self-interest that non-conformity is rejected because it does not serve the self-seeking ends of the individual. This is uncertain motivation, but it is clearly better than none, and occasional success will be encountered through this method.

The popular stereotype of the ex-mental patient, held even by many professionals in the mental health field, depicts the ex-patient as given to crimes of violence. A study of more than 10,000 male ex-patients over a five-and-a-half-year period (Staff, New York Department of Mental Hygiene, 1962) reflected that ex-patients had an annual arrest rate of 122 per 10,000 compared with 491 per 10,000 found in the general population. A pioneer study by Pollock (1938) had reflected the same conclusion regarding low incidence of crime among ex-patients, but the facts are ignored in the persistent stereotype.

Sex Offenders and Mental Illness

There is evidence also that sex offenders have a low rate of recidivism. A recent study of the sex criminal reflected that "not more than five percent of the convicted sex offenders are of the dangerous variety, . . . (and) sex offenders have one of the lowest rates as repeaters of all types of crime" (Staff, Philadelphia College of Physicians, 1960, p. 10).

Alcoholism and Mental Illness

Alcoholism may be symptomatic or causative or neuropsychiatric conditions. Regardless of setting—i.e., rehabilitation agency, hospital, local alcoholism council, etc.—the rehabilitation worker will need to have a high tolerance for failure and a consistent ability to maintain optimism without gullibility. The essential philosophy in the matter of rehabilitating alcoholics is brief: it is a firm belief that alcoholics deserve help, and that some alcoholics can be helped. If either leg of this philosophy is absent or weak, the rehabilitation specialist will be ineffective in dealing with alcoholism in its complex and frustrating manifestations. The basic task of the rehabilitation specialist in the alcoholic field is to restore or establish the alcoholic's self concept as being a worthy person, one who deserves to be helped, and one who can be helped. Once again, this is a seemingly naïve approach, but it is basic to the attitudes required to establish the relationship needed to be of rehabilitative help to the alcoholic.

PSYCHOLOGICAL ASPECTS OF GENERAL REHABILITATION

The degree to which emotional and mental illness contributes to the physical conditions, cannot be statistically stated, but it is certain that both factors are significant. Rehabilitation specialists, who work with any form of physical illness, therefore cannot overlook the emotional correlates—causes or results—in the physical conditions cited in the diagnosis. For this reason, clues to emotional disturbances must be alertly sought even when diagnostic data are silent on emotional involvement.

Behavior Clues to Emotional Conflict

Clues to emotional disturbances which may manifest themselves in the rehabilitation setting fall roughly into two main categories: first, clues in the actions of the client, and second, clues in the speech of the client. Each of these warrants a closer inspection than might be apparent on the surface.

Consider, for example, the *actions* of the client. In this area, the novice rehabilitation worker is quick to observe such culturally stereotyped clues as blushing, undue perspiration, undue fidgeting, or other such surface clues which frequently disclose feelings. All of these are good and will be observed by the specialist, but he will also need to observe other, perhaps more subtle clues, which escape common notice. Among these is excessive control which is manifested in a normally active or hyperactive individual, who begins very carefully to slow down his movements of smoking, knocking out ashes, squirming in his chair, and other such evidence of concern with the superficial signs of behavior disturbance. The implication is that the individual is trying to hide a disturbance by deliberately suppressing the culturally stereotyped signs of such disturbance.

Another clue is a change in the individual's habitual eye contact habits. This clue cannot be recognized very early, as first the individual's typical eye contact habits must be gauged. The individual who occasionally glances at the counselor has a very different pattern of eye contact habits from either the individual who habitually gazes at the counselor's eyes or who consistently avoids the counselor's eyes. During periods of emotional stress, individuals tend to change their eye contact habits, and once again the assumption is that a recognition of emotional disturbance causes the individual to be more aware of his interpersonal reactions. As the awareness of the interpersonal relations increases, the individual who typically avoids eye contact begins to force eye contact, and the person who typically maintains a steadfast eye contact begins to vary his approach. The first type of change is probably a conscious and a deliberate one whereas the second type of approach seems to be more unconscious and more readily explainable, in terms of avoidance impulses, than is the first.

Any change in body posture may tip off a controlled emotional disturbance. This change may be the easily apparent one whereby the counselee turns his chair and this trunk position away from the counselor, while maintaining his usual face-to-face and eye contact habits. The first reaction seems to be associated most often with persons who are experiencing feelings of dependency, along with emotional disturbance, whereas the second reaction is perhaps another indication of the avoidance impulse mentioned in the preceding paragraph

While not to be considered a clue to emotional disturbance, but certainly a clue to emotional tone, are such variables as the warmth of the handclasp at second and later meetings as compared to the warmth of the handclasp at the initial meeting; the honoring or keeping of appointment times on subsequent meetings as compared to that at the time of initial contact; the manner of settling down to subsequent discussions as compared to the initial session; and any other differences observed which might give an indication of whether the rehabilitation relationship is being actively accepted, passively accepted, actively resisted, or passively resisted.

Verbal Clues to Emotional Disturbance

The second main category of clues to emotional disturbance is that of the *speech* clues. The most superficial of these clues, of course, is found in the content, the *what is said* portion of the individual's speech behavior. This is almost too obvious to require discussion, but it should be noted that the content of the speech very frequently varies from other signs of emotional disturbance which seems to be present. For example, one individual might express a very strong statement of distress, anger, or other emotional disturbance; this content might not be supported by his manner of speaking and/or actions while speaking. In addition to the pure content, then the rehabilitation specialist must be alert to discrepancies between content and feeling.

In addition to the more or less apparent content implications, there are many other clues to emotional disturbance found in the speech behavior of the counselee. First, consider production or output of speech. An extremely high output of words may arise from any one of several reactions: some people are verbose to avoid silence, some people are verbose because the relevance of particular factors cannot be determined, and some people are verbose in a very effective attempt to cover up significant factors. The verbose counselee is by no means invariably the most revealing counselee: very frequently, the rehabilitation specialist will feel an initial satisfaction with the extremely high content and apparent good rapport which has been established with a verbose individual, but as time passes, he may experience less and less satisfaction with the session.

On the other side of the verbose counselee is the low-output or low-volume counselee. The individual is most likely one who is conscious of inferiority feelings, hostilities, and other negative feelings. This individual is also likely to be one who sees things as either black or white, with very little recognition of the shades of values or of meaning which are inherent in most of the complex and abstract concepts of our language.

The individual who is consistently verbose or consistently reticent thus gives some important clues to his emotional reaction, but much more dramatic is the individual who changes his speech habits during times of high stress. The verbose individual who has gone into great detail about every aspect of his life suddenly becomes reticent: the implication of emotional disturbance is very strong and the rehabilitation specialist should be quick to recognize this discrepancy in the normal output habits of the client. Similarly, the reticent individual who suddenly becomes verbose is also easily recognized as experiencing temporary emotional disturbances.

The habitual use of senseless questions, such as "Why did this have to happen to me?" or "What's the matter with everybody nowadays, anyway?" or other such unanswerable questions, seems to be definite indication of maladjustment. The occasional use of such unanswerable questions, as opposed to frequent or habitual use, serves to suggest an area or a time of heightened emotional disturbance or tension in the client.

The tone and loudness of the speech is an extremely significant indicator of emotional disturbance. The individual who maintains a steady, habitual loudness is probably one who is consciously or unconsciously aggressive toward his environment; the habitually softspoken individual may be the cultural ideal or may be utilizing soft tones as a means of agreeing with his environment; the lowspoken individual very frequently is seen to be one who is insecure and uncertain. In this matter of loudness and tonal quality, changes in the habitual speech behavior are seen as especially important with regard to identifying specific areas or times of heightened emotional stress.

TESTING CONSIDERATIONS

To what extent do neuropsychiatric symptoms or treatments affect the usual tests administered by rehabilitation specialists? It is obvious that testing of the psychotic individual in the acute phases of his illness is impractical and that such testing would provide seriously distorted information in many cases. Testing of highly depressed or anxious neurotics is also subject to distortions of results, but not to so great a degree as would be found for acute psychotics. Testing of personality-disordered clients will generally yield no serious distortions, and testing of the retarded should similarly be seen as appropriate. Testing in the improved phases of psychosis and psychoneurosis is acceptable, although the rehabilitation specialist must remain alert to possible idiosyncratic distortions which in many cases relate to the psychotic or neurotic symptomatology. For example, an individual considered to be in "good remission" from a psychotic condition may continue to be insecure and anxious with regard to his adequacy and accuracy insofar as tests are concerned. This individual may be so cautious and insistently careful during tests that his score is seriously depressed on any time-limited or time-bonusing tests.

Another individual may respond to the interpersonal warmth of treatment by reflecting higher scores on interests scales such as the Kuder Social Service or the California-Occupational-Interest Personal Social.

Tests involving time-limits may be expected to have individual disadvantages for neuropsychiatric clients. For measures of mental ability, the Wechsler Adult Intelligence Scale is desirable because it permits gauging the client's reactions to time-oriented tasks while still providing a satisfactory measure or estimate of his mental functioning.

For measures of such aptitudes as dexterity, more than one dexterity test is recommended, with the client compared, however, with the general populations norms. This is reasonable, as it is quite clear that competition in jobs requiring certain degrees of dexterity will be based on general population levels rather than on schizophrenic or other levels.

The extremely complex question concerning medication effects upon test results can be answered qualitatively but not quantitatively: there are significant effects, identifiable in carefully structured experimental approaches involving pre- and post-measures (pre-medication and post-medication) of dexterity, specific scales of the Wechsler Adult Intelligence Scale, and self-concept measures (Knape, 1958, pp. 195-198). This qualitatively confident answer, however, can merely serve to alert the rehabilitation specialist to possible distortions, since the experimental approach necessarily limits dosage and type of medication, length of time under medication, and other variables not controllable in the non-experimental situation. In general, individuals taking major tranquilizers may be expected to make less effective use of time on tests than other individuals, and those taking psychic energizers may be expected to work with great speed—but perhaps less accurately—than others. It is recommended, therefore, that rehabilitation specialists not blind themselves to the diagnostic implications of the tests, while at the same time avoiding the human temptation to present himself as a diagnostic expert as a result of the test data available to him. Diagnosis in neuropsychiatric fields is a vastly complex act and is the proper province of the physician, aided though he may be by other professions.

Rehabilitation specialists also use personality inventories of varying degrees of diagnostic ambition. The statistically impeccable Minnesota Multiphasic Personality Inventory and California Psychological Inventory are frequently used by the rehabilitation specialist in his attempt to understand the client more completely. Two cautions are to be strictly observed in the use of such inventories: their limitations for diagnosis must be recognized and the client must be told of results in non-psychiatric terms. The inventories can be very useful in the rehabilitation relationship if these cautions are observed. One of the most fruitful uses of the inventory is to provide a focus for discussion based on the reduced-threat approach of self-evaluation. For example, if the tests suggest a tendency to depression or low sense of well-being, the rehabilitation specialists can initiate discussion of this matter by stating, "You see yourself, at times, as not happy, perhaps even down-in-the-dumps more than you would like?" By stressing the self-view nature of the inventory, and by using non-threatening terminology, the rehabilitation specialist can usually lead the client into a non-directive counseling relationship around areas identified in the test.

JOB PLACEMENT PROBLEMS

The task of rehabilitating neuropsychiatric clients is made more difficult by public opinions concerning the mentally ill. In the now classic summary of the projected needs for improved and changed treatment plants for the mentally ill, *Action for Mental Health,* the Staff of the Joint Commission on Mental Illness and Health stated: "Mental illness . . . tends to disturb and repel others rather than evoke their sympathy and desire to help." (Staff, Joint Commission, 1961, p. 18). The literature is replete with surveys of the attitudes held toward mentally ill persons, most of which tends to support the viewpoint of the Joint Commission. Many organizations, however, have carried on active mental health educational programs, and there is evidence that the public is becoming more accepting of the mentally ill person.

The Client's Dilemma

A recent summary of many of the attitude surveys appeared in a pamphlet entitled "Public Opinions and Attitudes About Mental Health" (Halpert, 1963). The conclusion was drawn that "there has been forward motion during the past decade in terms of better public understanding of mental illness and greater tolerance or acceptance of the mentally ill" (Halpert, 1963, p. 19). Despite such admitted progress, however, there remains a substantial prejudice toward the neuropsychiatric client, and this is easily perceived by rehabilitation specialists and the clients themselves. The client, by definition, already experiences difficulty in the interpersonal sphere, and this additional tension in the relationships with others creates a very great psychological barrier to resumption of interpersonal effectiveness. Knowledge of the prejudice and expectancy of encountering it are strong reasons cited by clients who have reached the decision to conceal the history of neuro-psychiatric treatment. This decision is very incorrect, but it has persisted even among professionals, and it is fairly understandable.

The logic of the decision is clear: the client feels that opportunity for a normal job possibility and social life will be denied to him if he discloses the facts of his neuropsychiatric history—*ergo,* conceal the facts. While the logic seems sound, it represents distortion and will result in fear and unhappiness when concealment is extended to include the client's employer and close social contacts, especially those close enough to be considered "involved" in the client's life to a significant extent, such as a prospective mate, relatives, and very close friends. The neuropsychiatric client should not proclaim this fact to the world at large, but he should be helped to see that there is no shame attached to his illness, and that he can discuss it with prospective employers and close social contacts, the latter types of discussions being on those occasions when the subject arises naturally out of the conversation or the relationship proper.

The client who has had any medical problem other than a neuropsychiatric one generally is able to preserve a proper view of *when* and *with whom* he should discuss his condition, but the neuropsychiatric client quite often experiences great uncertainty in this matter. The rehabilitation specialist, accordingly, should help his client see his illness as a fact of history, to be disclosed to prospective employers routinely upon application, and to social contacts only when the subject would ordinarily be proper regarding any fact of medical history.

Interest in the job placement phase of the rehabilitation process has long been evidenced. Menninger (1956) stressed the importance of a prompt return to proper work, and the American Medical Association has published a useful "Guide for Evaluating Employability after Psychiatric Illness" (Staff, Joint Committee on Mental Health in Industry, American Medical Association). Lofquist, Siess, Davis, England, and Weiss (1964) stressed the usefulness of considering disability from the focus of work adjustment, and Olshansky and Unterberger (1963) emphasized the importance of work for the mental-hospital ex-patient. In an excellent pamphlet, Dorothy B. Thompson suggests that a rehabilitation specialist working with the mentally restored should have "three *C*'s . . . conviction, confidence, and common sense" (Thompson, 1965, p. 14).

Job placement of any handicapped worker is a challenging task for the rehabilitation specialist. The work of placement, from the initial determination by the counselor of just how much placement assistance is needed to the final closure of the case as an employed rehabilitant, poses substantial problems and difficulties at every turn. Some rehabilitation workers consider placement to be the most important phase of their work, whereas others try to relegate this phase of the placement process to other agencies, such as the public and private employment services. Neither approach represents a realistic attitude.

The theory that the individual should be counseled to the point where he is able to compete in the labor market by himself is a very persuasive argument. This argument proceeds from the fact that no job placement is permanent and that only preparation for flexible and effective competition in the labor market will solve the client's vocational problems. Essentially this is a restatement of the idea that the aim of counseling is to help the individual to solve his present and future problems by himself. However, the fallacy of this argument in rehabilitation is clear since it is used to excuse a blindness to the differing needs of clients.

There are some clients who will meet the challenge of self-placement and become effective, competitive participants in the economy. There are other clients, however, who will be able to meet the demands of a job only after varying degrees of placement help have been given. Experienced counselors recognize that the amount of placement help needed ranges from a pedagogic presentation of methods of job search to the ultimate intrusiveness in job placement—counselor location of an opening followed by active counselor participation and involvement in the application procedures. It is obvious to any counselor who has worked with a substantial number of rehabilitation clients that the idea of self-placement cannot serve as an adequate placement philosophy for the rehabilitation specialist in view of the widely variant needs of the clients.

The rehabilitation specialist who views the placement phase as the most important part of the rehabilitation process is likely to overestimate the amount of help which he should give to individuals in job search and placement. This counselor is likely to refer to successful clients by using such statements as "*I* placed him with a shoemaker", or "After *I* located a job for him", or "All he needed was *to be put* on a job and then he could make out fine." These and similar statements generally identify the counselor who takes great pride in the job-placement phase of rehabilitation. This pride may cause him to be blind to the individual needs of the cases to participate in the solution of their vocational problems. The avid placement enthusiast frequently finds himself trying to "convince" cases that a particular job is the sort of work for him, and he is likely to feel a sense of great frustration if the counselee does not wholeheartedly endorse his efforts to complete vocational placement for him.

The rehabilitation specialist who gives careful attention to the *extent* of placement help which he should render in each individual case, is likely to be a much more effective counselor than a counselor with either of the extreme positions just described. This philosophy of individualizing one's services to the client is not a new philosophy, but it needs restatement with reference to the placement phase of counseling, since the philosophies of the extremes have been advanced so energetically.

Overcoming Some Basic Difficulties

The neuropsychiatric client presents some very real job placement difficulties, perhaps problems more difficult than the placement of any other disability group. The generally favorable publicity which has been given to the physically handicapped worker for many years has still not had a decisive impact upon the prejudice, ignorance, and fear with which employers view the neuropsychiatric client. Hiring practices, based upon both written and unwritten policies of some employers, constitute a real block to re-employment. The neuropsychiatric case, however, has additional difficulties. It is almost the rule to find that the neuropsychiatric client has a poor employment record and a lack of current job skills. Since neuropsychiatric conditions are insidious in onset, the neuropsychiatric client has experienced a gradual deterioration in his patterns of work and education. The neuropsychiatric client will frequently have very poor recommendations as a result of long-felt development of his condition.

A third problem particularly pertinent to the neuropsychiatric client is the difficulty he finds in trying to fit in with a group, in *being* and *feeling* accepted by his fellow workers. The intensity of this problem in the interpersonal sphere is a distinguishing characteristic of the neuropsychiatric population, and while counseling and proper placement can reduce this factor, it will still have significance and bearing upon the individual's abilities to work effectively.

A fourth problem is the factor of special limitations with regard to the level of responsibility which can be tolerated, with regard to the soporific effect of some chemotherapies, with regard to the time-off requirements for out-patient treatments, etc.

A final problem relative to job placement of the neuropsychiatric client is the inadequate help and support which the client secures from his family in finding and holding a job. Family members frequently have the feeling that they have been disgraced by the illness which the case has been subject to and they do not render the help in finding jobs traditionally assumed by families in today's economy.

Job placement is not done by the rehabilitation specialist alone, but it is his responsibility—this thought summarizes a useful philosophy of placement, which may be expanded to increased usefulness. However, if rehabilitation specialists will recall this sentence as they carry out their job duties, it will surely aid them in placing a proper perspective on placement efforts.

Opportunities

Rehabilitation workers should be aware that there is no area of employment which should be considered closed to neuropsychiatric cases. The Veterans Administration recently published a pamphlet called "They Return to Work" (Staff, Department of Veterans Benefits, 1963). This pamphlet (of some 200 pages) describes the jobs into which rehabilitated neurotic and psychotic clients have been placed. These cover a broad range of occupations from professional positions to unskilled work. Similar findings are evidenced in the wide range of jobs in which the epileptic client has been successfully employed (Staff, Department of Veterans Benefits, 1960). The mentally retarded are similarly employable in a broad spectrum of jobs, as reported by Garrison and Force (1965, p. 118) and the staff of the President's Committee on Employment of the Handicapped (1963).

In the study relative to neurotics and psychotics, the job distribution compares favorably with that of all employed males in the labor force. The proportion of persons employed, however, does not compare favorably with the nation as a whole: 31 percent of non-hospitalized psychiatrically disabled veterans were unemployed as compared with the usual unemployed rate of about 5 percent of the civilian labor force. This indicates that further rehabilitation and readjustment services in behalf of the unemployed group is required.

Neuropsychiatric hospitals over the nation have been very energetic in trying many new post-hospital plans which do not involve the full and independent participation of the ex-patient in the economy. One of these plans which has become very popular is the Family or Foster Home Program. This program is usually administered by social workers, but close collaboration with the counseling psychologists is maintained to assure that the ex-patient has an adequate level of activity, either paid or unpaid in nature. The Foster Home Program simply involves the selection of a home in which the ex-patient can be placed, and the payment for such service generally is very little more than the usual room and board which anyone would pay in any independent arrangement. The personalities of the ex-patient and the foster family are carefully evaluated, and a follow-up program assures that adjustments and re-assignments will be made as required.

Other post-hospital programs serve similar purposes: the Day Hospital enables the ex-patient to return to the hospital for daytime activities and rehabilitation routines. He maintains his home in the community but "works" at the hospital. The Night Hospital enables the patient to live in the hospital while he works in the community. The Evening Hospital permits the patient to return to the hospital for evening social and recreational activities while maintaining his home and daytime activities in the community. Other variations of these programs are being devised as the attempt continues to return the patient to the community as soon as possible, even if such return, initially, is a partial one. Halfway houses permit a degree of sheltered living while the ex-patient functions in the community. Halfway houses also are used for alcoholics, as described by Thompson (1965).

Problems Involved in the Patient's Return to the Community

The philosophy of returning the patient to the community early has not evolved overnight. In the report to the staff of the Joint Commission on Mental Illness and Health (1961), the need for community involvement in the treatment of the mentally ill was stated again and again. Since 1955,

Federal legislation in this area has been extensive. The staff of the Public Health Service (1961) summarized some of the planning needs for community mental health facilities, and the staff of the Department of Health, Education and Welfare (1964) described the purposes and functions of an ideal community approach to mental health centers. Myers (1964) described improvement in the community approach to mental health. The staff of the Vocational Rehabilitation Administration (1965) has established guidelines for relationship of the vocational rehabilitation state services with the community mental health centers.

The need for full community understanding of the ex-mental patient was greatly increased when the new chemo-therapies began to be used extensively in the early and middle 1950's. During this period, literally thousands of neuropsychiatric patients underwent dramatic improvement in their condition. Many of these were able to return to the community as competing members of the economy. Others, however, no longer needing the hospital environment, were not yet ready to enter into competition at home. The return of these persons to the community for community acceptance and tolerance has sometimes been delayed because of the persistence of old prejudices back home as well as because of the fears of the mental patient himself.

Education of the community is proceeding, however, and employers, as a part of that community, are being informed as to the usefulness and potential value of employing ex-mental patients. Much more education is needed, as anyone who is involved in contacting employers will testify, in spite of techniques described above for providing information about hospitalization in a mental hospital. Surveys of the attitudes of employers are encouraging, and while there is a *public relations factor* which makes it easy to misinterpret survey responses, the *practices* of employers also seem to be improving relative to employment of the neuropsychiatrically handicapped. The "public relations" effect may be defined as the tendency to *speak* favorably but to *act* in a prejudiced manner.

Surveys of employer attitudes abound in the literature of rehabilitation and psychology. Bieliauskas and Wolfe (1960) made a telephone survey of large employers in a midwestern metropolitan area. They concluded that large employers have a highly positive attitude toward hiring former state mental hospital patients, with only a minority of the employers objecting to hiring former state mental hospital patients. These researchers described as untrue the general assumption that employers have an overall negative attitude toward hiring former mental patients. These researchers did not, however, mention the *public relations* effect cited in the preceding paragraph.

Olshansky (1961) found that three-fourths of two-hundred interviewed employers indicated they would hire ex-patients from mental hospitals, but in the three years covered by the study only 27 of these same 150 employers actually hired any known ex-patient. The public relations effect is evidenced by these findings, but again this factor was not pointed out by the researcher.

The author has completed a study in which the *public relations* effect is experimentally isolated and named (Knape, 1970). As a part of a larger research study conducted at Baylor University, supported in large part by a grant from the Vocational Rehabilitation Administration, a structured telephone survey was made of the attitudes *and* practices of employers in the Waco metropolitan area relative to the employment of handicapped persons, including neuropsychiatrically disabled. The survey was conducted by means of a telephone recorder, equipped with the usual "beep" signal, and accompanied by a request to permit the recording of the interview "for purposes of saving time." A control group, matched according to the type of enterprise and the size of the employed force, was also surveyed without the recorder. The experience of the employer with handicapped persons was surveyed, as well as his attitudes toward employing handicapped persons. Frankly negative attitude responses and disguised negative attitude responses were both counted.

Initial figures on this telephone survey reflect that of the 222 interviews, 118 of this group had had previous experience with employing handicapped persons of some category. Among this group of 118, 64 were recorded interviews and 54 were non-recorded interviews. Of the 104 employers which had not had previous experience with employing the handicapped, 47 were recorded interviews and 57 were non-recorded interviews. Employers who responded with openly non-favorable responses to two or more disability categories were distributed as follows:

Categories	*No.*	*Non-favorable Responses* *2 or more disabilities*
Previous experience with handicapped:		
Recorded group	64	18, or 28.1%
Non-Recorded group	54	31, or 57.4%
No previous experience with handicapped:		
Recorded group	47	24, or 51.1%
Non-Recorded group	57	43, or 75.4%

A follow-up replication revealed the same types of results, yielding confidence levels beyond .01 on chi-square tests of the date (Knape, 1970, p. 8).

One can see that experience in hiring the handicapped is related to stated attitudes, and that recording a telephone interview greatly increases the guardedness, the defensiveness or response—which the author chooses to call the *public relations* effect.

REHABILITATION MYTHS

In focusing upon the placement phase and discussing the desirable methods of accomplishing this phase, one is prone to lose sight of the actual experience which is encountered in the field. Accordingly, many new rehabilitation people feel quite inadequate in the placement phase because they have had to study placement in terms of several mythical ideals. Let us examine some of these mythical ideals and speak briefly to the facts as well as to the value of the myth.

Myth of Multiple Opportunity

First, there is the myth of multiple opportunity and the consequent selection of *the* job which best suits the client with regard to ability, disability, and personality. Any rehabilitation counselor knows, after his first week, that job openings are extremely scarce. Job development is not usually a matter of counselor persuasiveness, but in many cases is a matter of accidental time-liness of contact. Accordingly, the usual situation facing the rehabilitation counselor when a handicapped individual finishes a training program is that there is no known opening at all, much less multiple opportunity. The client becomes one of several persons awaiting job placement assistance so that when the counselor learns of an opening he has to select *among clients* rather than *among jobs* to effect the placement—herein is the actual value of the stress placed on "matching the man to the job." One is thus enabled to select from his clients persons who will be able to do the available job and who would be able to satisfy the employer to such a degree that later placement of other handicapped persons will be aided. Small adaptations of the job demands are possible, but major adaptations will not generally be made for new employees. Major adaptations are typically made in the event that an employee becomes disabled while employed, and this is quite obviously no advantage to the counselor who is seeking new employment opportunity for a seriously disabled client.

Myth of Ideal Employee

Secondly, there is the myth of the eager, efficient handicapped person who is well-trained and an ideal employee in every sense. By this myth reha-bilitation workers have somewhat fooled themselves in their attempt to secure non-prejudicial treatment of the handicapped. There has been drawn a picture of the handicapped which is much distorted by our wishes. Most workers who deal with the handicapped any length of time soon find that the handicapped persons are very much like anyone else—that they have their moods, their disinclinations to work, their gaps in skill, and various crochets and eccentricities. Clients who look very good in the rehabilitation office frequently will make a very poor appearance before a personnel officer. A rehabilitation worker may have had some experience along this line but it never fails to surprise him to see the variation between the rehabilitation-worker view of the client and the personnel-office view of the client. This myth, however, is an important one in maintaining worker morale and the morale of the handicapped person. The author would rather expect too much of a handicapped man and have to adapt his expectations to reality than to expect too little of the client and cause the client to feel that even the professionals in the field are discouraged about his opportunities.

Myth of the Ideal Employer

A third myth deals with the viewpoint that employers are generally anxious to give the handicapped person a chance if one can establish the fact that the handicapped person can do an adequate job. Any experienced rehabilitation man will know that this attitude is not at all the rule. A substantial number of employers have deep-rooted psychological rejections of handicapped persons, and consciously or unconsciously reduce the chances of such persons to be employed. Other employers have less-than-mentally-healthy attitudes and reasons for employing the handicapped, and some may seek to establish more than the usual amount of dependency on the part of the handicapped employee. Once again the myth serves a useful purpose, however, in that counselors must maintain the expectancy that employers are reasonable beings, subject to logic and open to the persuasion of the counselor. One bit of philosophy which the author has found very useful in dealing with employers is to recognize that they are in business to make a profit, but if they can make a profit they are not averse to adding to their business self-concept a philanthropic hue.

Counselors of the handicapped may resent the thought that employers occasionally hire handicapped persons out of pity. Many rehabilitation workers feel that this is bad for the handicapped worker and bad for the cause of the handicapped as a whole. The author shares this feeling wholeheartedly in a theoretical sense, but pragmatically he recognizes that many employers, convinced that the client would do an adequate job, employ a handicapped person on the basis that "he needed a chance." It has not been the author's experience that this type of employment situation was any less desirable than the hiring of a handicapped person by an employer who said that all he considered was whether the man could do the job.

Techniques of Approaching a Prospective Employer

This topic leads one to consider the various techniques which may be used when approaching employers about the placement of a handicapped person. The author has very little patience with the philosophy which advances the theory that employers should be required to hire a certain proportion of handicapped workers, as is done in England and a few other countries. It seems that this requirement is quite detrimental to the cause of handicapped workers as a whole, since employers will say, "But I have hired my *quota* of handicapped persons." The philosophy in this country is much more wholesome in that it is believed that the handicapped worker should not be employed unless he is able to do the job. Stress is placed on the fact that hiring the handicapped is not a sacrifice but is a good business endeavor.

This same stress upon the profit motive must be maintained by the rehabilitation counselor as he considers the selection and training phases with the client as well as the placement phase of the rehabilitation process. Once the fact is granted, however, that the handicapped person must do an adequate job and must earn his salary, there is still much opportunity for the employer to feel that he is being a "good man" by employing the handicapped person. Counselors should not use this fact in *persuading* employers, but can use it in the closing phases of the placement process when the employer has already indicated that he is going to employ the client. The counselor can then bring in this factor by statements such as the following:

> Now you are getting a good man here, Mr. Jones, and he will earn his salary, but it's very good of you to recognize this. Many employers would be blind to the value of this man because of his handicap.
> This man will earn his pay, Mr. Jones, and you will be glad you hired him. He will also be grateful to you for not turning him down because of his disability—many employers never look beyond the fact of disability.

Statements such as this are very important as a subtle reward to the employer, as most employers will be feeling at the time they employ a handicapped person that they have done something worthy of praise. This should not be overlooked by the counselor as he completes his contacts with the employer. It will also enable the counselor to have a warm re-entry into the employer's office for follow-up visits and later placements.

CONCLUSION

Tennyson told us, "A man's reach should exceed his grasp, or what's a heaven for?" This is particularly applicable when one considers the frustrating, challenging job of the rehabilitation worker. It is always necessary for the rehabilitation worker to try to reach some of the ideals embodied in the "myths" just enumerated. While he continues to do what can be done with the dross and the reality of his day-to-day job, it is most important for him to maintain his hope that he can reach some of these ideals and actualize some of these myths.

REFERENCES

Ausubel, D.P.: Personality disorder *is* disease. *American Psychologist, 16*:69-74, 1961.

Bieliauskas, V.J. and Wolfe, H.E.: The attitude of industrial employers toward hiring of former State Mental Hospital patients. *Journal of Clinical Psychology, 16*:256-259, 1960.

Crawford, F.R.: *Mental Illness in Texas—A Morbidity Report for 1964.* Austin, Office of Mental Health Planning, Texas Department of Health, 1965.

Crump, W.A. and Harry, W.M.: Foster homes help mentally retarded. *Rehabilitation Record, 5*:3, 23-25, 1964.

Garrison, K.C. and Force, D.G.: *The Psychology of Exceptional Children* (4th ed.). New York, Ronald Press Co., 1965.

Goldman, L.: *Using Tests in Counseling.* New York, Appleton-Century-Crofts, 1961.

Halpert, H.P.: *Public Opinions and Attitudes About Mental Health* (Public Health Service Publication No. 1045). Washington, Government Printing Office, 1963.

Knape, C.S.: *The Dynamics of Placement in the Vocational Rehabilitation Process* (Condensed Final Report, Project Number RD-746-61-G). Waco, Baylor University, 1970.

Knape, C.S.: *The Effect of Certain Chemotherapeutic Agents upon Vocational Counseling Services in a Neuropsychiatric Setting.* (Microfilm.) Austin, University of Texas, 1958.

Lofquist, L.H., Siess, T.F., Davis, R.V., England, G.W., and Weiss, D.J.: *Minnesota Studies in Vocational Rehabilitation* (XVII. Disability, and Work). Minneapolis, Industrial Relations Center, University of Minnesota, 1964.

Menninger, W.C.: Mental patients can be cured. *Reader's Digest, 69*:13-16, 1956.

Milt, H.: *Basic Facts About Mental Illness.* Fair Haven (New Jersey), Scientific Aids Publications, 1959.

Mowrer, O.H.: "Sin," the lesser of two evils. *American Psychologist, 15*:301-304, 1960.

Myers, Evelyn S. (Ed.): *Community Mental Health Advances* (Public Health Service Publication No. 1141). Washington, Government Printing Office, 1964.

Olshansky, S.: Employer receptivity. *Journal of Rehabilitation, 27*:5, 35-36, 1961.

Olshansky, S. and Unterberger, Hilma.: The meaning of work and its implications for the Ex-Mental Hospital Patient (Personnel Information Bulletin No. IB 05-172). Washington, Veterans Administration, 1963.

Pollock, H.: Is the paroled patient a menace in the community? *Psychiatric Quarterly, 12*:2, 236, 1938.

The President's Committee on Employment of the Handicapped: *Guide to Job Placement of the Mentally Retarded.* Washington, Government Printing Office, 1963.

Rinkel, M. (Ed.): *Biological Treatment of Mental Illness.* New York, L.C. Page and Co., 1966.

Rothaus, P. and Hanson, P.G.: *Community Attitudes Toward the Mentally Ill:* Implications of Current Experimental Investigations (Mimeographed). Paper presented at the American Psychological Association Annual Meeting, Chicago, 1965.

Rothaus, P., Hanson, P.G., Cleveland, S.E., and Johnson, D.L.: Mental illness and employment. *American Psychologist, 19*:200-201, 1964.

Schlaifer, C.: *Report and Recommendation of the Joint Commission on Mental Illness and Health* (Proceedings of the Mental Health Assembly, 1961). New York, National Association for Mental Health, 1962.

Staff, Council on Mental Health, American Medical Association: *Proceedings, National Congress on Mental Illness and Health.* Chicago, The Council, 1962.

Staff, Department of Veterans Benefits: *Occupations of Epileptic Veterans of World War II and Korean Conflict* (VA Pamphlet 22-6). Washington, Government Printing Office, 1960.

Staff, Department of Veterans Benefits: *They return to work* (VA Pamphlet 22-9). Washington, Government Printing Office, 1963.

Staff, Joint Commission on Mental Illness and Health: *Action for Mental Health.* New York, Basic Books, 1961.

Staff, Joint Committee on Mental Health in Industry, American Medical Association: Guide for evaluating employability after psychiatric illness. *Journal of the American Medical Association, 181*:146-149, 1962.

Staff, National Committee Against Mental Illness: *What are the Facts About Mental Illnesses?* Washington, The Committee, 1961.

Staff, National Congress of Parents and Teachers: *Children's Emotional Health.* Chicago, National Congress, 1964.

Staff, National Institute of Mental Health: *Research Activities of the National Institute of Mental Health* (Public Health Service Publication No. 1291). Washington, Government Printing Office, 1964.

Staff, New York State Department of Mental Hygiene: Criminal Acts of Ex-Mental Hospital Patients. Mental Hospital Service, No. 153 (Supplementary Mailing), August 1962.

Staff, Philadelphia College of Physicians: *A Symposium on the Problem of the Sexual Criminal.* Philadelphia, Pennsylvania Mental Health, 1960.

Staff, Public Health Service: *Planning of Facilities for Mental Health Services* (Public Health Service Publication No. 808). Washington, Government Printing Office, 1961.

Staff, Texas State Hospitals and Special Schools Board: *Annual Report for Fiscal Year September 1, 1962, to August 31, 1963.* Austin, The Board, 1964.

Staff, Vocational Rehabilitation Administration: *Rehabilitating the Mentally Ill.* Washington, Government Printing Office, 1965.

Staff, World Health Organization: *The International Classification of Diseases, Eighth Revision.* New York, WHO, 1968. Also available, adapted for use in the United States, as Public Health Service Publication No. 1693. Washington, U.S. Government Printing Office, 1968.

Szasz, T.S.: The myth of mental illness. *American Psychologist, 15*:113-118, 1960.

Thompson, Dorothy B.: *Guide to Job Placement of the Mentally Restored.* Washington, Government Printing Office, 1965.

Woolley, D.W.: New insight into mental illness—Philosophical implications. *Atlantic Monthly, 216*:1, 46-50, 1965.

Woolley, D.W.: *The Biochemical Basis of Psychosis.* New York, John Wiley and Sons, 1952.

(PART EIGHT)

THE CANCER CLIENT

MEDICAL AND PSYCHOLOGICAL PROBLEMS
IN THE REHABILITATION OF THE
CANCER PATIENT

Chapter 21

MEDICAL AND PSYCHOLOGICAL PROBLEMS IN THE REHABILITATION OF THE CANCER PATIENT*

A. Beatrix Cobb

INTRODUCTION

CANCER is perhaps the most baffling and challenging disability now referred for rehabilitation. It is baffling on two counts: medical and vocational.

On the medical side, cancer is surrounded by many unknowns. Despite recent dramatic advances in treatment and research, the cause of cancer is not clearly understood; the course of the disease varies extremely from organ to organ and from individual to individual; and the prognosis, although always guarded, now carries a hope for longer and longer, but uncertain, survival time.

The vocational frustration arises from two diverse sources. First, even when physical restoration seems successful, the nature of the disease still leaves the client and the rehabilitation counselor living under the very real threat of recurrence. Even if the individual seems physically able to cope with his previous or a new job, the question is always present, "For how long?"

The second vocational placement dilemma appears when the prospective employer is approached. If obvious physical mutilation or limitation due to the disease or treatment is present, it can pose a problem. Many are loath to accept an individual whose appearance may detract from business, or whose work may be interrupted by recurring illness.

As the survival time of the cancer patient has increased in more recent years, thought and effort have been turned to the "quality" of that survival (American Cancer Society, 1969). No longer is it sufficient to point with pride to the fact that more and more cancer patients are alive five or ten years after initial treatment of the disease. The questions now arise: How are they alive? Are they invalids depending on others for emotional care and physical comfort? Are they living the life of a recluse, hiding from family

---

*Special appreciation is here expressed to Malcolm J. Thomas, Jr., M.D. for invaluable assistance in the medical approach to cancer.

and friends? Is the disease still under control? Have they picked up the pre-diagnosis threads of their lives and returned to gainful employment and rich personal existence?

No longer are physicians content to save a life; now they ask, "What kind of life?" In May of 1968, a national award-winning program, "Quality of Survival of the Cancer Patient," was held in Hartford, Connecticut. This conference was co-sponsored by the Connecticut Division, Inc., American Cancer Society; the American Society of Surgeons; the Connecticut Society for Crippled Children and Adults; and the Vocational Rehabilitation Branch, United States Department of Health, Education, and Welfare. At that conference, Dr. Charles Rogers, Memorial Hospital, New York City, epitomized the past and pointed to the future in these words;

> I am saying that in our zealous endeavor to make more people survive longer, we have to a degree, lost sight of a very necessary part of survival, and that is quality.
> I offer you a quotation from the Bible . . . Matthew 16, verse 26: "For what do it profit a man if he gain the whole world, but suffer the loss of his soul?" In the case of the cancer victim, I say to you: And what do we gain if we save a larger number, only to have them lead a life which for them is living hell? (p. 17).

The *quality* of survival—is that not what rehabilitation is all about? The return of the disabled to meaningful personal and vocational self-sufficiency is the rehabilitation goal in any disability.

What is meant by "quality of survival?" In the referenced conference (1968), five pertinent factors were enumerated as essential to a quality survival (W. Bradford Patterson, p. 1). These five included health, functions, comfort, emotional response, and economics.

The **Health** quality of survival encompassed not only recovery from onslaught and treatment of the disease, but also the general physical condition of the client five to ten years later. Is he up and around, with energy to live abundantly and to pursue gainful employment? Or, is he bed-fast or without enery and motivation?

The topic of **Functions** included the ability of the patient, in the follow-up period, to carry on with personal living chores and work assignments. Has he resumed pre-diagnosis work responsibilities, or is he limited in performance?

Comfort involved freedom from pain or the distress of limited activity. The quality of survival cannot be high if the patient endures debilitating pain or if he is constantly hampered in movement.

An often overlooked factor in the quality of success is that of **Emotional Response.** If the ravages of the disease or treatment have left the individual disfigured, his emotional reaction may interfere with his acceptance of the altered self. Included in this area are such items as his successful adjustment back into family and community living as opposed to having become a recluse. Here, too, we must come to grips with the presence or absence of *undue* anxieties and fears centered around his future.

Finally, the **Economic element** in the quality of survival is a pressing one. Even the initial expense of diagnosis and treatment is phenomenal. When there is added to this sum, the cost of follow-up observations and treatment, plus the loss of income due to necessary absences to accomplish this treatment, the financial drain is considerable. If survival has meant bankruptcy for his family, the patient is not likely to look upon that survival as a "quality" one.

So, the role of rehabilitation in ensuring a quality survival in cancer is indeed a challenging one. Once the *initial* treatment is concluded and the patient is able to think in terms of picking up the joys and responsibilities of his life, rehabilitation can add much to the quality of that living. A return to the world of work brings emotional relief and financial assistance. It allows the patient to focus on overcoming physical limitations and psychological anxieties in the process of preparing for return to gainful employment. The pain becomes more bearable; the limitations become more acceptable; the health status improves; and the emotional fears lessen as he once again assumes even partial financial responsibility for himself and for those he loves.

Little is known, however, as to the ways and means to employ to ensure this "quality of survival". In many instances, the patient can return to his old job when he is physically and emotionally ready. In some cases, although he is physically and psychologically capable, the employer and his co-workers are not ready to accept him. In other cases, new jobs with pre-placement training are indicated. In a few circumstances sheltered work situations are needed.

More well-planned experience and much action research are needed before this challenge can be adequately met. Agency and medical personnel alike are still in early exploratory stages of rehabilitation work with cancer patients. Communication between the two groups is still difficult, though in their own way, representatives of each are earnestly trying to work with the other. Agency personnel are understandably unfamiliar with the medical parameters involved in this complex disability. Medical members of the team too often are not aware of the availability of services or of legal procedures guiding the work of the agency. Before much progress toward an integrated effort to enhance the "quality of survival of the cancer patient" can be accomplished, some concerted effort must be made to establish a pool of common knowledge (medical and rehabilitative) and to then systematically expand this information in both directions.

Toward that goal, this chapter will seek to bring together pertinent medical and psychological data which may assist the rehabilitation counselor, or the family member, in a better understanding of the physical and emotional problems the cancer patient must endure. Through this understanding it is hoped that communication between the counselor and the physician (or the family member) can improve, and that through this improved communication and insights, the quality of survival for the cancer patient will be enhanced in his home and his community.

DEFINITION OF CANCER

One of the many baffling factors surrounding cancer is the difficulty of defining the term precisely. Cancer is a collective term used to describe all malignant neoplasms arising in the body tissue (WHO, 1966). Since cancers differ widely when associated with diverse organs, or structures, of the body, it is not possible at present to formulate a specific cause of cancer. The Medical Dictionary (Dorland, 1957) defines *cancer* as "a cellular tumor the natural course of which is fatal and usually associated with formation of secondary tumors" (p. 223). The Report of a World Health Organization Expert Committee (1966) defines cancer as a "protean disease" and further states that a proper understanding of its many manifestations is essential to good clinical management" (p. 5).

Such definitions give little satisfaction to one experiencing cancer, or one seeking to help an individual who has the disease. So much mystery and dread, so many unknowns surround the term that it is understandable that the diagnosis strikes terror to the hearts of those stricken and those who love them.

Perhaps following a comparison that leads from known factors to less known ones, could bring a clearer understanding of this disease to all concerned. It is accepted that the normal cell grows in connection with that part of the body in which it has specific function. For instance, as the body develops in the uterus of the mother, the cells that make up the arms, hands, etc., take food, multiply, and grow in harmony with other cells and organs until the arm, hand, or other members of the body is complete. Upon completion of the body member, and from that time forward, the cells continue to take food and multiply but also *die* according to a regular cycle. In this way the body member is maintained, but does not continue to grow to massive size.

Cancer cells, however, do not grow in harmony with the cells from which they are derived or with the organs in which they arise, but operate in a lawless, unorthodox manner. So instead of maintaining order and coordination among the body organs, the cancer cells continue to grow and multiply. They relentlessly invade the body structures, "taking over" the food supply by diverting the blood and lymph channels to supply themselves rather than allowing the normal delivery of oxygen and food to the essential organs of the body. Thus they damage the organs adjacent to, or containing, the new invading mass. The result is body weight loss, anemia, and decreased tissue function; so the savage cancerous horde sweeps over the weakened body much as a plundering army spreads over a conquered land.

Once the cancer cells have set up operations within the body, they spread through the blood-stream, the lymph channels, and locally to adjacent structures. Again like an invading army they divide, conquer and colonize. When the cancer cells are carried by blood-stream or lymph channels to parts of the body distant from the original site, the new colony of spread is referred to as "metastasis".

Under a microscope, this rebellious cancer cell resembles the normal cell but appears to be immature (not fully developed). It looks like embryonal cells. The younger the appearance of the cell, the more vicious seems its power of tissue invasion. This accounts for the fact that cancers differ in rate of spread. Some are said to be "fast-growing" and spread over the body rapidly. Others are termed as "slow-growing" and may take years to overwhelm the body functioning.

Since the term *cancer* includes all malignant tumors, the usual practice is to speak of "different cancers affecting different organs or structures" (WHO, 1966, p. 5). Because this is true, cancer has been said to be not one disease, but many. The symptoms, course, treatment, and prognosis are related specifically to the organ invaded and its normal function. All of this seems to add up to a fatal condition surrounded by dangerous unknowns or little knowns. The picture is not as dark as these facts would seem to indicate. Indeed, "it has been estimated that one cancer in every three is of a type for which cure by the best existing method is feasible" (WHO, p. 5).

Perhaps further clarification of the meaning of the disease known as cancer will develop as the discussion continues to the complex procedures of medical diagnosis of the condition. The emotional impact of the diagnosis of cancer on the patient and his family will also be considered.

MEDICAL AND PSYCHOLOGICAL IMPLICATIONS IN THE DIAGNOSIS OF CANCER

In cancer perhaps more than any other disease an early diagnosis is significant. Speaking of cancer, medical experts have coined a prophetic saying, "The first chance to cure is the best chance to cure" (WHO, 1966, p. 6). Far too often, and contributing considerably to the fatality of the disease, the diagnosis is not made until the malignancy is widespread. This fact is not usually due to inept medical service, but to the insidious nature of the disease itself. In many instances, the cancer has reached advanced stages before the patient becomes aware of a difficulty sufficient to take him for medical advice.

The Importance of Early and Accurate Diagnosis

The urgent need for early diagnosis is also centered in the complexity of the disease. Cancers not only differ in tissues of origin and structural appearances, they arise from different causes, have varying clinical courses, and appear in individuals of divergent sex, age, and of differing physiological and psychological characteristics. Proper treatment for the specific cancer can be initiated only when correct and comprehensive information is available to the treating physician.

Again, cancer is said to be not one disease, but many diseases, as deter-

mined by the organ (site) in which it originates. These diversified malignancies respond in specific ways to various treatments. Effective diagnosis, therefore, is concerned with the identification of a specific type of cancer (histological), affecting a certain organ (site) or structure, of a particular individual of a specific sex and age, and who has unique physiological and psychological characteristics. The extent of the onslaught of the malignancy, and
the presence or absence of metastasis must also be known. All of these factors
are of extreme importance in the diagnosis and prognosis (medical prediction of the course and termination of the disease). Only with this information
can definitive treatment be instigated.

It is readily obvious that this comprehensive evaluation can be done best
in a well-equipped center where cancer-trained physicians and ancillary staff
members are available. The fact is, however, that most cancers are first ten-
tatively diagnosed by a family physician. The patient may not suspect the
presence of cancerous material and the family physician uncovers the possibility in routine examinations or in exploratory procedures. Such a patient
is referred *immediately* to a center or clinic where adequate equipment and
medical specialists are available. The lives of many have been saved, or
lengthened, by such prompt referrals.

One of the most treacherous traits of cancer is its ability to remain hidden
until the functioning of a vital organ is interrupted. This gives the malignant
growth opportunity to establish itself firmly in the primary site, and even set
up colonies in adjacent organs or tissues (metastasis) before its presence is
recognized. Often the symptoms mask the true condition by assuming physical signs peculiar to other diseases. For instance, cancer of the breast may
appear as the cystic mass sometimes present in mammary tissues; or cancer
of the lung has at times been honestly diagnosed as tuberculosis. Cancer of
the cervix often mimics menopausal indications, etc.

Lay people, puzzled by the intricate peculiarities of the disease, sometimes ask, "What does a cancer look like?" Or, "Why do you need a biopsy
(a surgically excised bit of tissue from the suspected site) before a diagnosis
can be made?" If you will review the section on definition of cancer, the
answer is obvious. It is *only* when the tissues can be studied under a microscope in order to determine the structure of the cells themselves that definitive
diagnosis can be made. Even then, this study must be done by a highly
trained, skillful pathologist, or errors may arise.

Psychological Impact of Diagnosis of Cancer

All of the intricate medical procedures mentioned above are being carried
out on a person. Even the most stoic individual dreads the discomfort and
indignity of a thorough physical examination when it is a routine procedure.
When the patient realizes that something serious is going on, anxiety looms
and permeates his being.

Threat of the Intimate Meaning of the Diagnosis

When the diagnosis has been made and it is cancer, the patient is precipitated into a state of biological defenselessness that is almost intolerable. There is no simple physiologic explanation of cancer, and there can be no firm assurance of recovery. So the patient comes face to face with a threat that is consistent with his own intimate knowledge of the meaning of cancer.

Cancer means many things to many people (Cobb, 1959). In a study of forty patients with a known cancer diagnosis, there seemed to be a continuum of anxiety experienced, ranging from "no appreciable threat" through a vague non-specific fear to a verbalized specific menace, and ending in what seemed to be an intelligent, controlled anxiety.

No appreciable threat at the diagnosis of cancer was reported by 12.5 percent of the sample Cobb studied. An evaluation of the reasons for no anxiety given by this group indicated that they were not informed about cancer. Several individuals simply were from uneducated families where their life styles precluded their having been reached by cancer education literature. They said such things as: "I thought it was just one of them little old tumors," or "I didn't see how it could be serious; it didn't hurt me none." A few well-educated members of the group were lulled into a false security by such specific medical names as "melanoma" and "Hodgkin's Disease" and did not at first connect these names with malignancies.

Approximately 25 percent of the population investigated reported vague non-specific fears focused around the diagnosis of cancer. When their reports were analyzed, it was obvious that for the most part this one-fourth of the group really went into "shock" when the diagnosis was revealed to them. There seemed to be a lack of anxiety that was really an inability to verbalize fears. Several said such things as: "It just seemed like one of those things that you think can't happen to you," or "I had mixed emotions about it." Others simply repeated, "I was scared to death." One gave an exquisite description of acute shock (Cobb, 1959).

> I guess I was just petrified when he (the doctor) told me. I came through the operation in a stage of what seemed like exaltation, or joy, and felt completely unafraid. I seemed at peace with the world, but didn't seem attached to it. I made up poetry all the time, and fell back on religion. I was living in a world above earthly woes. . . . Then, it wore off and I came back to earth with a bang. Now, I realize that I was simply in a daze. I was so petrified, I didn't know what was happening to me really (p. 276).

More than half (52.5 percent) of the sample reported a specific, personal threat. This specific menace was *Death*. To them cancer was synonymous with death. One man expressed the consensus:

> If you get it, it ain't no use to run to a doctor, for he can't do nothing for you anyway. . . . You're gonna die. I seen my old daddy die of the same thing, just like I got . . . . I know (p. 277).

Another younger man described the feeling he had by saying, "It was just like walking up to a sleeping man, shaking his hand and saying to him, 'You're gonna die right now!' " One spinster in her late fifties was precipitated into a psychotic episode by the diagnosis. She said,

> I want to go home. I no can get well. I have chickens and a cow at my house. I have flowers. . . . They are so pretty (voice breaks, tears threaten, then she sat up suddenly rigid and claws violently at the lump in her throat—thyroid cancer). I have cancer. I have cancer here. I die. I die. I know, I die (p. 278).

The patient was hospitalized in a mental institution several days later. After treatment there, a successful operation was performed and the thyroid cancer excised.

To a small number in this specific threat category, the menace was not so much death *per se* as it was punishment for prior sins. They said such things as, "I've been wicked all my life. I had it coming to me." Or, "It's a disgrace sent on me for my sins."

> One black woman was convinced that God had sent cancer of the breast upon her because she sold beer at her "eating place." She had sent for a "prayer cloth" through the mail and waited nine weary and painful months, while the tumor in her breast fulminated and broke into a running sore, hoping that God would forgive and heal her (p. 278).

Only 10 percent of the group studied accepted the diagnosis of cancer with intelligent, controlled anxiety. Proper knowledge of the course of cancer and the medical advances toward its control seemed to determine this reaction. One man put it simply.

> I know about malignancies. My wife had one. You face such things, get the best possible medical care, and keep it controlled (p. 278).

One patient expressed her reaction succinctly:

> I was absolutely petrified when this friend told me I had cancer, but I had the good sense to call my doctor, and after I had talked to him, I felt so much better. He was blunt, but he gave me courage and hope. He said you have met hard problems before and this is just another one. You are an adult, and I know you would want to know. I want you to put your house in order before you go down there for treatment. . . . I mean your spiritual house as well as your mental and physical house, and then go down there and give those doctors everything you have in you to help them get you well. You know the doctor can do only so much and then it's up to you. I appreciated that so much in the days to come. I talked with other doctors; I read; and, I found out what my chances were, what they had to offer in the way of treatment; and then I set myself to help the doctors help me (p. 279).

To be told you have cancer, then, may mean different things. The counselor, or family member, must know the specific fear the patient visualizes if he is to give maximum emotional support. Often, the anxiety experienced is realistic; in some instances, it is based upon misinformation which can be corrected. As has been reported, a picture of no appreciable threat may be based upon ignorance of the course and prognosis of the disease. What seems to be stolid acceptance or cheerfulness may be shock that defies verbalization. Often some of this discomfort can be relieved by talking about realistic risks of the disease and what can be done for the patient. The focus of the debilitating anxiety may be death *per se* or guilt over past sins. If so, correct information and exposure of the fancied fears to the light of scientific advances and hope may push this individual over into the desired category of controlled fear of the disease. A controlled, intelligent fear is to be desired. It assists the patient in resisting the onslaught of the disease by intelligent cooperation with the physician in the treatment schedule. It also assists in alleviating debilitating anxiety and converting it into a mobilizing energy which may be used to combat the disease.

Psychologic Meaning of the Organ Involved

The emotional significance of the organ involved (which may be destroyed by the disease or treatment) adds to the impact of the diagnosis. This trauma is especially debilitating when the organ or structure has symbolic impact. A woman faced with the loss of a breast feels that her sexual attractiveness is threatened. Often a young woman feels she is losing the right to love and marriage with the loss of a breast. She cannot countenance the possibility of the look of admiration turning to repulsion in the eyes of the man she loves.

Married women often fear they will lose their husbands as a result of the body mutilation. In fact, a number of divorces, and separations, have occurred for this reason. It is plausible, however, that the break in the marriage relationship was as much due to the attitude and fear of the wife, as to the change or repulsion in the husband. With proper talking and "feeling" through the projected loss and clarification of the symbolic meaning of the organ, the marriage may have been saved. On numerous occasions, when the husband and wife were led to discuss the problem candidly with the guidance of the counselor, the marriage relationship was actually reenforced. One brave young man, whose initial reaction was one of horror and distaste (because the scar offended his esthetic sense) came to the counselor, worked through his emotions, and arrived at his own basic decision that love was stronger than any disfigurement. With his support and the knowledge of the depth of his love, the wife made a remarkable recovery. They weathered the threat and left the hospital more secure in their relationship than ever before.

Cancer of the cervix carries a deep symbolic significance also. Cobb (1959) reported a case wherein the patient felt the radical surgery essential to control of the cancer was a violation of her womanhood. She told of a poignantly sad episode of the last night before her operation. Feeling that this was to be her last night as a whole woman, she wore her wedding gown (she had only been married a short six months). Her husband, she said, scoffed at her, but

> That is the way I felt. You go in there, knowing that when you come out you can no longer function as a normal woman. It's like taking away your womanhood (p. 280).

When the husband places great value on a large family, cancer of the cervix carries an added threat to the patient. Often a woman needs reassurance that normal physical marital relationships are possible following treatment.

Emotional reactions related to the symbolic meaning of the organ invaded are not limited to women. Men see cancer of the prostate and of the genitalia as a menace to their manhood as well. The loss of sexual potency is often even more traumatic to a man than to a woman.

The counselor, family members, and the medical team all could profit from knowledge of the possible emotional impact of the diagnosis of cancer to the patient. This information should include the intimate meaning of the word "cancer" to the patient, as well as the symbolic significance of the organ or structure involved. Medical management may be facilitated by this knowledge and much of the emotional trauma of the patient ameliorated. As the physician, the counselor, and the family members listen to the patient and respond to his verbalized and unspoken fears, the way is paved for acceptance of the diagnosis and intelligent participation of the patient in treatment.

TREATMENT OF MALIGNANT TUMORS

Treatment of cancer is complex and varied. As has been stated, often the treatment itself is a frightening experience for the patient. This phase of the management of patients with a malignant disease will be approached from two directions. First, the complicated choices of techniques for medical treatment will be presented. Second, the emotional impact on the patient, of experiencing the treatment, will be explored.

Medical Treatment of Cancer

Once the diagnosis is made, the preparation of an individual plan for management of the disease becomes the first and most important step in treatment. The extent and form of treatment should be devised in light of the specific circumstances of the patient and in his best interest. This plan must be flexible to the point that modifications may be made in an expedient manner if surgical or pathological examinations so indicate. This is a major reason that it is unwise to start treatment if the hospital is not equipped and professionally manned to cope with any emergency that might arise.

So complex is cancer that it is prudent that the plan be devised and treatment be carried out by a team of specialists. This team should include a surgeon, a radiotherapist, an internist (or family physician), a pathologist, a psychologist or psychiatrist, and a rehabilitation counselor. Figure 21-1 is an extension of the chart carried by WHO (1966), adding the services related to emotional comfort and return to work.

The emotional response of the patient to the disease must be given careful attention by a physician (or a psychiatrist or psychologist if the reaction is severe) in order to enlist the confidence and cooperation of the patient and his family in the treatment plan. The effect the disease and/or the treatment

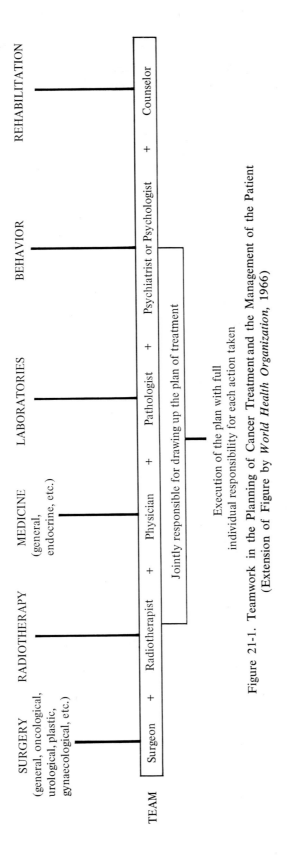

Figure 21-1. Teamwork in the Planning of Cancer Treatment and the Management of the Patient (Extension of Figure by *World Health Organization*, 1966)

will, or may, have on the career of the patient should be frankly discussed, and the rehabilitation counselor be brought into the team prior to initial treatment, if feasible. This gives the patient a hope for a return to normal wage earning upon recovery which can add to motivation to overcome the disease and decrease the degree of depression during the critical days following radical surgery or extensive radiotherapy.

Again prior to initiation of treatment, the team needs to review the precise clinical extent of the disease, the anatomical site of the original tumor, and presence or absence of distant spread (metastasis) of the disease. In deep-seated cancers (i.e., cancer of the stomach, lungs, breast, etc.) specific assessment can be made only through surgical exploration and pathological examination of the tissues involved.

The pathologist, then, is a most essential member of the treatment team. Pathological examination of the cells makes possible a definitive diagnosis of cancer. Through pathological examination the type of cancer is determined. It should be pointed out that although cytological and clinical examinations may *indicate* the presence of cancer, the diagnosis cannot be *confirmed* until completion of the histo-pathological examination has been reached and the structure of the tumor clarified.

For instance, when cancer of the breast is suspected, immediate histological examination of sections obtained by limited resection is accomplished. While the patient is still on the operating table, the report of the pathological findings (benign or malignant) determines whether or not radical mastectomy is to be done.

In all instances, the pathologist should examine the entire specimen removed during surgery. This examination gives the treatment team essential information as to the histological characteristics of the tumor, the type of reaction in the surrounding tissues, the extension of the cancerous growth to surrounding structures, and something of the adequacy of the excision.

A full microscopic examination should also be made of any lymph nodes removed in order to determine whether or not there is metastatic spread of the disease. This evidence may determine whether or not radiotherapy and/or chemotherapy should follow the surgery.

The treatment plan should also take into consideration several biological characteristics of the client. The physical fitness and the age of the patient must be considered. Again, in cancer of the breast, such conditions as pregnancy and lactation demand extreme caution in treatment since some tumors seem to evidence extremely rapid growth at that time.

Taking into consideration all of these factors, a team decision as to the preferred treatment is made. The patient then becomes the major responsibility of the specialists (surgeon, if surgery is decided upon; radiotherapist, if radiation is chosen; or the internist or endocrinologist, if chemotherapy is indicated). Stehlin and Beach (1966), a surgeon and a psychiatrist, writing on the topic "Psychological Aspects of Cancer Therapy" spoke of the plan in terms of the emotional needs of the patient.

> A reasonable plan is one in which optimism and hope for cure are combined with reality. Too little optimism is more reprehensible than too much (p. 101).

TYPES OF TREATMENT

Five types of treatment may be utilized in the battle to save the life of an individual diagnosed to have cancer. Usually, the treatment of choice is surgery. Radiotherapy is used extensively in combatting cancer, sometimes as the initial treatment, and often as supplementary to surgery. Recently, chemotherapy, although not considered able to produce a permanent cure, has been found to have considerable application in cancer treatment (WHO, p. 22). Also quite recently hormone therapy (particularly in instances of cancer of the breast, cervix and prostate) has been utilized successfully in the control of cancer. The fifth form of treatment is known as combined therapy. Combinations of surgery, radiotherapy, chemotherapy and even hormone therapy have been used in the over-all management of the patient through the course of the disease. Each of these forms of treatment will be briefly discussed.

Surgery

Because of the vicious nature of the disease, surgery is the preferred treatment (WHO, 1966). Particularly is this true if the patient presents himself for medical care early in the history of his disease, while the cancer is still encapsulated in the primary site (no metastasis to distant parts of the body). Three types of surgery are performed in cancer: diagnostic, curative, and palliative. The nature of each will be reviewed.

Diagnostic Surgery

Diagnostic surgery is performed in order to establish a correct diagnosis. This procedure may be a simple biopsy or an exploratory operation.

A biopsy involves the incision and removal of tissue from a lesion (tumor) for pathological examination. As previously mentioned, the pathological examination of the biopsied material helps to establish a correct diagnosis, and gives essential facts which may determine the nature and extent of treatment needed.

When all medical investigations fail to establish a definitive diagnosis, when malignancy is suspected or must be ruled out, surgery is sometimes recommended.

Curative Surgery

It was the consensus of the members of the Expert Committee of the World Health Organization (1966) that,

> The value of surgery in the treatment of cancer lies in the fact that in the great majority of cases the neoplasm is unicentric in origin. This being so, there is every prospect of cure if the tumour can be extirpated before its has metastasized (p. 13).

Palliative Surgery

The purpose of palliative action is to relieve pain and discomfort or to prolong life. This type of surgery is carried out to help the patient, but it is not expected to cure. Surgical procedures are employed to resect infected, foul, bleeding or obstructive cancer tissues. Severance of sensory-nerve tracts or alcohol nerve blocks are used to relieve intractable pain. By-pass operations in cancer-infiltrated gastro-intestinal and urinary tracts are utilized to relieve obstructions. Palliative surgery may also be employed to enhance the degree of freedom from distress experienced by the patient found to be inoperable for cure upon exploratory operation. It has been shown that the removal of a primary tumor, in some cases, will cause regression of distant metastasis, relieving the patient of symptoms and complications and prolonging life.

In case of bone sarcoma, or soft-tissue malignancies, an amputation of an extremity may be considered a palliative operation. It should be pointed out, however, that a palliative resection can be useful only when the general condition of the patient is fairly good, and when the goal is to prolong life. If no sign of disemination is present, procedures not palliative but curative may be carried out.

Radiotherapy

It has been estimated that radiotherapy is indicated in the management of at least 50 percent of all cancer patients (WHO, 1966).

> Radiotherapy depends for its action on the biological response if ionizing radiation. The immediate effect of ionizing radiation on tissue is a specific kind of physically induced inflammation, the degree of the reaction depending on the dosage of radiation to which the tissue has been exposed (WHO, 1966, p. 18).

The radiation works to damage the cancer, not through a cauterizing effect, but by selective damage of the malignant cells. Cancerous tumors are classified as radiosensitive, radioresistant, and intermediate. Radiosensitivity implies rapid regression in response to radiotherapy. Radioresistant tumors are those that evidence limited or no regression when irradiated.

Radiotherapy, like surgery, is used as a palliative procedure as well as a curative process. When the size of the tumor is considered feasible for cure, every effort is expended to that end. Radiotherapy may be used before surgery to reduce the tumor to operable size. Surgery is then carried out to remove the primary site. Radiotherapy may also be utilized following surgery as a precaution against scattered malignant cells that could be left.

If the patient is considered incurable, relief from pain, ulceration, etc., may be secured through irradiation. It may also be used in conjunction with drugs in such cases.

Chemotherapy

Treatment of cancer by drugs alone is not indicated when there is hope the tumor can be cured by surgery or irradiation. However, around 50 percent of malignant diseases are known to respond to chemotherapy, either used alone, or in combination with other forms of treatment. In the lymphomas, Hodgkin's Disease and the retinoblastomas, chemotherapy is often used in combination with other treatment when the disease is limited in extent. In the treatment of acute and chronic leukemia and multiple myeloma, chemotherapy may be used (WHO, 1966). When cancer is advanced and generalized, and other treatment cannot be accomplished, chemotherapy is widely used.

Intrapleural and intraperitoneal chemotherapy have been utilized successfully with patients with pleural or ascitic effusions resulting from cancer. The fluid is drawn and the drug is introduced into the pleural or peritoneal cavity. This procedure often reduces the rapidity of the recurrence.

Regional chemotherapy (extracorporeal circulation to perfuse the organ attacked with the chemotherapeutic agent) has been used in treatment of intractable cancer. This method is complicated.

Intra-arterial infusion in localized areas appears to have more promise in certain cancers. Both of these procedures need further research (WHO, 1966).

Hormone Therapy

The first physiological substances known to influence the course of cancer are hormones. Hormone therapy is used both as additive and as suppressive treatment. Over the past twenty years, sex hormones have been used as additive treatment in cancer of the breast in females and prostate in males. Progesterone has been used in endometrial cancer and in acute and chronic leukemia. In malignant lymphoma, corticosteroids have proven of value.

Side effects of hormone administration represent a complication that required medical consideration. Research to find a hormone free from these effects is underway. Investigations are also in progress attempting to identify hormone-dependency in types of cancer other than in the breast and prostate.

Combined Therapy

Many combinations of forms of treatment for cancer have been used through the years. Surgery plus radiotherapy, surgery plus chemotherapy, radiotherapy plus chemotherapy and other combinations have been tried.

Surgery Plus Radiotherapy

Surgery may be preceded or followed by radiotherapy, or both may be performed. Pre-operative radiotherapy may be used when the bulk of the tumor makes surgery difficult. The irradiation not only decreases the size of the malignancy, it reduces the risk of dissemination of cancer cells during the operation, by the obliteration of blood and lymphatic vessels surrounding the malignant site. Post-operative radiotherapy is based on the theory that isolated malignant cells may be left following operation, that can be killed more readily as isolated than when in mass.

Breast cancer irradiation post-operatively is well established. Intra-uterine radiation before hysterectomy for adenocarcinoma of the corpus uteri is often used. Radon seeds and radioactive isotopes are widely used in combination with surgery.

Surgery Plus Chemotherapy

This combination seems advantageous in the management of some cancers (i.e., cancer of the ovary, breast). The drug may be given preceding, during, or following the operation. Chemotherapy is used in conjunction with surgery on the same premise that radiotherapy is utilized. First, it could be used to reduce the size of the tumor. Second, it could attack remaining cancer cells left in the body following operation. Much research should continue in this area.

Radiotherapy Plus Chemotherapy

The management of malignant lymphoma often requires the use of radiotherapy and chemotherapy combined. Radiotherapy is used as a curative treatment when the extent of the disease is limited. Chemotherapy assumes an important role when the cancer is widespread.

Surgery, Radiotherapy and Chemotherapy with Hormone Treatment

Inasmuch as breast cancer has been demonstrated to be hormone dependent, the use of hormone therapy has been added to the massive attack on this disease. Even more recently, knowledge relative to steroid excretion and the growth of breast cancer has also improved patient survival in cancer of the breast. Treatment for this disease, if it is widespread, then, may include surgery, radiotherapy, chemotherapy, and administration of hormones.

Team Treatment in Cancer

Treatment for cancer is a complex and challenging problem. The Expert Committee of WHO (1966) pointed out that cancer is definitely a team responsibility.

> The plan of treatment should be determined, not by a single specialist, but by a team, and the team approach should be adopted as widely as possible. The aim should be to employ, often in combination, techniques that will give the best results with the least upset to the patient. The team should have the necessary facilities for the proper diagnosis of cancer, including a well-equipped pathology laboratory capable of dealing with biopsies, urgent surgical biopsies, pathological examination of specimens taken at operation, and necropsies (p. 39).

PSYCHOLOGICAL IMPACT OF TREATMENT FOR CANCER

When the patient has accepted the diagnosis and agreed to treatment recommended, his emotional trauma is not ended. The very nature of the treatment poses the greatest threat of all. Radical surgery is usually advocated, and this sometimes means the loss of portions of the body that the patient has not associated with his problem. For instance, a patient with sarcoma may lose an entire leg, when to him the trouble seems localized on the ankle. A woman who has a small mass in her breast may awake from anesthesia to find that her breast has been removed. Intellectually, she knows this radical procedure was carried out to save her life, but an unreasoning emotional grief results.

Many patients are deathly afraid of surgery. Often this fear is based on the loss of consciousness under anesthesia and the horror of the knife cutting into their defenseless bodies. Sometimes it is realistic anxiety arising from having known someone who experienced the same procedure and being too keenly aware of what to expect.

Radiotherapy is also approached with uneasy anticipation. It is difficult for the lay person to understand how heavy dosages of irradiation can be delivered to the body without literally destroying it. The sound-proof rooms in which extensive irradiation is usually administered give an eery "feeling" to the treatment. Often the patient experiences nausea following irradiation. At times this nausea is a result of the physical impact of the therapy, but it may also be intensified or even a result of the emotional reaction to the unknowns of the radiotherapy.

Radioactive iodine seems an awesome mystery to most patients. They are asked to drink what appears to be a glass of strange tasting water. Then they are warned of the presence of the radioactive substance in their bodies and may be isolated, or restricted as to visiting time. The next day, the geiger counter buzzes over them in an alarming manner. This is boring routine to the physicians and technicians, but it is dangerous magic to many patients.

Chemotherapy and hormone treatments precipitate psychological concerns. Anxiety-producing side-effects of the drugs used heightens the psychological discomfort of the patient. Hormones and the cortisones bring about personality, as well as physical, changes that alarm the patient and his family.

Supportive Needs of the Patient During Treatment

During treatment, the cancer patient needs open communication lines between his physician, his family and himself. He needs to know *what* is going to be done, *how* it is going to be done, and *why*. If he has the answers to these urgent questions, he can relax and use his energy to meet the aftermath of the treatment.

Cobb (1962) reported a case where a young woman yanked the needle from her arm and refused to allow blood to be drawn for a laboratory test. She had not been told what was going on or why it was being done. An older man refused prostatic treatment because he did not understand how the procedure was to be accomplished. Much debilitating anxiety can be avoided by carefully laid and maintained communication channels between the doctor, nurse and patient.

After surgery is over, the physician has a responsibility to discuss the results with the patient. Stehlin and Beach (1966) address themselves to this obligation.

> Initially, he (the patient) should be told merely "you came through the operation fine, and as soon as you feel more comfortable, we shall go over the whole matter." . . . When the appropriate time arrives, the operative findings and procedures should be briefly and simply described.
> The surgeon should therefore be prepared for such questions as "Did you get it all?", "Had it spread?", "Will it come back?", and "What are my chances?" Again he (the doctor) must appreciate the patient's extreme anxiety and attempt to cope with it in an intelligent and realistic manner (p. 101).

Psychological Needs of the Incurable Cancer Patient

The course of incurable cancer is usually a series of remissions, during which time the patient feels much better, only to be followed by a recurrence which precipitates treatment again. The patient needs consistent emotional support to assist him toward an acceptance and enjoyment of the period of remission when he can live fairly normally, as well as an acceptance of the surety of recurrence, and relief that he has a medical haven to which to return when that time comes. Many patients make remarkable adjustments to these cycles of health and illness. They seem to place the responsibility in the hands of the medical team, relax and enjoy the pain-free days, and with faith return for another miracle when the cycle turns against them.

Faith in the medical team and hope for a cure "around the corner" seem to be major ingredients that make for a cooperative attitude and good mental health in the patient. Stehlin and Beach (1966) state:

> If the incurable patient is to gain the utmost benefit from the surgeon's care, their relationship must be a close one, and this is possible only in an atmosphere of mutually free and open communication (p. 101).

Speaking of hope, they continue:

> We surgeons who are constantly dealing with the physical aspects of cancer should realize that the words "incurable" and "hopeless" are not synonymous. To tell a patient that his condition is hopeless is both cruel and technically incorrect. Incurability is a state of the body, whereas hopelessness is a state of mind, a giving up—a situation that must be avoided at all cost. A patient can tolerate knowing he is incurable; he cannot tolerate hopelessness (p. 102).

One might well question the source of hope upon which the incurable patient may draw. Again Stehlin and Beach (1966) have a meaningful theory.

> The answer is simply that he can hope things will be better. The nature and the quality of his hope will be influenced by (1) the patient's attitude toward cancer, (2) the physical factors associated with his disease and the method available for treatment, (3) his attitude in general toward life and his will to live, and (4) the attitude and personality of the physician (p. 102).

There can always be hope for control of the disease, if cure is not feasible. Even when hope for control of the disease is no longer reasonable, there is still hope for comfort. These hopes may be met through medical management.

> . . . By a change of narcotics, or the addition of a tranquilizer, an adjustment of electrolyte imbalance, measures to improve hydration and nutrition, transfusions, attention to malodorous ulcers, stabilization of fractures, physical therapy and, if feasible, efforts directed toward ambulation (Stehlin and Beach, p. 103).

It is within the parameters of the third quality of hope (attitude toward life and the will to live) that the contribution of the psychiatrist, the psychologist, clergyman, social worker and/or rehabilitation counselor is most pertinent. It is at this point that the patient and the team members must come to terms with the intimate meaning that death has for each of them. If the team member in the supportive role has not made a personal peace with the concept of death, he may be threatened and ill at ease with the patient. Cobb (1962) speaks of the dilemma in which the inexperienced psychologist finds himself at such times.

> Paradoxically, the most devastating and at the same time the most rewarding experience of working with cancer patients comes from the relationship leading to an acceptance of the inevitability of death. It is devastating because no sensitive person can work with the deep emotional problems of another human being in the process of preparing for death without reeling at times under the impact of stark separation trauma. It is rewarding because there is never a greater need for emotional support, for emphatic understanding, even for moments of diversion, than one finds in the patient getting ready for death. Between devastation and reward, it takes courage, tenacity, and humility to maintain a counseling relationship when the goal is acceptance and adjustment to the finality of death (pp. 151-152).

Too often the supportive team member (professional or family) hesitates because he doesn't know what to do or say. Three comforting rules-of-thumb may reassure him. First, the most important rule is to listen. Listen not only to the words but to the feelings made apparent by a tone of voice, a sad look, a tear. Many times the patient only needs a sympathetic ear to work through his own problems. These problems may have to do with his family. What will happen to them when he is gone haunts his waking hours.

Here a family member, or members, can give more comfort than anyone. It is, however, one of the most difficult things a person may ever do to talk quietly and with as little emotion as possible about closing the family circle when the patient is gone. One farmer worked out a dated diary during this period, in which he went through a year, writing in the dates that cotton should be planted, the hogs sold, the wheat planted and harvested, the insurance and taxes paid, etc. When he had finished it, he went through it carefully first with his wife, then with their two teen-age children. He gained relief from the planning and discussion and the family lived by it for a number of years.

Putting his "house in order" financially and spiritually are urgent questions to many. The helper can assist by contacting individuals who can help, such as a lawyer for financial planning, or a clergyman for spiritual comfort.

This is done only if the patient wishes it to be done, but settling these affairs often brings a peace of mind that eases the confrontation with death.

Second, the individual in the nurturing role may give information that concerns the patient. For instance, he may want to know how much longer the treatment he is enduring will continue, and if something else will be done when it is discontinued. With close contact with the physician these questions can be answered. He may wish to see a child or a friend but wonders if they could or should come. He may just need to be reassured that the medical team is not going to give up, that as Stehlin and Beach (1966) have said, even beyond hope for control there is hope for comfort, and *always* there is the consideration and dignity to which he is entitled as an important human being.

Third, and most important of all, though it is part and parcel of the first two, the supporting person can "stand by" physically and emotionally. Waiting for death is the loneliest time a person can experience. A warm, human contact brings surcease from desolation for a time. Cobb (1962) puts it this way.

> Often patients yearn for physical contact, and a touch on the hand or shoulder soothes and reassures the weary wanderer between two worlds (p. 155).

It is not so much what one says as it is that he is there, and says something that diverts the patient's thoughts to more cheerful topics, or allows the patient to lose himself in the happenings of the day.

If a family member is to become his emotional "Rock of Gibraltar" for the patient, he must have guidance and support. If the husband or wife can talk through approaches with the counselor, some of the anguish is drained off and he or she can meet the needs of the spouse with sensitivity and concern for the patient, rather than anxiety relative to his own grief. A supportive member should always remember to keep the patient involved in the activities of the family. If there is a problem, the patient senses it and may imagine it to be worse than it is. Even a worry over a problem may relieve the nagging anxiety of his illness for a short while, and he feels that he is still an important part of the family.

Sometimes, the family members feel that they must keep a cheerful face regardless. The patient sometimes interprets this false front as indifference. Let the patient know you love him, that you are aware of his pain and his condition, but share with him your "hope that things will be better." Listen to what he has to say; let him talk. It is hard to hear one you love talk about dying, or his discouragement, but he needs to talk about his feelings to someone who cares.

The relationship that grows during this sharing of grief and hope is the most beautiful an individual ever experiences. It is the epitomized expression of love. On numerous occasions the husband or wife of a cancer patient, who had lingered for a number of months before death claimed them, communicated with the counselor afterward to say that the last few months of sharing had been the deepest expression of love and happiness of their marriage. One man said,

> We went home (from the hospital) and I sold our house and bought a trailer-house. She (the wife) had always talked about seeing the ocean, and the mountains. She was feeling pretty good after treatment, but we both knew and had discussed our knowledge that her days were limited. So we set out to see as many of the things she had dreamed about as we had time to make. We traveled slow and rested a lot. She bloomed. For a while, it was like she was well again!
>
> We made it. We saw the mountains and we went on over to the ocean side and stayed there for as long as she wanted. She got brown as a berry.
>
> Then one day, she said she was ready to come home. We worked our way back another route and both enjoyed it, but we rested more.
>
> Yesterday, we brought her back into the hospital. We both know this is it. But we are so grateful for the most wonderful days of our lives, and we are prepared for whatever comes *(Case Notes).*

ILLUSTRATIVE MEDICAL AND PSYCHOLOGICAL PROBLEMS SPECIFIC TO TWO DIVERSE CATEGORIES OF CANCER

The preceding sections have dealt with cancer diagnosis and treatment on a general basis. Inasmuch as this disease entity is a multifaceted one, it is deemed helpful to the new counselor, or the family member, to outline specific problems associated with the medical and psychological course of two diverse types of cancer. Because cancer of the head and neck is probably the most mutilating type of cancer, this category has been chosen for presentation. The type that most often involves the younger age group (from ten to thirty years) is cancer of the bone and soft tissues; therefore, a discussion of this category has been included.

Cancer of the Head and Neck

The reported incidence of cancer of the head and neck has increased in the past twenty-five years. It is possible that the incidence has remained stable, but the reporting has improved. This improvement in reporting could be due to improved diagnostic methods, increase in the population, increased longevity of the population, or to the fact that cancer registries are being kept in more hospitals and medical centers than before.

Cancer of the head and neck is probably the greatest ego threat of all malignancies because of its visibility. The disease and its cure are both highly mutilative, and even at best the body image is damaged.

Medical Factors Involved in Treatment of Cancer of the Head and Neck

The primary goal of treatment of malignancies of the head and neck is, of course, cure. The diagnostic process is designed to determine the possibility of cure. Treatment is then planned, in accordance with the diagnosis, to be curative, palliative, or both.

The treatment of choice for cancer of the head or neck is surgery. This involves surgical resection of the primary tumor and regional lymph nodes.

This surgery may be followed by irradiation of the primary site plus regional lymph nodes, or the physician may wish to do irradiation first as indicated by the specifics of the case. A combination, then, of irradiation and surgery may be prescribed. Adjuvant chemotherapy may be used (Healey, 1970).

In this category of cancer, the physician and the patient are interested not only in the cure, but also in functional and cosmetic results as well. This complicates the procedures and the results in that many of the curative and/or palliative procedures produce either functional or cosmetic defects—or both. For example, treatment for cancer of the maxillary sinus may require enucleation of the eye-ball, with partial or total blindness. Radical surgery on the nasal cavity may result in an impairment of the sense of smell. Paralysis of the muscles of the face may follow parotid gland surgery. Removal of the tongue and mandible damages the process of mastication. Cancer of the tongue may result in destruction of taste buds as well as impairment of speech. Removal of the larynx results in loss of speech. If the spinal accessory nerve is severed, movements of the neck and shoulder are limited. In addition to these functional problems, the patient must cope with the accompanying cosmetic disfigurement.

In malignancies of the head and neck, then, the patient must have an important role in decisions of treatment. The physician must first determine the curability or incurability of the case. This is often made by presence or absence of distant metastasis. If the cancer is deemed curable, the patient and his family must not only be made aware of the meaning of the proposed cure in terms of mutilation, but also briefed on possible cosmetic reconstruction available. These choices will often depend on the physician himself and the resources he has available. The age of the patient must be considered as well as the time element involved. Factors such as time for the slow procedures, in terms of remaining life-span and energy out-put of the patient, must be weighed. Such procedures are very expensive; therefore, the economic situation of the patient should be considered and the case referred to one of the available research centers where medical care can be provided at no cost or at minimal expense, if the patient so desires.

Often, the pain the patient is experiencing leads him to grasp at any hope for betterment. At times the odor from the fulminating abscesses makes radical surgery acceptable to the patient just to eliminate the sickening smell.

If the case is deemed incurable, the physician and the patient may decide on resection for relief of pain or odor. Irradiation is often prescribed as a palliative measure in such cases.

Psychological Aspects of the Treatment and Course of Cancer of the Head and Neck

Because of the visibility of the mutilation associated with cancer of the head and neck, this type of malignancy, probably more than any other type, poses the greatest emotional threat to the patient and his family. Too often, even with excellent medical care, the patient is left with an eye, part or all of a nose, ear or other portion of the face and neck missing. Despite giant strides in the areas of plastic surgery and prosthetics, the disfigurement is still grossly apparent. It is traumatic to experience mutilation of the body image by loss of a limb, but to endure the agony of a face made grotesque to the point that even friends and family members avert their eyes while speaking with the patient, or betray repulsion in other ways, is excruciating punishment. To live with the knowledge of the presence of foul odors arising from some of the fulminating tumors, and to realize how abhorrent the smell is to others is another step into emotional hell. To lose the ability to speak and be forced to communicate in a Donald Duck type esophageal speech is psychologically offensive, especially to younger women. This patient needs and deserves the unconditional regard and emotional support of the entire medical team (including an empathic psychiatrist or psychologist), as well as the encouragement of a loving and understanding family.

The psychological services essential to the good mental health of the patient with head or neck cancer will be discussed under three topics. First, the emotional pre-operative preparation of the patient and his family will be considered. Second, the psychological reaction to the post-operative disfigurement by the patient, his family, and sometimes his surgeon, will be weighed. And, finally, the special problems posed by loss of speech will be reviewed.

Psychological Preparation of the Patient for Unavoidable Disfigurement

When the onslaught of the disease process and the results of the treatment essential must result in facial disfigurement, the patient and his family have a right to know the expected extent of the damage. When this knowledge is made known, it would require super persons to accept the realistic facts without reeling emotionally. In these instances, both the patient and his family need not only the empathic support of his physician, but the opportunity to work through the ego-blow with a competent psychiatrist, psychologist, or social worker. They need exact medical information concerning the surgical procedures, what to expect, and what can be done to reconstruct the area mutilated. They need emotional support to work through the depression and real fear of rejection that must arise from the loss. The patient will want to discuss not only his own emotional reactions, but how he can make the impact easier for those he loves.

The family members will need to work through their own repulsive reactions and deep grief in order to protect the patient and make it easier for him. Preparation for treatment includes accurate medical information and hopeful emotional support for both the patient and his family.

Reaction to Disfigurement

No matter how carefully the patient and his family have been prepared for the results of treatment, the accomplished fact is always a shock. To know it will happen is one thing, to live with it is another. The emotional support needed in the early post-treatment days is great. The courage and optimism of many of the patients under the most trying and painful circumstances are humbling.

The physician, the psychiatrist, psychologist, or social worker will be struck with the terrible courage that rises to meet this disaster in many cases. Cobb (1959) speaks of one dauntless woman who continued to operate a village grocery store, with apparent good mental health, even though she had lost one eye, all of her nose, part of one cheek, and her upper lip. She wore a cloth patch over the invaded portion of her face and carried on as if this were the fashion of the day.

Family members also need a listening ear, and someone who can help them learn to accept the damage and rise above their grief. Usually, it is the unconditional acceptance of the patient by his family that makes it possible for him to accept himself, and to seek the acceptance of others in his social world.

One must never forget that the physician, too, is deeply involved in these cases. He entered the profession with the desire to heal, not mutilate. His emotional gratification comes from cures of disease not controls. When the cure, or control, leaves a disfigured individual, despite his every effort, the emotional impact on the physician is tremendous. The patient and his family, as well as other members of the medical team, should remember this fact, and also give subtle emotional support and understanding to the doctor in charge.

Special Problems Encountered in Loss of Speech

Removal of the larynx brings about loss of speech. This is a threat to communication that is painful to consider. The patient, however, has four methods of communication left him. He may write his thoughts for meaningful persons in his world to read. He may communicate by hand signals. He may learn esophageal speech, or he may have an artificial larynx installed.

The medical consensus seems to be that every effort should be expended toward the development of esophageal speech (Healey, 1970). Psychologically, the raspy texture of the new voice seems unpleasant to most women patients. Indeed, one younger woman (probably in her early thirties) withdrew into a psychotic episode when a man who spoke esophageal speech came to talk with her prior to her operation. The intent was to reassure her; the Donald Duck quality of his voice repulsed her.

The psychological significance of the loss of voice could be explored, and preparation for the loss built around this intimate meaning. In the young woman referred to above, the prospect of loss of her natural voice and the acquisition of the raspy sound, was tantamount to loss of sexual attractiveness. When her husband assured her of his love, and when other laryngectomized patients, who spoke more naturally, were brought in (following treatment for the psychotic episode), she was able to face the radical treatment essential to cure of the disease.

Careful medical consideration should be given when the patient is not motivated to attempt esophageal speech, or if the individual is elderly. Improvements in the artifical larynx are needed, but with rapid advancements in biomedical-electronic fields, improvements should be forthcoming, and could solve some of the problems of those who cannot master esophageal speech.

Surgical attempts to create an air tunnel to facilitate speech in the laryngectomized patient have not been entirely successful (Healey, 1970). The development of an artificial larynx, or pseudo-larynx, by surgical measures seems to be a new challenge to experimental surgery replacing work on the air tunnel.

Cancers of the Bone and Soft Tissues

In 1968, the American Cancer Society estimated that the incidence of cancer of the extremities ran over nine thousand per year (Healey, 1970). Tumors of bone and soft tissues most commonly involve the younger age group (from ten to thirty years). Bone and soft tissue tumors frequently affect children and adolescents. The overall prognosis of these patients is more guarded than for those with cancer of the breast or thyroid. The variety of tumor types and anatomic sites involved make the rehabilitation process complex.

Medical Factors Involved in Treatment of Cancer of the Bone and Soft Tissues

Cancers of the soft tissues arise from structures such as fibrous tissues, fat, fascia, muscles, tendons, nerves, lymphatics, and vascular structures. Bone cancers develop in any anatomical part of the bone, producing either a bone destruction or the formation of new bone.

Treatment of choice for both soft tissue and bone malignancies is usually surgery. In cancer of the soft tissues when diagnosis is early an "en bloc dissection" (c.f. Martin in Healey, 1970, p. 85) is recommended. This is a surgical procedure in which large muscle groups are removed, leaving enough limb to be useful to the patient. In many instances, however, amputation is indicated.

Irradiation may be used for palliative purposes when surgery is not feasible. It is sometimes used post-operatively also for palliative reasons.

The treatment of choice for cancer of the bone is also surgery. Following a lower extremity amputation, the major muscle group involved is sewn together over the severed end of the bone. When possible, a three-ply sock is applied, and a rigid plaster-of-paris bandage contoured to the stump. The prosthetic unit is then incorporated into this stump bandage. This unit then receives the temporary pylon which permits ambulation within forty-eight hours (c.f. Dr. Burgess in Healey, 1970, p. 86).

Radiotherapy is utilized as an adjunct to surgery. It lessens pain and seems to slow the growth of the malignant cells. It is considered a temporary measure.

Pain in Cancer of Bone and Soft Tissue

Pain is a major problem in bone cancer. Lawrence J. Pool, M.D., Director, Rehabilitation Project, Memorial Sloan-Kettering Cancer Center, New York, has suggested that the two main types of pain encountered in bone cancer are phantom limb pain, or awareness, and the painful stump (Healey, 1970). Doctor Pool states that, although all amputees probably experience phantom pain or awareness, only around 3 percent report the sensation. Dr. Pool's explanation of the phantom limb awareness is that the experience results from "upsetting the feedback balance to the cortex and thalamus."

> Nobody knows for sure what the mechanism is, but I think it's the upsetting of the sensory feedback balance to the thalamus and cortex sensory association areas; not the primary sensory cortex but just beyond it where the sensations are synthesized and put together in a recognizable form. This electrical circuit, if you will, is disturbed by the cutting off of the limb (Healey, 1970, p. 93).

Other explanations of the cause and treatment of phantom pain may be found in Dr. Roy C. Grzesiak's contribution to this volume (Chapter 18).

Dr. Pool described a neurological procedure he performed to relieve phantom pain in cancer. The physicians of the cancer conference on Cancer of the Bone and Soft Tissues (Healey, 1970) were in consensus that neither narcotics nor chordotomy can successfully control phantom limb pain. The use of hypnosis to alleviate intractable pain has been documented (cf. Miller in Healey, 1970, p. 94).

Doctor Miller also mentioned at the conference the work of a group of anesthesiologists who taped the conversations in the operating room at time of surgery. Six months later, according to this report, the patient would be hynotized, age-regressed to time of the operation, and asked to recall the conversation heard during his surgery. Memory recall was checked against the tapes. Recall was phenomenal. As an outcome of this experiment, while the patient was still under anesthesia, he was given the suggestion, "You will not feel any pain." This technique was reported to work in almost 80 percent of the patients. These patients had no need for narcotics following surgery.

Surgeons and psychiatrists (Healey, 1970) agree that the immediate post-operative application of the elastic stump sock and plaster to immobilize the stump for early prosthetic fitting lessens both wound and phantom pain.

The painful stump (neucoma pain) develops in the post-amputation period. This trauma may often be prevented by early proper treatment of the stump. It can also be corrected by a resectioning and capping of the nerve end. This is true nerve pain while the phantom may be due to brain distortion.

Cousalgia results when a nerve is only partially injured. Partial injury to a nerve will induce disturbance of the autonomic system leading to excessive perspiration and vascular changes in the extremity.

Psychological Implications of Loss of an Extremity

Strong emotional stress results from the loss of an extremity. The individual is called upon to give up a part of himself and to modify his body image. This brings into focus fears of pain, of mutilation, of social unacceptability, and of death. Anxiety is present. If the patient is to be able to accept and respond maximally to treatment, these fears and his mourning must be recognized and dealt with.

The anxiety experienced varies with the age of the patient. In the young child, the trauma of the parent must be considered as well as the apprehension of the child. The stress experienced by the adolescent is specific to his stage of development. The adult's concerns are intensified by his apprehension relative to possible impairment of his ability to earn a livelihood, and the emotional reaction to his family, as well as the stress of the financial burden he visualizes. To the older patient the trauma is specific to fears of body deterioration and the burden he may become to his children, or spouse. Each will be reviewed briefly.

When a young child is faced with amputation the major psychological stress will be experienced by the parents. If the child is seen as an extension of the parents, loss of a limb and threat to his life become a greater stress than the same loss to the parent himself, would be. If there has been some ambivalence, or hostility, toward the child on the part of the parent (or parents), guilt reactions are likely. This guilt often results in overprotection of the child and undue demonstrations of love. The anxiety of the parents must be dealt with, or the child will suffer vicariously from their contagious fears. Once the parents have reached some acceptance, the child should be told what to expect. If the parents are mature and loving, they may wish to break the news to their child themselves. If they are not, a relaxed physician, psychiatrist, or psychologist should be called in to perform this service in such a way as to give the child some reassurance and the security of trust in his doctor and parents.

Amputation of an extremity during the adolescent period is probably the greatest blow of all, coming at a time when the ego is particularly sensitive, and when the body image is just crystallizing. The young patient may need constant emotional support in order to adapt and rebuild his self-concept. This is a time when youth seeks to be like everybody else in his group. To suddenly have only one leg, or hand, sets him apart in a damaging way. Often young boys view amputation of a leg as castration. Girls sometimes feel that with a damaged body they will never be able to marry.

On the other hand, adolescents are individuals too, and many times their acceptance of the loss of an extremity is exemplary. Cobb (1959) tells the story of a thirteen year old girl who was faced with a hip disarticulation. She had been in considerable pain. The psychologist was requested to talk with her regarding the impending operation. The patient listened intently, asked several questions, was reassured she would be up on crutches and walking in a very few days, and reminded that the removal of the primary tumor would alleviate the pain she was enduring. When the surgeon came by to see her later in the day, he reported (with some emotion) that she reassured him! This patient did walk on crutches a few days post-operative; she returned to school and, despite the availability of a life-like artificial limb, continued to use her crutch. It seemed more like her own leg, she said.

When the patient who is to endure an amputation is an adolescent, then care should be taken that the reason for the operation is explained fully. Questions should be carefully answered. The ability to walk, or use of the arm or hand, should be emphasized, and the intelligence and sensitivity of the individual recognized and respected. Most of the time, adolescents will respond beautifully to this adult approach. At the same time, it must not be forgotten that in many ways the adolescent is still a child; so mood swings should be expected and the needs expressed met.

The adult man who faces an amputation feels an emotional brunt that is three-fold. The first reaction may be one of deep concern at the loss of a limb, and the symbol that loss becomes of possible impending death. The second impact is so strong that often the first is submerged. "How will this amputation affect my ability to make a living for my family?" he asks himself and the doctor. Financial security for his family has been his major concern through the years; what will happen now? Finally, he wonders how his family will feel about him as a part of a person, rather than a whole. Will they love him and respect him as before? Will he become a financial and emotional burden to them?

These debilitating conflicts must be explored and met, to some extent at least, if the patient is to utilize his energy effectively in getting well.

The mourning at the loss of a part of his body is a natural reaction that he should not be ashamed to express. Once he has explored his feelings about this loss, and has been told by his doctor of his ability to walk again (with crutch or prosthesis), he is ready to move on to coping with the financial problems and the emotions of the family. This is the reason that instant fitting of the prosthesis following surgery is advantageous. The motivation of the patient is provided and maintained by this early effective ambulation.

The pressing financial problems can most effectively be dealt with by the rehabilitation counselor. If he is called in to see the patient even before the surgery, it prevents much anxiety. In fact, he may be able to supplant it with healing hope. The patient is reassured that if he can return to his usual means of earning a living, he will have help to do so. If he finds this impossible, he is told of training and support until he is ready for, and placed in, a new job.

This training along with early ambulation keeps motivation high and depression minimal.

The family reaction to his loss of a limb should be approached first by work with the family members. The patient's condition and prognosis should be discussed by the physician to the point that the family members are aware of the limitations and emotional qualms of the patient.

The rehabilitation counselor may then assist the family in assuming a supportive and reassuring role. If the wife and children do not minimize his loss but make him feel that he is loved, and needed to guide and to provide, the patient seems able to rise above anxiety and pick up the responsibilities and joys of a full life. If the family overprotects him, or leaves him out, they hinder his recovery.

The problems of the working woman facing amputation are very similar to those of the man just discussed. She, however, must also cope with the perceived loss of beauty and femininity at an even deeper level than does the man. Her worth as a woman is threatened. She needs all the emotional support mentioned above plus almost constant (for a while), but subtle, reassurance of her charm and ability to inspire love.

The housewife will experience the same traumas. Her concern will center more around her ability to care for her family, but she will need the same sincere reassurance of the love and understanding of her family and friends.

Amputation in the older patient (sixty-five years and above) seems to reinforce his fear that his body is deteriorating. This fear, of course, leads immediately to thoughts of death, and depression sets in. This depression often is not so much anxiety at approaching death as it is concern for the financial burden he is, or may become, to his children. He may be caught in an ambivalent situation where he, on the one hand, lashes out at this dependency because he has for so long assumed the supportive role.

Here again, the physician and the rehabilitation counselor must work together to interpret the patient to the family, and the family to the patient in such a way as to bring harmony and understanding. Often, the children do not accept, or understand, this changing of the roles. They tend to think of father and mother as always adult, always coping, always equal to any emergency. When they are led to understand that the time has come that mother, or dad, needs to look to them for protection and comfort, they usually respond. Illness, or the amputation, may hasten this change of roles. On the other hand, as with the adolescent, the older person is an individual. He may accept the body loss with equanimity, walk in a few days, and return to independent living.

Rehabilitation counselors and family members who work, or live, with the geriatric patient should read carefully some of the recent research in the area. A panel discussion of medical management, energy *conservation,* nerves and proprioceptive problems, and rehabilitation of the geriatric population, prepared by the National Research Council's Committee on Prosthetic Research and Development (WHO, 1966), is recommended.

REHABILITATION SERVICES IN CANCER

Prior to 1966, the problem of rehabilitation of the cancer patient was more academic than realistic. In the first place, many physicians were still unaware of the availability of rehabilitation services for individuals with malignant disease. Some of those who knew of the agency and its work, because of the uncertainty of the prognosis, failed to refer cancer patients for services. On the agency side, two eligibility requirements made it difficult to accept cancer patients for service. First, to be eligible for rehabilitation services prior to 1967, the client was required to be eighteen-months post-operative without evidence of metastasis. Second, feasibility for full-time employment was also a prerequisite for eligibility. Combine these facts with the prevailing feeling of despondency as to the outcome of cancer treatment and it is really surprising that the question of services to the cancer patient even came under discussion.

Recent Developments

However, as the medical world became more and more interested in the quality of survival, and as the improved knowledge and techniques made possible a longer, more comfortable life expectancy for the cancer victims, rehabilitation came into focus. In the meantime, a change in the definition of rehabilitation made full-time employability no longer demanded. Under the new regulations, the client could be served when he had only part-time work potential and/or if she were a housewife. The eighteen-month waiting period was removed.

As the need for services and the vocational potential of the surviving cancer patient were recognized, federal funds were allocated to initiate and carry out services to the cancer patient. Clark and Moreton (Healey, 1970) of The University of Texas M.D. Anderson Hospital and Tumor Institute of Houston, Texas, reviewed the early history of the rehabilitation program there.

> However, it was not until 1965 that national legislation established the Regional Medical Programs for Heart Disease, Cancer, and Stroke. Through the efforts of Miss Mary Switzer, legislation made grant funds available in 1966 from the Vocational Rehabilitation Administration of the Department of Health, Education, and Welfare for the rehabilitation of victims of cancer; interest then began to refocus from the primary concern of 5-year survival rates to the possibilities of rehabilitation of these cancer patients (p. 1).

Even with money available and the new mandate on eligibility, the rehabilitation of this new clientele did not progress rapidly. Clark and Moreton explain.

> Even after attempts were made to establish programs, as was the case at M.D. Anderson Hospital, the facilities were so fragmented there was often little patient benefit. Adequately trained personnel and space were often not available. Too

few of the services, such as the Medical Social Service Department which assisted with socio-economic problems of the patient and the family, vocational counseling, ministerial and volunteer services, were activities independent of the medical staff.

Other than one or two institutions that had programs oriented toward the physical rehabilitation of the cancer patient, such as Dr. Howard Rusk's program at New York University, initiated in 1946, there were no institutions in the country that were directed toward the total rehabilitation of the cancer patient (p. 1).

M.D. Anderson Hospital did offer a number of rehabilitation services prior to 1966, however. The first program to be established there followed the close of World War II when a war veteran who had lost his larynx was employed to work with laryngectomized cancer patients to teach them to speak again. Eventually, this program became a cooperative venture with the Houston Speech and Hearing Center.

By 1952, a program of maxillofacial and dental restoration for head and neck patients was established through the collaboration of the University of Texas Dental Branch, Rice University, and the University of Houston with M.D. Anderson Hospital. Programs were also initiated to restore shoulder function following radical mastectomy and neck surgery and to prevent the "frozen shoulder syndrome" following pre-operative irradiation for breast cancer. Occupational therapy, "which had previously been little more than craftwork, was expanded to include functional therapy and muscle reconditioning particularly of the upper extremities and hands, the design of adaptive equipment to encourage self-help activities, and much attention to the psychological as well as the physical needs of the patient" (Clark and Moreton in Healey, 1970, pp. 2-3).

> Patients were not solicited by the rehabilitation personnel of M.D. Anderson Hospital. Referral was strictly at the discretion of the attending physician. . . . In 1960-61 there were 280 new patients referred. . . . In 1966-67 there were 762 new patients referred. . . . (Clark and Moreton in Healey, 1970, p. 3)

In 1966, four grants were awarded to M.D. Anderson Hospital to increase cancer rehabilitation services. Neuromuscular effects of drug treatment in pediatric leukemia patients and initiation of early physical restoration for all neurosurgical patients were studied. The Regional Maxillofacial Restorative Center was established to serve a five-state region. Finally orientation and instructional courses for vocational rehabilitation counselors and other ancillary personnel were conducted by the hospital staff. Also during that year, a cooperative program to expedite early post-operative fitting of prostheses for cancer patients undergoing limb amputation was initiated with the Texas Institute for Rehabilitation and Research.

Since 1966, all rehabilitation programs at M.D. Anderson Hospital have been centralized under the direction of Dr. John E. Healey, Jr., in the Department of Rehabilitation Medicine. Under his leadership, a comprehensive rehabilitation center for cancer patients was opened in late 1972.

It will provide medically-supervised housing and vocational rehabilitation for the patients who no longer need to occupy a hospital bed but are not yet ready to return to their communities, or who require ambulatory therapy (Healey, 1970, p. 5).

Future Availability of Services

Despite the more liberal rehabilitation eligibility policies, a number of problems still prevent adequate service coverage of the cancer cases. First, attending physicians are still predominantly unaware of, or indifferent to, the availability of rehabilitation services. Second, the medical prognosis is still quite guarded. Third, when a patient is referred, the rehabilitation counselor is still uncertain of the vocational feasibility of the client. He needs much more information relative to the disease process and treatment as well as experience and research in effective placement of these clients. Finally, and this is probably the most urgent factor, there is the need of the prospective employers of controlled or cured cancer patients for information as to the life expectancy and vocational potential of these individuals.

It would seem, then, that improved rehabilitation services are dependent in great measure on comprehensive educational programs. First, and perhaps foremost, is the education of the physician himself. Healey (1970) states:

> When medical students and physicians are better informed regarding the value and availability of rehabilitative measures, more progress can be anticipated in the field of rehabilitation (p. 169).

A second, and a challenging, educational goal is the dissemination of correct information to the public. Much effort has been, and is being, expended in this direction. More emphasis should be placed on the rehabilitation potential of the cancer patient. When the public becomes aware of the need and the availability of services, pressure will be exerted that will produce more effective procedures, and more referrals.

The family constellation is another important target area for cancer education. The major emotional support to the patient and cooperative agent to the physician is the family. In order to be of maximum assistance to the patient and to the medical team in the treatment effort, the family must have accurate and complete information relative to the disease process and the treatment employed. The busy physician may not have time to instruct each family group personally. He should, however, arrange for adequate written or verbal instruction to insure the emotional support of his patient. Written information should be prepared by professionals under medical guidance. Verbal instructions and support could be given the family by experienced social workers, nurses, psychologists, or rehabilitation counselors, again working in collaboration with the attending physician. This one educational area could result in significant improvements in the emotional and career rehabilitation of cancer patients.

Fourth, and finally, the patient himself has tremendous educational needs. He needs to know the what's, how's, and why's of each phase of his treatment.

His education should begin during the pre-treatment phase upon diagnosis. Throughout the treatment period he must have continued instruction and emotional support. During post-treatment, if the disease is under control, he needs reassurance and assistance in re-establishing his career. If the disease is deemed incurable, the patient needs added information as to the final stages of the disease process, and emotional support to come to grips with the encounter with death.

The closing comments of the Proceedings of Three Interdisciplinary Conferences on Rehabilitation of the Patient with Cancer, summarized the critical medical challenge yet to be met in the rehabilitation of the cancer patient (Healey, 1970).

> It was the consensus that the medical profession should alter its concept of cancer. We should emphasize the successes, rather than the failures as we have in the past. We should take a positive approach in handling and controlling, as well as curing, this disease. The cancer patient should be regarded in the same way as any patient who is afflicted with a chronic disease. We need not always wait for a cure before starting rehabilitation measures. . . . We must develop a positive, hopeful and eventually successful outlook among the medical profession as well as the public in dealing with all aspects of the disease—cancer (p. 184).

The vocational rehabilitation challenge in cancer is just as critical as the medical. So little is known of the work-related problems of the cancer patient as he returns to employment. Much action research through carefully planned experience will help to open the world of work to these clients. The rehabilitation counselor's knowledge of the course and results of treatment for this disease is far too limited. Expanding educational endeavors on the part of cancer research and treatment centers will bridge that gap. Continued efforts to make employers aware of the work potential of cancer patients will lead to greater acceptance, not only of the disease but also of the client in the business world. The greatest challenge of all lies in the preparation and support of the patient and his family as they face the diagnosis, treatment, control and/or the knowledge of the incurability of the disease.

Doctor Healey (1970) said it beautifully, quoting a participant of a conference.

> The first principle of rehabilitation, I believe, is not to be satisfied with life-saving but to be equally as concerned with the quality of living and not merely the quantity of the not-yet dead (p. v).

Doctors Clark and Moreton (Healey, 1970) spoke of rehabilitation as opening "a door long closed to the cancer patient. To give these patients hope for a useful remaining life is a worthy goal . . ." (p. 5) The quality of survival—this is the goal and the challenge of rehabilitation in cancer today.

REFERENCES

Clark, Randolph Lee and Cumley, Russell W.: *The Year Book of Cancer*. Chicago, Year Book Publishers, 1957.

Cobb, Beatrix: Emotional problems of adult cancer patients. *Journal of the American Geriatrics Society, 7*(2):274-283, 1959.

Cobb, Beatrix: Psychological impact of long illness and death of a child on the family circle. *Journal of Pediatrics, 49*(6): 746-751, 1956.

Cobb, Beatrix: Cancer. In Garrett, James F. and Levine, Edna S. (Eds.), *Psychological Practices with the Disabled*. New York, Columbia University Press, 1962.

Dorland, W. A. Newman: *Medical Dictionary,* 23rd Edition. Philadelphia, W. B. Saunders Company, 1957.

Healey, John E., Jr.: *Ecology of the Cancer Patient*. Washington, D.C., The Interdisciplinary Communication Associates, Inc., 1970.

Kuehn, Paul G.: *Quality of Survival of the Cancer Patient*. Hartford, The American Cancer Society (Connecticut Division), 1969.

Stehlin, John S., Jr. and Beach, Kenneth H.: Psychological aspects of cancer therapy, a surgeon's viewpoint. *Journal of the American Medical Association, 197*:100-104, July 1966.

World Health Organization Expert Committee: *Cancer Treatment, Report of a WHO Expert Committee*. Geneva, World Health Organization Technical Report Series, No. 322, 1966.

AUTHOR INDEX

A

Adler, 347, 363
Agras, 135, 139
Alexander, 333, 341
Alkane, 177
Alumbaugh, 176
Ammons, 168, 178
Anastasi, 250, 263
Armstrong, 173, 176
Aronfreed, 21, 38
Aronson, 138, 139
Arrell, 160
Atwell, 176
Ausubel, 370, 394
Ayer, 348, 350, 363
Ayers, 144, 149
Ayllon, 340, 341

B

Bacon, 177
Baer, 42, 55
Bahn, 138
Bailey, 169, 170, 177
Ballis, 363
Bandura, 20, 21, 39
Barber, 313, 341
Bard, 315, 333, 341
Bardach, 334, 342
Barger, 177
Barlow, 135, 139
Barrell, 366
Barrett, 276
Barron, 89, 96
Barry, 351, 363
Barten, 334, 342
Battle, 105, 135, 138
Bauman, 275, 276, 284, 285, 296
Beach, 410, 416, 432
Bean, 88, 96
Beck, 81
Belfer, 170, 177
Bell, 176, 177
Bellak, 334, 342
Benda, 263
Bergin, 138
Bernstein, 177
Berzon, 135, 138
Bettis, 135, 138
Bibring, 347, 363
Bieliauskas, 390, 394
Biggs, 174, 180

Bill, 177
Bills, 55
Binet, 263
Birch, D., 354, 363
Birch, J., 264
Blanchard, 23, 39
Blane, 174, 177
Block, 163, 170, 171, 177
Bloeser, 17, 19
Bloxom, vii, 98, 140
Bobey, 338, 342
Bolman, 164, 171, 177
Boring, 249, 263
Borow, 276
Bowden, vii, 213
Braceland, 90, 96, 342
Brandt, 138
Brill, 103, 138
Bronfenbrenner, 103, 138
Burk, 301, 302, 309
Burke, 89, 90, 309
Butler, 348, 350, 363
Bychowski, 144, 149

C

Cantor, 252, 263
Carkhuff, 41, 55, 106, 140, 145, 146, 150
Carrell, 173, 296
Carroll, 170, 177
Cartwright, 135, 138
Cattell, 177, 347, 353, 363
Caylor, vii, 279
Chambers, 171, 177
Charles, 263
Chittenden, 22, 39
Cholden, 276, 278, 280, 281, 282, 283, 284, 296
Clancy, 171, 173, 177
Clark, G., vii, 153
Clark, R., 428, 431
Clarke, A., 259, 263
Clarke, G., 179, 263
Clinebell, 155, 156, 160
Cobb, vii, ix, 335, 336, 342, 405, 407, 415, 417, 422, 425, 432
Cohen, A., 90, 96
Cohen, I., 177
Čohen, J., 61, 81, 139
Collingwood, vii, 14, 19, 41
Combs, 347, 363
Cooper, A., 343

433

Cooper, I., 312, 338, 342
Coopersmith, 169, 177
Cope, 70, 81
Corotto, 177
Cowan, 357, 366
Cowen, 24, 39
Crasilneck, 332, 342
Crawford, 27, 378, 379, 394
Cristol, 139
Cruikshank, 257, 263
Crump, 10, 14, 15, 19, 394
Culclasure, 308, 309
Cull, ix
Cumley, 431
Cummings, 366
Cutsforth, 292, 296

D

Daniels, 341, 342
Danielson, 348, 364
Darling, 348, 350, 364
Davidson, 338, 342
Davis, D. P., 135, 138
Davis, H. G., vii, 161, 173, 176, 177
Davis, R., 386, 395
DeLateur, 321, 338, 342
Demone, 173, 177
DeMonn, 348, 364
Deutsch, 335, 342
DeWolfe, 23, 39
Dickerson, 366
Di Francisca, 51, 90, 96
Di Michael, 259, 263
Di Scipio, 338, 342
Distler, 170, 177
Dittman, 173, 174, 177
Doll, 252, 263
Dominick, 159, 160
Dorland, 402, 432
Drasgon, 348, 364
Dreher, 348, 364
Dubrow, 261, 263
Duvall, 170, 178
D'Zmura, 138

E

Eckhardt, 308, 309
Edwards, A. A., 177
Edwards, A. E., 167, 180
Edwards, W., 313, 342
Edwards, 313, 342
Ehrle, 348, 364
Ellis, 359, 364
Engel, 260, 263
England, 386, 395
English, 307, 309
Erickson, 42, 55, 83, 96
Ewalt, 321, 323, 328, 342
Eysenck, 337, 342

F

Farrell, 276
Feldman, 328, 342
Felzer, 138
Fenichel, 317, 322, 327, 328, 342
Fenoglio, vii, 299
Filer, 364
Fink, 353, 366
Finley, 31
Fischer, 325, 328, 342
Fishman, 336, 342
Fitzhugh, 165, 177
Fleiss, 145, 149
Flescher, 321, 342
Force, 389, 394
Fordyce, 321, 338, 342
Fowler, 321, 338, 342
Fox, 164, 172, 177
Fraenkel, 261, 263
Frank, 105, 118, 133, 136, 138
Frankl, 347, 364
Frantz, 352, 364
Freeman, 342
Freud, A., 316, 342
Freud, S., 315, 317, 343
Fromm, 141, 149
Furst, 338, 343

G

Gannon, 338, 343
Ganzer, vii, 14, 19, 20, 23, 24, 25, 27, 39, 40
Garfield, 135, 138
Garrett, 299, 309
Garris, 307, 310
Garrison, 389, 394
Geer, 23, 39
Gentry, 338, 343
Gibbins, 168, 178
Gladden, viii, 246
Gladwin, 250, 264
Glass, 38, 39
Glasser, 14, 19
Gliedman, 138
Goddard, 247, 264
Goldin, 68, 81
Goldman, 394
Goldstein, A., 138
Goldstein, J., 178
Goodenough, 174, 178
Gordon, 332, 343
Goslin, 38, 39
Gowman, 276
Gracanin, 310
Greene, vii, 267
Griener, 169, 178
Griff, 178
Griogy, 64, 81
Grzesiak, vii, 311
Guntrip, 337, 343

H

Haberman, 177
Hall, C., 326, 343
Hall, J., 332, 342
Halpert, 385, 394
Hamlin, 357, 364
Hansen, 64, 81
Hanson, H., 276
Hanson, P., 395
Hardy, ix
Harley, 85, 86, 87, 88, 96
Harmatz, 170, 177
Harriman, 278, 280, 282, 296
Harrison, vii, 161
Harry, 394
Hartmann, 316, 326, 343
Healey, 423, 424, 428, 429, 430, 431, 432
Heartzen, 166, 178
Heath, 353, 364
Heber, 230, 244, 252, 254, 259, 264
Hegge, 231, 244
Heilbrun, 348, 364
Helm, 180
Henderson, 89, 96
Herring, 355, 364
Hershenson, 165, 178
Herzberg, 351, 364
Hightower, 332, 343
Hill, 166, 178
Hoehn-Saric, 105, 133, 135, 136, 138
Hoffer, E., 362, 364
Hoffer, W., 309, 343
Holland, 180
Hollingshead, 103, 139
Holtzman, 81
Hooper, 366
Houston, 81
Houts, 140
Hoyt, 173, 176
Hughes, 351, 364
Hurwitz, 90, 96

I

Imber, 105, 118, 133, 135, 136, 138
Irelan, 36, 88, 96
Irwin, xii
Itard, 246, 264

J

Janzen, 91, 96
Jastak, 251, 264
Jellinek, 164, 178
Jenkins, 353, 365
Jennings, vii, 5
Jenson, 168, 171, **179**
Jesness, 42, 55
Johnson, D. E., 348, 364
Johnson, G. D., 229, 244, **263**
Jones, 22, 39
Jordan, 348, 364

K

Kaisar, 178
Kanner, 252, 264
Kapner, 171, 178
Karp, 174, 178
Katz, 352, 364
Keller, 157, 160
Kelly, F., 42, 55
Kelly, G., 22, 39
Kelly, J., 229, 244
Kelman, 352, 364
Kirk, 229, 244
Kir-Stimon, 336, 343
Klein, 177
Knape, vii, 343, 384, 391, 395
Kodman, 106, 140
Kolb, 321, 328, 343
Kotkov, 139
Kramer, 39
Krause, vii, 83
Krumboltz, 39
Krupp, 311, 312, 343
Kuehn, 432
Kunce, 70, 81
Kurzhals, 286, 296

L

Lamborn, 66, 81
Lamotte, 81
Lawlis, vii, 346, 353, 356, 358, 359, 364
Lazarus, 22, 39
Lehew, J. L., III, 332, 343
Lehmann, 321, 338, 342
Leitenberg, 135, 138, 139
Leitner, 309, 310
Lesh, 348, 364
Lesser, 348, 350, 364
Levitt, 135, 139
Lief, H., 353, 364
Lief, V., 353, 364
Lillesand, 23, 39
Lindner, 311, 343
Lindsley, 337, 343
Litman, 351, 364
Little, 353, 364
Littman, 346, 364
Locke, 170, 178
Lofquist, 386, 395
Loughmiller, 42, 55
Lovaas, 23, 39

M

MacAndrews, 166, 167, 178
MacGuffie, 91, 96
Machover, 135, 139, 168, 178
Macland, 250, 264
MacLeod, 334, 344
Maddux, vii, 213
Madison, 355, 364
Magers, 276
Maglry, 348, 365

Malamud, A., 135, 138
Malamud, R., 135, 138
Malinovsky, 351, 363
Mannie, 142, 148, 149
Manson, 166, 178
Margolin, 307, 310
Marlatt, 23, 39
Martin, H., 135, 139
Martin, P., 81
Maslow, 347, 364
Mason, 356, 364
Massie, 299, 310
Matkom, 170, 171, 178
Maxwell, 191
May, 170, 177
McDaniel, 325, 326, 343
McDonald, 146, 149
McFall, 23, 39
McGowan, 276, 299, 300, 308, 310
McLean, 55
McMahon, 364
McNemar, 250, 264
McPhee, 348, 364
McWhorter, 81
Mead, 320, 343
Meadow, 139
Meares, 330, 335, 343
Mechanic, 165, 178
Meer, 168, 178
Melzack, 314, 321, 343
Menninger, 386, 395
Merrill, M., 264
Merrill, S., 64, 81
Meyer, 264
Meyers, 174, 177
Michael, 313, 321, 337, 340, 341, 344
Miller, G., 178
Miller, N., 321, 339, 344
Miller, S., 103, 134
Milt, 375, 395
Mindlin, 171, 179
Mischler, 103, 139
Moles, 106, 140
Moore, 165, 173, 179
Moreton, 428, 429
Morgan, 21
Morris, 321, 342
Morrow, 170, 178
Mowrer, 370, 395
Murdough, 334, 344
Murphy, D. G., 164, 173, 179, 335
Murphy, W. F., 342
Myers, 390, 395

N

Nadolsky, 91, 96
Nash, 105, 118, 133, 135, 138
Neff, 336, 339, 344
Nemo, 352, 364
Newell, 140
Norman, 138

Nunnally, 135, 139

O

Obermann, 59, 60
O'Brien, 55
O'Connell, D., 356, 364
O'Conner, J., 309, 310
Oliveau, 135, 139
Olshansky, 386, 390, 395
Olson, 23, 39
O'Neill, 64, 81
Orne, 104, 107, 139
Osgood, 55
Overall, 135, 139

P

Pande, 136, 139
Patterson, C., 364
Pattie, 330, 344
Pattison, E., 171, 179
Paul, 338, 344
Paulos, 179
Pearl, 139
Pepeinik, 139
Perdue, vii, 227
Perlman, 349, 350, **364**
Peterson, G., 170, 179
Peterson, L., 55
Pfeifer, 11, 19
Pfonts, 353, 364
Phillips, 364
Pierce-Jones, 81
Place, viii, 59
Plumeau, 168, 178
Pollock, 380, 395
Porter, 296
Poser, 23, 39
Postman, 364
Puzzo, 168, 178

Q

Quay, 55

R

Rabinowitz, 26, 348, 350, 364
Radcliffe, 363
Ramseur, 165, 179
Ramsey, 168, 171, **179**
Rand, 140
Randall, 321, 342
Rangell, 316, 333, 344
Raskin, 277, 296
Redkey 261, 264
Redlich, 103, 139, 329, 334, 344
Reilly, A., 348, 350, 364
Reilly, D., 177
Reimonis, 352, 364
Reinhart, 171, 179
Reisel, 135, 138
Rhoades, viii, **181**

Rich, vii, 177
Riessman, 139
Rinkel, 371, 395
Rioch, 148, 149
Risley, xii, 267, 276
Ritter, 23, 39
Roberts, 11, 19
Robson, 179
Rogers, C., 145, 150
Rogers, D., 149
Roman, 88, 96
Rosen, 166, 179
Rosenberg, viii, 192
Rosenthal, 139
Roth, 86, 88, 96
Rothaus, 395
Rotter, 55, 264
Rubin, 359, 364
Rusk, 299, 300, 310, 311, 312, 344
Russell, R., viii, 5

S

Sacerdote, 313, 344
Saggerman, 179
Samuelson, 350, 365
Sandness, 365
Sankowsky, 348, 349, 350, 365
Sarason, 250, 254, 264
Sarazon, 14, 19, 23, 24, 25
Saunders, 144, 150
Schilder, 317, 344
Schlaifer, 378, 395
Schlien, 145, 150
Schneck, 330, 344
Schultz, 171, 179
Schwartz, 93, 94, 96
Scott, 286, 296
Seeman, 86, 87, 97
Senter, 144, 149
Serafetinides, 321, 344
Shader, 170, 179
Shapiro, 106, 140
Shell, 294, 296
Shoben, 145, 150
Shontz, 339, 344
Shorr, 334, 344
Shumaker, 138
Siess, 386, 395
Siller, 89, 97
Simmel, 301, 325, 328, 344
Simon, A. J., 227, 244
Simon, T., 263
Singer, 23, 40
Skeels, 250, 264
Skelton, viii, 141, 146, 150
Skinner, 346, 365
Slicer, 170, 171, 179
Sliden, 167, 179
Sloan, 264
Sloane, 134, 136, 139
Small, I., 334, 342, 352, 366

Small, L., 344
Smart, 171, 179
Smith, J., 353, 366
Smith, R., 245
Snygg, 347, 363
Solomon, 135, 138
Sommers, 168, 179
Soulairac, 313, 344
Spangler, 310
Spencer, 305, 310
Spern, 170, 179
Staples, 139
Stehlin, 410, 416, 432
Stein, E., 334, 344
Stein, M., 329, 344
Steinbach, 338, 343
Stokvis, 331, 344
Stone, 105, 118, 135, 136, 138, 139
Storm, 171, 179
Storrow, 103, 138, 355, 364
Strayer, 171, 173, 179
Strickland, 241, 245
Strupp, viii, 98, 140
Suci, 55
Super, 352, 366
Sussman, 87, 88, 97
Sutherland, 91, 97
Sweney, 176, 178, 356, 361, 363, 366
Swinn, 366
Switzer, 6, 19, 60
Szasz, 140, 312, 314, 315, 317, 318, 319,
   320, 321, 322, 323, 324, 325, 328,
   332, 336, 344, 370, 396

T

Tannenbaum, 55
Terman, 264
Thomason, 276
Thompson, 386, 389, 396
Thorenson, 39
Thoreson, 348, 350, 363
Thorsen, 90, 96
Tiebout, 162, 176, 179
Tiffany, D., 356, 357, 360, 366
Tiffany, P., 356, 357, 360, 366
Tizard, 264
Tomlinson, 338, 344
Tredgold, 251, 264
Trice, 88, 96
Truax, 106, 140, 145, 146, 150
Tuma, 170, 177
Turney, 89, 97
Turteltaub, 23, 39

U

Ullman, 39
Unterberger, 386, 395

V

Vance, 55
Vernier, 352, 366

Veroff, 354, 363
Viaille, 165, 179
Vogel, 168, 175, 179
Volksdorf, 106, 140
Voth, 169, 170, 171, 180

W

Wadel, 171, 180
Wadsworth, 73, 81
Wagner, 338, 344
Waldman, 335, 344
Walker, 299, 310
Wallace, 353, 364
Walloch, 140
Walpin, 135, 138
Walters, 20, 21, 168, 178
Wardlow, 348, 366
Wargo, 166, 136, 140
Warnick, 288, 296
Warren, 353, 364
Watson, 250, 264, 337, 345
Weber, 42, 55
Wechler, 264
Weinstein, 325, 326, 327, 328, **345**
Weiss, 336, 339, 344, 386, 395
Weller, 277, 296

Wells, 176
Wender, 104, 109, 139
Whitcraft, 16, 19
Whitten, 59, 82
Williams, 167, 180
Wilson, 180
Windle, 264
Wine, 167, 180
Wispe, 360
Witkin, 174, 178
Wolberg, 334, 345
Wolfe, H., 390, 394
Wolfe, R., 12, 14, 19
Wolff, 180
Wolpe, 145, 150, 337, **345**
Woody, 339, 345
Woolley, 371, 396
Wright, 63, 82

Y

Yalom, 134, 140
Yepsen, 242, 245

Z

Zelhart, 355, 366
Zox, 24, 39, 174, 178

SUBJECT INDEX

A

Addiction, 153-223
  alcoholic, 153
    challenge, 189
    counseling of, 156
    counselor's characteristics, 158, 190
  alcoholism, 161
    definition and drinking patterns, 163
    history and philosophy, 161
    rehabilitation of, 153
      eligibility, 154, 186
      process of, 188
      prognosis, 173
      treatment and results, 170
      variables associated with, 165
  chemical (drug abuse), 181-223
    characteristics of drug abuser, 183
    drug abuse programs in Texas, 181
    effects of mood altering drugs, 192-223
    parameters of drug problem, 182, 185
    types of drugs used and results, 182
      depressants, 210
      hallucinogens, 193-204
        LSD, 193
          acid experience, 194
          changes in direction, 195
          clinical use, 198
          flashback psychosis, 196
          panic and "bummers", 194
          physiologic considerations, 198
        marijuana and hashish, 200
          adverse reaction, 204
          physiologic effects, 202
          psychological change, 203
  drug dependence, 213
    compulsive use, 215
    first use, 214
    intermission and relapse, 216
    symptomatic use, 214
      anger, 215
      anxiety, 214
      depression, 214
      interpersonal inhibition, 215
      pain, 215
      pleasure, 215
    termination of, 216
  therapy or counseling challenge, 218-223

    attitude of counselor, 218
    continuing to care, 223
    hidden meaning of language, 220
    motivation for treatment, 217
    pessimism, dealing with, 221
    reality focus, 220
    role modeling, 219
    specific problems of methadone maintenance, 222
    values, 222
    mescaline, 199
    peace pill, 200
    psilocybin and psilocin, 199
    STP, 200
    inhalants, 211-212
      aerosol spray, 212
      asthmador, 212
      gasoline, etc., 212
      glue, cement, etc., 211
    stimulants, 204-210
      amphetamines, 204
        pharmacological effects, 205
        syndrome, 205
        treatment, 206
      cocaine, 207
        physiological effects, 207
        use of, 207
      narcotics, 208-210
        heroin, 208

C

Cancer, 399-432
  definition of, 402
  medical aspects
    diagnosis, importance of, 403
    treatment, 408
      chemotherapy, 412
      combined therapy, 413
      hormone therapy, 413
      radiotherapy, 412
      surgery, 411
        diagnostic, 411
        curative, 411
        palliative, 412
      team treatment, 414
  psychological considerations, 414
    diagnosis, impact of, 404
      meaning of, 405
      organ involved, 407
    treatment, emotional problems, 414
      need for support, 415

terminal psychological needs, 416
faith, 416
hope, 416
information, 418
listen, 417
stand by, 418
support family, 418
psychological and medical problems
illustrated by two categories
of cancer, 419-428
head and neck cancer, 419
medical factors, 419
psychological aspects, 420
speech, loss of, 422
unavoidable disfigurement, 421
soft tissues and bone cancer, 423
medical factors, 423
pain, role of, 424
psychological implications, 425
extremity, loss of, 425
rehabilitation services, 428
history of recent developments, 428
resume of future potential, 430
educational goals, 430
comprehensive approach, 430
dissemination scope, 430
family instruction, 430
patient instruction, 430
vocational rehabilitation
challenge, 431

D

Disabled Disadvantaged, 59-150
characteristics of, 83-91
compared with normal adults, 83
care, 85
competence, 84
fidelity, 84
hope, 83
love, 84
purpose, 84
wisdom, 85
psychological characteristics
of poor, 85-88
emotional isolation, 86
helplessness, 86
low achievement motivation, 87
poor health orientation, 88
present-time focus, 87
psychological needs of
disabled, 88-91
for life goals and
self-determination, 91
for security, 99
to be interdependent, 90
to be individual, 90
to be same, 89
rehabilitation of, 91-150
approach for rehabilitation, 93
assumptions, 93
role of agency and worker, 94

tasks of worker, 94
contributing data, 95
defining limits, 95
identifying obstacles, 95
lending a vision, 95
searching out common
ground, 94
goals for the disabled poor, 91-93
development of
faith, 93
perspective on life, 93
self-acceptance, 92
self-determination, 92
strengths, 92
partialization of objectives, 92
utilization of resources, 92
history of movement, 59-67
joint rehabilitation—welfare
efforts, 74-81
examples,
Pruitt-Igoe Project, 61
San Antonio Project, 62
West Texas Project, 73
Wood County Project, 63
operational procedures, 67-81
eligibility, 70
monitoring role of DPW,
79-80
pre-vocational evaluation-
adjustment, 71
special groups served, 70
staffing patterns, 69
philosophy of, 67
techniques of working
with, 98-150
motivation of, 141-150
nature of problem, 141
role of counseling, 144
characteristics of
effective counselors, 148
search for meaningful
techniques, 98-156
concept, 105
development of
instruments, 107
need for, 98-105
procedures, 112-138
effects of role induction
procedures, 119-131
relative effects of
two induction
techniques, 131-134
work implications, 134

E

Emotionally disabled
mentally and emotionally
handicapped, 369
categories of, 369
mental retardation, 370
neurotic

symptoms, 373
  primary, 373
    anxiety, 373
    compulsions, 374
    conversion reactions, 373
    obsessions, 373
    phobias, 374
  secondary reactions, 374
    depressive, 374
    dissociative, 374
    somatization, 374
personality disorders, 374
  criminality and mental
    illness, 399
  alcoholism and mental
    illness, 380
  sex offenders and mental
    illness, 380
  instability reactions, 375
psychotic, 369
  symptoms, 371
    emotional disorders, 372
    motor function disorders, 372
    perception disorders, 372
    thought disorders, 371
causes of, 378
medical treatment of, 375-377
psychological aspects of
  rehabilitation, 381
  behavior clues to conflict, 381
  verbal clues to conflict, 382
  rehabilitation of, 385
    job placement, 385
      basic difficulties, 387
      opportunities, 388
      return to community, 387
    myths of, 391
      ideal employee, 392
      ideal employer, 393
      multiple opportunity, 392
    techniques of approach
      to employment, 393
    testing considerations, 383

M

Mentally retarded, 227-264
  classifications of, 254
    educational, 257
    medical, 254
  definition of, 229,251
    considerations of, 249
  habilitation of, 230, 260
    determination of adjustment, 232
    establishing disability, 232
    planning services (state agency),
      232
      counseling, 232
      evaluation, 233
      follow-up, 234
      job placement, 233

      other, 233
      physical restoration, 233
      rehabilitation of, 258
      training, 233
    counselor, 240
    misconceptions of, 259
    plan, 234
    prediction of success, 234
    resources in Texas, 235
      cooperative school
        programs, 237
      extended living, 237
      federal employment, 235
      halfway houses, 236
      National Association, 236
      state schools, 236
      role of sheltered workshop, 261
      social factors in, 262
  history and philosophy, 228
    scope and problem, 249

P

Public Offender, 5-55
adult offender, 7
  characteristics of, 13
juvenile offender, 8
rehabilitation of, 9-55
  delivery of services, 12
  essentials of, 9
    disability, 9
    evaluation, 11
    physical restoration, 16
    placement, 16
    training, 15
  history of movement, 5
  techniques of, 13-15
    counseling, 13
    modeling, 20
      behavior modification in, 21
      concept of, 20
      development of procedures, 25
      example of, 24
        Cascadia Project, 24
          role modeling material, 28
          results and effects, 35
    survival camping
      example of, 44
        Camp Challenge, 44
        aim of, 44
        assessment of, 49
        campstages, 46
        organizational
          considerations, 48
        participants, 45
        program development, 46
        process, 47
        staff, 45
          selection, 45
          training, 45
      role of survival camping, 52

S

Severely disabled, 299-366
  background, 299
  developmental ideology, 301
  rehabilitation of catastrophically
    disabled, 303
    eligibility (state agency), 304
    program expectations, 307
    program philosophy, 303
    supportive programming, 305
      hospital referral, 305
      job development, 306
    unsolved problems,
  special problems of, 346-366
    motivation, 346
      background, 346
      correlates of, 348
      counseling for, 351
        remotivation tactics, 354
          conceptual model, 357
      rehabilitation application, 360
        basic misconceptions, 360
        research, utilization, 361
        some new approaches, 362
  pain, 311-345
    chronic, 311
    psychological approach to, 315
      need for, 313
      pain as effect, 317
      pain as ego orientation, 317
      symbolic nature of, 319
    psychological problems of
      phantom, 322
      theoretical overview, 325
        central theory, 325
        fantasy theory, 326
        peripheral theory, 325
        other, 329
        psychodynamic
          exploration, 326

psychological management
  of, 330
  behavioral, etc., 337
  counseling or
    psychotherapy, 333
  hypnosis, 330

V

Visually disabled, 267-296
  definition of, 268
  psychological implications, 277
    adjustment, patterns of, 278
      acceptance, 283
      anxiety, 278
      contra-indicated hope, 281
      denial, 278
      depression, 282
    interfering personality
      manifestations, 284
      attitude toward blindness, 269
      distrust, 286
      feelings of inadequacy, 286
      recurring depression, 286
      sensitivity, 284
      social competency, 285
      somatic symptoms, 285
  special family problems, 287
    crisis, 291
    fear, 291
    first realization of blindness, 288
    impact of final diagnosis, 288
    peer rejection, 290
    separation from family, 287
    sex problems of adolescent
      blind, 292
    sibling relationships, 290
  vocational problems, 269, 293
    placement, 271, 293
    process of rehabilitation, 269
    marriage as vocational problem, 294
    separation from family, 294